LEUKEMIA-LYMPHOMA

Proceedings of the Annual Clinical Conferences on Cancer
sponsored by The University of Texas M. D. Anderson Hospital
and Tumor Institute at Houston, and published
by Year Book Medical Publishers, Inc.

TUMORS OF THE SKIN
TUMORS OF BONE AND SOFT TISSUE
RECENT ADVANCES IN THE DIAGNOSIS OF CANCER
CANCER OF THE GASTROINTESTINAL TRACT
CANCER OF THE UTERUS AND OVARY
NEOPLASIA IN CHILDHOOD
BREAST CANCER: EARLY AND LATE
LEUKEMIA-LYMPHOMA

LEUKEMIA-
LYMPHOMA

*A Collection of Papers Presented at the
Fourteenth Annual Clinical Conference on Cancer, 1969
at The University of Texas M. D. Anderson Hospital
and Tumor Institute at Houston, Houston, Texas*

YEAR BOOK MEDICAL PUBLISHERS, INC.

35 EAST WACKER DRIVE, CHICAGO

Library of Congress Catalog Card Number: 74-119578

International Standard Book Number: 0-8151-0207-0

Table of Contents

5

Acknowledgments

FOR THEIR SUPPORT in making possible both the Fourteenth Annual Clinical Conference and the publication of this monograph, the staff of The University of Texas M. D. Anderson Hospital and Tumor Institute at Houston gratefully acknowledges the assistance of the Texas Division of the American Cancer Society; the Division of Continuing Education of The University of Texas Graduate School of Biomedical Sciences at Houston; and the Regional Medical Program, United States Public Health Service.

The program was arranged and organized by a committee composed of the following staff members of M. D. Anderson Hospital: C. C. Shullenberger, chairman; Lillian M. Fuller, co-chairman; and members Raymond Alexanian, James J. Butler, Leon Dmochowski, Emil J Freireich, Evan M. Hersh, W. W. Sutow, Sidney Wallace, and Jordan M. Wilbur. Special thanks are due Mrs. Anita Miller for secretarial efforts and Mrs. Mary McCracken for editorial arrangement of the panel discussion.

This volume was prepared for publication by the following members of the M. D. Anderson Hospital Department of Publications: R. W. Cumley, Joan E. McCay, Wendelyn White, Judith James, Barbara Gail Arnold, Lynda Burgner, Carol Lee Dimopoulos, Janina Ely, Shirley Hartman, Judith Letteney, Lucinda Marinis, Carol Thompson, and Kathleen Yacuzzo.

Many of the illustrations in this volume were prepared by members of the M. D. Anderson Hospital Department of Medical Communications.

Introduction to the Fourteenth Annual Clinical Conference

R. LEE CLARK, M.D., M.Sc., D.Sc. (Hon.)

President, The University of Texas M. D. Anderson Hospital and Tumor Institute at Houston, Houston, Texas

As an integral part of The University of Texas and its widespread educational programs, we at the M. D. Anderson Hospital and Tumor Institute at Houston continue to be proud of the increased interest shown in our Annual Clinical Conference on Cancer. The gratifying attendance each year reinforces our conviction that physicians welcome the opportunity to continue their education in current treatment modalities for the patient with cancer and to exchange freely their findings with others having mutual interests. Through analysis of our own experiences and comparison with reports from other research and clinical centers offered by the outstanding guest lecturers, our desire to provide increasingly better care for all cancer patients will be realized more quickly.

The registrants of this conference will confront the problems of neoplasia of the lymphatic and blood-forming systems, *i.e.,* lymphomas and leukemias. These malignant conditions account for less than 10 per cent of deaths from cancer and approximately 1.5 per cent of deaths from all causes; yet paradoxically, they command a major proportion of the attention of students of neoplasia.

The American Cancer Society estimated that during 1969, 19,000 new cases of leukemia would be diagnosed and 15,000 deaths would result from this disease. Leukemia accounts for approximately one half of cancer deaths in children between the ages of three and 14 years. With increasing age, the percentage of deaths caused by leukemia drops considerably.

It is estimated that there will be 22,000 new cases of lymphoma and 17,000 deaths caused by this disease in the United States in 1969. Although deaths from leukemia and lymphoma are essentially equal in number, there are far fewer deaths in childhood attributed to lymphoma than to leukemia.

9

Significant advances in the chemotherapy for these neoplastic disorders have been made in the past 20 years, particularly in the past five years. In major treatment centers, more than 90 per cent of children with acute lymphocytic leukemia achieve complete remission; six years ago, the complete remission rate was 50 per cent. Although the median survival figures for these patients differ somewhat at various institutions, some recent reports have indicated a median survival of at least 33 months. In 1963, the median survival figures were in the range of 12 to 19 months.

Members of the Acute Leukemia Task Force, organized by the National Cancer Institute and composed of oncologists from throughout the country, have compiled a registry of more than 150 long-term survivors with acute leukemia, an increasing number of whom are living more than five years following diagnosis of leukemia. The Task Force reported an apparent justification to discontinue leukemia treatment seven years after diagnosis if there had been no evidence of disease for at least four years. This strongly suggests cure in at least some of the cases.

The first significant development in the chemotherapy for acute leukemia occurred in 1947 when Dr. Sidney Farber observed that folic acid antagonists induced remissions. The development of new and more effective drugs and their use, individually and in combinations, as well as the use of protected environments, platelet transfusions, and more effective antibiotics to combat infection have been the major factors in improved treatment for acute leukemia.

Chronic leukemias continue to pose serious challenges. Because of their basic nature and tempo, it is difficult to devise studies which will show well-delineated increases in survival which are directly attributable to specific therapy. However, chronic granulocytic leukemia has furnished a starting point for the fascinating application of cytogenetic studies to the clinical problem of leukemia. There is evidence to substantiate the belief that a selected chromosome constitution endows other cancer or leukemia cells with the capabilities for proliferative growth, but the mechanisms by which one particular chromosomal combination is selected in preference to another and by which the selected combination allows the neoplastic cells to maintain their growth rate are presently unknown.

Malignant lymphoma represents a basic neoplastic process of the reticuloendothelial system which often overlaps the clinical patterns of leukemia and which may assume various appearances. Basic scientists and clinical investigators are challenged to explain the relatively benign course of follicular lymphomas as opposed to the relatively aggressive course of reticulum cell sarcoma. Hodgkin's disease also presents challenging clinical and therapeutic problems. Recent concepts of histological classification, correlated with clinical staging and the nature of spread of the disease, have resulted in close collaboration between chemotherapists and radiotherapists. The Anderson Hospital experience with malignant lymphomas and Hodgkin's disease indicates that the concepts that radiotherapy should be restricted to treatment for localized disease and that chemotherapy should be reserved for generalized disease are somewhat rigid. For example, our preliminary experience in controlling advanced stage III Hodgkin's disease with a combination of radiotherapy and chemotherapy confirms the encouraging results from other institutions.

In studies on leukemia and lymphoma today, the fundamental problems of etiology and etiologically oriented therapy begin to emerge. The possibility of viral etiology is a compelling concept, and the contributions of investigators of African Burkitt's lymphoma, beginning with Dr. Denis Burkitt, lead us to concentrate heavily on studies in virology, epidemiology, and immunology. There are now over 60 viruses known to cause a wide variety of cancers in every major group of animals, including subhuman primates. There is conclusive evidence in experimental systems that virus-induced, chemical-induced, and even spontaneous tumors contain new antigens which resemble weak transplantation antigens that are not shared by host tissues. These provide a selective target for chemotherapy.

Application of this knowledge to the disease in human beings has revealed that viruslike particles can be detected and, in some cases, isolated from patients. Burkitt's lymphoma is frequently associated with a herpes-type virus (HTV), and many patients with Burkitt's tumor exhibit high levels of antibodies to HTV antigens. These findings are responsible for a resurgence of interest in immunotherapy. However, much laboratory and clinical investigation remains to be done before any cause-and-effect relationship between viruses and cancer in human beings can be substantiated.

Preliminary studies of techniques designed to assist a patient's natural immune mechanisms appear to have achieved positive results. Reports from Russia of a "positive therapeutic effect" after injection of live leukemia cells into children acutely ill with leukemia, trials in France with adjuvant therapy with BCG vaccine combined with therapy with pooled allogeneic leukemia cells pretreated with formalin or radiation, and similar investigations and clinical trials here in the United States give us potentially rewarding approaches to the control of these diseases. Other attempts which have produced some objective benefit include the use of spleen cells from normal donors to reduce a patient's immune response following chemotherapy, and the use of bone marrow grafts from normal individuals to reduce leukemic cells and the host immune response following irradiation. Also, there is some evidence that serum antibodies can affect tumors, but the potential for use of these has not been fully explored.

Although these research avenues are compelling and fascinating to all of us, the primary over-all objective of the Annual Clinical Conference is the presentation to the practicing physician of current ideas and methods in the diagnosis, clinical investigation, and management of cancer in its various forms. It is our hope that physicians attending this conference will return to their practice with a clear and useful picture of the current activity of the scientific community at large and of this institution as it applies to increased understanding and, therefore, better treatment of the patient with leukemia or malignant lymphoma. We welcome the opportunity to present our distinguished guest speakers and the members of Anderson Hospital who represent the various fields of basic science, diagnosis, and therapy, all of which contribute to the total effort essential for the effective management of malignant disease.

Our thanks are extended to the Texas Division of the American Cancer Society and to the United States Public Health Service for their assistance in making this Clinical Conference possible.

The GUY H. HEATH *and* DAN C. HEATH
Memorial Lecture

Problems in the Evaluation of Chemotherapy for Lymphomas*

DAVID A. KARNOFSKY, M.D.†

Medical Oncology Service, Memorial Hospital for Cancer and Allied Diseases, and Division of Chemotherapy Research, Sloan-Kettering Institute for Cancer Research, New York, New York

THE SEARCH for more effective antilymphoma drugs involves: (1) the clinical trial of potential antilymphoma drugs, (2) development of a methodology for the evaluation of therapeutic activity, (3) studies on the mechanisms of drug action, and (4) investigations into the nature of lymphomas.

In the treatment of patients with cancer, two important situations require a decision on the part of the physician. First, in what situation is therapy of practical value? This question must surely be answered differently for patients with advanced cancer and for those with disease for which there is more satisfactory treatment. Patients with advanced cancer may be desperately ill, or they are aware of the inevitable course of the disease with its increasing servere symptomatology, disability, and deterioration. Table 1 presents a list of those forms of cancer in which benefit has been obtained with some degree of regularity by using anticancer drugs, in contrast to other forms of cancer for which useful results are less frequent and incon-

*Supported in part by Grant No. 08748 from the National Cancer Institute, National Institutes of Health, United States Public Health Service.

Based in part on a lecture given at an International Conference on Leukemia-Lymphoma, The University of Michigan, Ann Arbor, Michigan, October, 1967.

†Dr. David A. Karnofsky died on August 29, 1969. The Guy H. Heath and Dan C. Heath Memorial Award was bestowed on him posthumously on November 6, 1969. Accepting the award for his former colleague was Irwin H. Krakoff, M.D., Attending Physician, Memorial Hospital for Cancer and Allied Diseases, and Member, Sloan-Kettering Institute for Cancer Research, New York, New York. Dr. Krakoff also delivered The Guy H. Heath and Dan C. Heath Memorial Lecture, which had been prepared in large measure by Dr. Karnofsky before his death.

TABLE 1.—COMMON NEOPLASTIC DISEASES WHICH SHOW AN APPRECIABLE
INCIDENCE OF THERAPEUTIC RESPONSE TO ANTICANCER DRUGS

LEUKEMIAS AND LYMPHOMAS

Acute lymphoblastic and myeloblastic leukemia	Reticulum cell sarcoma
Chronic myelocytic and lymphatic leukemia	Multiple myeloma
Hodgkin's disease	Polycythemia vera
Lymphosarcoma	

OTHER CANCERS

Breast	Lung
Prostate	Carcinoid
Endometrial	Adrenal cortical
Trophoblastic tumors in females	Wilms' tumor, children
Ovarian	Neuroblastoma
Testicular	Soft-part tumors
Large bowel	

stant. The lymphomas and leukemias are prominent among those neoplasms which respond to chemotherapeutic agents as well as to radiotherapy.

Second, if a reasonably useful form of therapy is not available, or if the patient has become resistant to previously effective therapy, it is necessary to decide if an experimental form of treatment should be offered the patient. The use of investigational drugs or procedures is often justified in clinical situations for which no effective form of treatment is known. Such procedures can be undertaken, not necessarily with the promise of producing important benefits to the patient (although this is conceivable), but with the clear necessity of learning more about the mechanism of action of the drug and its pharmacological and therapeutic effects. It is important to note that we are not talking about isolated drug trials by untrained individuals, but about studies conducted in a setting where there is a thorough understanding of the state of the disease and where one has the facilities and skills to obtain a great deal of information about the effects of the drug.

The clinical evaluation of the therapeutic activity of a drug effective against lymphomas or other forms of cancer when used alone, in combination with other drugs, or by various routes of administration is a complicated problem. If agents were available that caused a substantial cure rate for certain forms of cancer at nontoxic doses, the assessment of therapeutic effects would be easy. Many of the anticancer drugs available today, however, are highly toxic and have a weak or negligible therapeutic action against most forms of cancer. These drugs are given, often at maximum tolerated doses, with the expectation that a significant therapeutic response will be obtained in only a small proportion of the treated patients.

There is no simple end point which permits one to measure the partial and temporary therapeutic responses that occur in most patients with cancer. There are many kinds of cancer which behave differently; even within a particular group, the disease may evolve differently in each patient and may respond differently to the various forms of treatment used. It is difficult to make consistent generalizations. In this complex setting, it is tempting to develop arbitrary and easily applied methods of grading therapeutic responses and to avoid the more complicated, controversial, and broader aspects of the evolution of the patient's disease and its control by the treatment under evaluation. Thus, in many reports of drug trials, it is stated that a certain percentage of responses occurred to a particular agent as measured by shrinkage of selected palpable masses. Careful examination of other relevant data (not necessarily included in the published reports) may reveal, however, that there was steady deterioration of the patient's condition caused by progressive disease, drug toxicity, or both; in some cases, the maximum regression of the tumor masses coincided with the death of the patient.

To avoid this type of pitfall in our clinical evaluations, each patient is studied in a detailed manner with the purpose of obtaining clinically meaningful results from a drug trial. Investigators experienced in the evaluation of anticancer drugs recognize the need to test them against a background of the behavior of cancer in general and a thorough understanding of the disease in the individual patient. For each patient, this includes an analysis of the primary site, extent, clinical pattern, and rate of progression of the cancer, the stage of the disease, and the types and results of previous treatment. After this baseline is established and the new agent, or procedure, is administered in an adequate dosage, we are then concerned with a careful analysis of the anticancer effects obtained. These effects relate not only to the ability of the drug to cause tumor regression, but also to its effect on the patient's symptoms and signs and functional activity. We must assess whether we are merely causing minor regression of selected nodes or nodules, alleviating symptoms without prolongation of survival, or interrupting tumor growth with a significant increase in survival time. We must determine if significant therapeutic responses occur in a small number of patients at the expense of life-threatening toxicity and concomitant worsening of the general condition of a majority of the patients treated. We must also concern ourselves with the consistency of the therapeutic responses in a large number of patients who have a uniform type of disease, as far as classification is possible. A single magnificent result, which may be coincidental, in the study of 100 patients with a particular problem is probably of little importance except to that individual patient.

If the therapeutic activity of a drug proves to be weak and brief, even

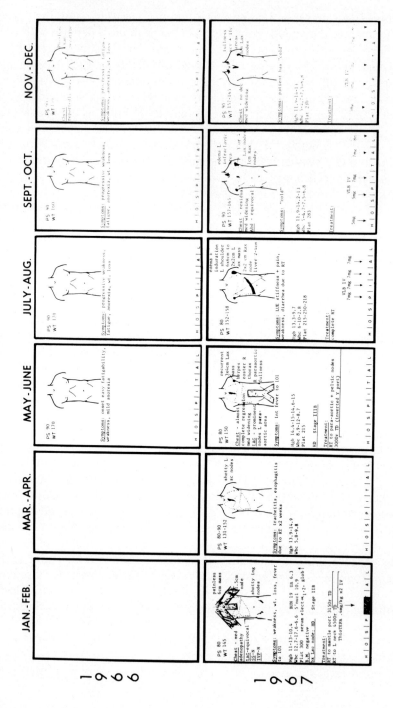

FIG. 1.—This placard depicts the clinical course of a 20-year-old male with Hodgkin's disease. Symptoms were present for eight months before a diagnosis was made in January 1967. Because of an equivocal abdominal lymphangiogram and the findings of weight loss, fever, and anemia, the patient was classified in stage IIB. He was treated with Thio-TEPA followed by radiotherapy to a mantle port (3,150 R tumor dose). He showed excellent local tumor regression and symptomatic improvement, but within two months, fever recurred and the abdominal nodes were found to be enlarged. He received 3,000 R tumor dose to an inverted Y abdominal port. He was weak and complained of diarrhea after radiotherapy, and recurrent masses developed in the left and right axillae. It is not clear to what extent his symptoms were caused by the course of abdominal radiation or by recurrent disease. Nevertheless, he was started on vinblastine (VLB) and improved steadily, although the left axillary mass persisted. This is not a clear-cut response to vinblastine since the drug was started shortly after abdominal radiotherapy was completed. Improvement has continued for six months thus far, with weight gain and a normal performance status (PS), and he is on maintenance vinblastine therapy.

after a prolonged and painstaking analysis, the conclusions must be consistent with the detailed clinical data, no matter how disappointing this may be to the investigator. It is essential to progress in cancer chemotherapy that we observe the need for this type of practical and objective analysis.

The Medical Oncology Service of Memorial Hospital, in cooperation with the Division of Chemotherapy Research of the Sloan-Kettering Institute, has developed a number of record-keeping techniques which permit an orderly and detailed analysis of the course of disease in the individual patient and the response to anticancer drugs. These techniques will be presented briefly to illustrate the variety of procedures that enter into the analysis and evaluation of a response to an anticancer drug.

Figure 1 represents a calendar placard which has been developed to chart the over-all course of illness in each patient. At two-month intervals, a

FIG. 2.—A single 3 × 5-in. card on the calendar placard shown in Figure 1 which shows the relevant physical findings, laboratory data, and forms of therapy during the first two months of 1967.

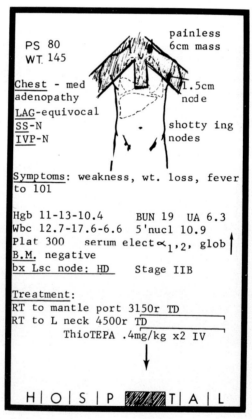

TABLE 2.—CRITERIA OF PERFORMANCE STATUS

CRITERIA	%	STATUS OF PATIENT
Able to carry on normal activity; no special care is needed	100	Normal; no complaints; no evidence of disease
	90	Able to carry on normal activity; minor signs or symptoms of disease
	80	Normal activity with effort; some signs or symptoms of disease
Unable to work; able to live at home; cares for most personal needs; a varying amount of assistance is needed	70	Cares for self; unable to carry on normal activity or to do active work
	60	Requires occasional assistance but is able to care for most of his needs
	50	Requires considerable assistance and frequent medical care
Unable to care for self; requires equivalent of institutional or hospital care; disease may be progressing rapidly	40	Disabled; requires special medical care and assistance
	30	Severely disabled; hospitalization is indicated, although death not imminent
	20	Very sick; hospitalization necessary; active supportive treatment necessary
	10	Moribund; fatal processes progressing rapidly
	0	Dead

3 × 5-in. card is prepared which outlines the patient's status in a concise form during that period (Fig. 2). These cards are pasted in correct chronological sequence on a 20 × 30-in. cardboard which has sufficient space for a three-year period (Fig. 1). The placards permit a rapid survey of the course of the disease, its pattern, methods of treatment, and the therapeutic responses. The placards are available in the outpatient clinic at the time of each patient's visit and in the wards. Techniques are being developed to introduce the data on the placards into computers so that it will be possible to retrieve the appropriate placards which display our experience with specific clinical problems, drug responses, or toxicity within the context of the course of the disease in individual patients.

An additional technique which we have found useful in evaluating the effect of the disease on a patient and the influence of therapy is classification by "performance status" (Table 2) (Karnofsky and Burchenal, 1949). At each clinic visit, grading the performance status is a routine part of the evaluation of each patient, and it provides a quantitative estimate of his competence within his environment.

TABLE 3.—CATEGORIES OF RESPONSE

CATEGORY 0	No CLINICALLY USEFUL EFFECT ON THE COURSE OF THE DISEASE
0 - 0	Disease progresses–no objective or subjective benefit
0 - A*	Subjective benefit without favorable objective changes
0 - B*	Favorable objective changes without subjective benefit
0 - C	Subjective benefit and favorable objective changes in measurable criteria, but of less than 1 month's duration; then the disease progresses
CATEGORY I	CLINICAL BENEFIT WITH FAVORABLE OBJECTIVE CHANGES IN ALL MEASURABLE CRITERIA OF THE DISEASE
I - A*	Distinct subjective benefit with favorable objective changes in all measurable criteria for 1 month or more.
I - B*	Objective regression of all palpable or measurable neoplastic disease for 1 month or more in a relatively asymptomatic patient who is able to carry on his usual activities without undue difficulty. The observed tumor regression should be unequivocal, and it is suggested that all lesions be reduced at least 50% in bulk. This category applies as long as the regression persists and ends if any old lesion recurs or new lesion appears.
I - C	Complete relief of symptoms, if any, and regression of all manifestations caused by the active disease for 1 year or more. The relation to the frequency of therapy is not relevant if the disease does not recur between courses of therapy.
CATEGORY II	INTERRUPTION OR SLOWING IN THE PROGRESSION OF THE DISEASE WITHOUT DEFINITE EVIDENCE OF SUBJECTIVE OR OBJECTIVE IMPROVEMENT (No criteria are presently available to classify this type of response. Statistical evidence of prolongation of survival time in specific patterns of cancer may be applicable some day.)

ADEQUATE THERAPY

The adequacy of the course of treatment should be defined in the patients who complete the course of treatment. In most cases, therapy is given to the point of toxicity in order to give the maximum opportunity for an anticancer effect. If the patient can be observed for signs of benefit for at least 2 weeks following treatment, this ordinarily represents an adequate trial.

If tumor regression and a satisfactory clinical response occur before any signs of toxicity appear, this is also considered an adequate trial.

LEVELS OF TOXICITY

1+ —Slight
2+ —Moderate
3+ —Life threatening
4+ —Directly lethal or a proximate contributory cause of death

---

*Categories apply as long as improvement from baseline persists. Superscript time in months of duration of response. Examples: O-A^4 or I-B^3.

Following a clinical trial, the "categories of response" method (Table 3) (Karnofsky, 1961) is used to classify in a brief and comprehensible manner each patient's response to therapy, the duration of response, and the degree of toxicity produced by the treatment. Classification by categories of response presents in a meaningful way the degree of benefit produced by specific therapy in each patient.

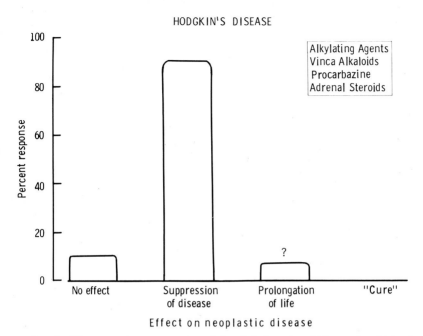

FIG. 3.—Diagrammatic representation of the clinical results which may be obtained with available chemotherapy for advanced Hodgkin's disease.

Another graphic method has been used to present a practical view of the therapeutic activity of a method of treatment within a defined context. Figure 3 (Young, 1967) summarizes the therapeutic activity of the available chemotherapeutic agents for stages III and IV Hodgkin's disease. These drugs suppress the manifestations of disease in a large percentage of patients and may cause some prolongation of life in some. If one were to consider stages I and II Hodgkin's disease and to include radiotherapy in the treatment regimen, a different summary would be necessary. The graph can be made more precise and useful by narrowing the framework of the analysis to a specific pattern or stage of disease or specific types of therapy.

These formal procedures for interpreting the course of the disease and the pattern of response to each type of therapy are essential in order to evaluate new agents and procedures, to define their role in the practical management of cancer, and to provide a vocabulary understandable to all investigators in the field of cancer therapy. These methods of data analysis and presentation do not simplify therapeutic trials, but they are mandatory if we are to present reliable and useful data on the indications and the effectiveness of anticancer drugs.

The therapeutic response is defined in relation to the patient's clinical status, the degree and duration of improvement, the adequacy of treatment, and the order in which the new agent was used in the therapeutic sequence. Although these factors are evident to all investigators, two matters require comment. (1) A distinction must be made between a brief or single course of treatment given to elicit evidence of the therapeutic activity of a drug and the prolonged use of a drug until resistance develops to determine how long it will be effective. Although both procedures are therapeutic studies, the effectiveness of a drug over a period of time is obviously of greater importance. (2) We have tried to make a distinction between suppression of the manifestations of disease, that is, temporary relief of symptoms and signs, and the interruption in the progression of the disease as reflected in appreciable prolongation of life. That treatment has the latter effect on acute lymphoblastic leukemia has been amply proved, but such effect on lymphomas is far more difficult to demonstate. The term "complete remission" (a carry-over from clinical studies on the acute leukemias), which implies that all evidence of disease has disappeared, should be avoided in evaluating lymphomas. In patients with lymphoma, no direct effort is made to prove the disappearance of all signs of disease following chemotherapy, since this would require the rebiopsy of areas of known involvement. In fact, an "incomplete remission" with persistence of measurable disease may be as effective as a "complete remission" in terms of relief from symptoms and the duration of response. Radiotherapy to localized disease may cause a "complete remission," indicating that the lymphomas are not necessarily systemic diseases; in this sense, remission may be equated with surgical cure. For systemic lymphomas (where the term is applicable), it seems appropriate to use a less specific description of a therapeutic response, *i.e.,* a "complete or partial suppression of manifestations of disease," until such time as there is a valid definition of "complete remission."

In this context, what is the practical meaning of the response rate to an antilymphoma drug? It cannot be of fundamental therapeutic significance if there is no evidence to show that the therapeutic activity of the drug is responsible for an increase in the cure rate or survival time. Operationally, the chemotherapeutic trials are at the level of "temporary suppression of manifestations of the disease." Thus, Spurr, Carbone, and Schneiderman (1966) report that vinblastine is superior to cyclophosphamide in producing remissions in patients with Hodgkin's disease; this report was supported by Stutzman, Ezdinli, and Stutzman (1966), although Fairley, Patterson, and Scott (1966) found no difference in the two agents. DeVita, Serpick, and Carbone (1969) have demonstrated a large number of "remissions" in Hodgkin's disease managed with combination chemotherapy, but this has not yet been interpreted in terms of total remission time or over-all survival.

Cyclophosphamide gave a higher percentage of remissions than vincristine in patients with lymphosarcoma, whereas there was no difference between the two drugs in patients with reticulum cell sarcoma. If these agents merit comparative studies in this limited context, similar studies are required for other antilymphoma drugs such as chlorambucil, nitrogen mustard, methyl ester of streptonigrin, and procarbazine.

But what is the relevance of these therapeutic trials and their comparative response data to the practical management of a patient's disease? The great difficulties in drawing useful conclusions are apparent when cure rates and prolonged survival time, attributable to the drug, are not part of the equation. Despite data revealing measurable differences when two drugs are compared, when the patient becomes refractory to the more active drug, the other will be tried; an individual patient, despite the statistical pressure to conform, may respond better to the less effective drug. In addition, the factors of convenience in the use of a drug, patient acceptability, and toxicity must be taken into consideration. Currently, it is suggested that the effects of an antilymphoma drug be interpreted in relation to the pattern of the disease in the individual patient, and from the detailed, organized, but largely empirical experience, insights may result which will be important in the management of specific clinical situations.

The mechanisms of action of an antilymphoma drug at a subcellular and cellular level in normal and neoplastic systems are under detailed investigation. These studies may explain in time the therapeutic effects of a drug and, in addition, may provide clues to the etiology and pathogenesis of the disease itself. The available antilymphoma drugs act on biochemical processes present in both normal and cancer cells, and they do not, with the possible exception of L-asparaginase, show a qualitatively selective action on neoplastic cells. In favorable situations, however, for reasons not as yet understood, the antilymphoma drugs may destroy or inhibit the growth of some lymphomas and suppress systemic symptoms at doses not causing serious host toxicity. The anticancer drugs act principally by damaging the structure of deoxyribonucleic acid (DNA), by interfering with DNA-dependent ribonucleic acid (RNA) synthesis, and by blocking biosynthetic pathways involved in the production and interconversions of the purines and pyrimidines. The vinca alkaloids are spindle poisons which inhibit cell division, and the steroid hormones, including the adrenocortical hormones, act on responsive cells by a variety of postulated mechanisms (Karnofsky and Clarkson, 1963). In adults with lymphoma, the most useful agents damage DNA (polyfunctional alkylating agents and procarbazine), inhibit mitosis, and perhaps, have additional effects (vinca alkaloids) or destroy lymphoid tissue and proliferating mesenchymal cells by mechanisms as yet unclear (adrenal steroids). Lymphosarcoma in children, and to a lesser extent in adults, may respond to the purine and pyrimidine antagonists (methotrexate, 6-mercaptopurine, and arabinosyl cytosine). For the lymphosarcomas and reticulum cell sarcoma, effective drugs appear to destroy susceptible cells directly, but their action against Hodgkin's disease is less certain. They may act not only on the neoplastic cells, but also on the cellular reaction in the involved node which appears to be an integral part of the process.

The etiology of lymphoma in man is not understood, and knowledge of the pathogenesis of systemic signs and symptoms related to the disease is incomplete. Based on animal models, the possibilities that the disease may be of viral origin or caused by disturbances in the immunological reactivity of the host have been considered (Obstacles to the Control of Hodgkin's Disease, 1966). In the absence of known causative factors or of the demonstration of a continuing pathogen or metabolic disturbance in the host or in the neoplastic cells, attempts at effective chemotherapy remain empirical.

There are numerous systemic disturbances in patients with lymphoma, particularly Hodgkin's disease; these include fever, anemia, itching, weight loss, lymphopenia, serum protein abnormalities, and immunological defects. Many of these effects, at least at a clinically detectable level, do not appear to precede the diagnosis of localized or asymptomatic disease, but may become progressively more severe as the process advances and becomes more generalized (Brown et al., 1967).

There are techniques to study these disturbances; examples are serum electrophoresis and immunoelectrophoresis, tests for delayed hypersensitivity, erythrocyte survival, cytological and histochemical studies of the neoplastic tissue, correlation of the histological findings of the involved node with the clinical course, and analysis of the mechanism of hyperpyrexia. The results of these studies will be important in providing explanations for some of these consequences of active disease, but not necessarily of the basic process itself. Chemotherapeutic agents temporarily alleviate many of these specific systemic manifestations, presumably by inhibiting functional processes or destroying neoplastic cells. Their effects may suggest methods of studying the pathogenesis of the systemic disturbances.

A more specific approach is to study the effects of drugs with a more precise or limited mechanism of action. Cycloheximide, for example, suppresses the fever associated with Hodgkin's disease during the period of infusion; the associated rise in plasma amino acid levels during infusion is supportive clinical evidence that the drug is acting by inhibiting protein synthesis (Young and Karnofsky, 1967). This suggests that the fever associated with Hodgkin's disease is caused by a specific nonantigenic protein, and it is hoped that the characteristics of this postulated substance can be determined. If the mechanism of the production of these systemic disturbances and the proximate factors can be determined, it may be possible to discover specific drugs for the alleviation of symptoms, even if they do not act against the basic processes of the disease.

Summary

It appears likely that studies which clarify our understanding of the clinical nature of the lymphomas and their pathophysiology may lead to more effective therapy and that studies of the mechanism of drug action may permit us to use the available drugs in optimal ways.

REFERENCES

Brown, R. S., Haynes, H. A., Foley, H. T., Godwin, H. A., Berard, C. W., and Carbone, P. P.: Hodgkin's disease: Immunologic, clinical, and histologic features of 50 untreated patients. *Annals of Internal Medicine*, 67:291-302, August 1967.

DeVita, V. T., Serpick, A., and Carbone, P.P.: Combination chemotherapy of advanced Hodgkin's disease (HD): The NCI program, a progress report. (Abstract) *Proceedings of the American Association for Cancer Research*, 10:19, March 1969.

Fairley, G. H., Patterson, M. J. L., and Scott, R. B.: Chemotherapy of Hodgkin's disease with cyclophosphamide, vinblastine, and procarbazine. *British Medical Journal*, 2:75-78, July 9, 1966.

Karnofsky, D. A.: Chemotherapy of the lymphomas. In Zarafonetis, C. J. D., Ed.: *Proceedings of the International Conference on Leukemia-Lymphoma*. Philadelphia, Pennsylvania, Lea & Febiger, 1968, pp. 409-422.

_____: Meaningful clinical classification of therapeutic responses to anticancer drugs. (Editorial) *Clinical Pharmacology and Therapeutics*, 2:709-712, November-December 1961.

Karnofsky, D. A., and Burchenal, J. H.: The clinical evaluation of chemotherapeutic agents in cancer. In MacLeod, C. M., Ed.: *Evaluation of Chemotherapeutic Agents*, Symposium Held at the New York Academy of Medicine, New York, New York, 1948. New York, New York, Columbia University Press, 1949, pp. 191-205.

Karnofsky, D. A., and Clarkson, B. D.: Cellular effects of anticancer drugs. *Annual Review of Pharmacology*, 3:357-428, 1963.

Obstacles to the Control of Hodgkin's Disease (Symposium Sponsored by the American Cancer Society and the National Cancer Institute Held at the Westchester Country Club, Rye, New York, September 13-15, 1965). *Cancer Research*, 26:1047-1312, June 1966.

Spurr, C. L., Carbone, P. P., and Schneiderman, M. A. (Acute Leukemia Group B and Eastern Solid Tumor Chemotherapy Group): Comparative evaluation of cyclophosphamide and vinca alkaloids in lymphomas. (Abstract) *Proceedings of the American Association for Cancer Research*, 7:67, April 1966.

Stutzman, L., Ezdinli, E. Z., and Stutzman, M. A.: Vinblastine sulfate vs cyclophosphamide in the therapy for lymphoma. *Journal of the American Medical Association*, 195: 173-178, January 17, 1966.

Young, C. W.: Cancer chemotherapy: New agents and new applications of established agents. *Academy of Medicine of New Jersey Bulletin*, 13:46-59, March 1967.

Young, C. W., and Karnofsky, D. A.: The necessity of protein synthesis for fever in Hodgkin's disease. (Abstract) *Proceedings of the American Association for Cancer Research*, 8:75, March 1967.

Leukocyte Kinetics in Leukemia and Lymphoma*

HOWARD E. SKIPPER, Ph.D.

Kettering-Meyer Laboratories, Southern Research Institute, Birmingham, Alabama

I AM DEEPLY INTERESTED in the subject of leukocyte kinetics in leukemia and lymphoma. However, my interest may not be purely basic. I want to know everything that I can learn about the kinetic behavior of neoplastic and normal cell populations because I believe that such information is vital to the optimal design of therapeutic trials against cancer in animals and man and to the translation of knowledge gained in studies on animal cancer to those on human cancer and vice versa. I state this in advance because I have learned that I cannot talk about kinetics without talking about therapy and I cannot talk about therapy without talking about kinetics.

In Figure 1, I have tried to illustrate variables and relationships worthy of consideration in the design of a therapeutic trial against any type of disseminated cancer. Almost every box in Figure 1 implies biochemical, pharmacologic, toxicologic, and kinetic overlap. Two goals are implied also: (1) Selection of agents with knowledge of their mechanisms of action, for control of specific neoplastic diseases with differing growth rates and proliferative states and (2) optimal scheduling of dosage intervals to provide the concentrations of the drug in the blood which will kill neoplastic cells faster than they are being replaced without toxicity to the host.

One can design experimental or clinical trials using any one or a combination of several strategic approaches: (1) intuition with faith in luck, (2) stepwise trial and error, (3) guidance from certain quantitative information such as is indicated in Figure 1, and (4) learning how to alter and translate known optimal regimens for high growth–fraction neoplasms to lower and lower growth-fraction neoplasms. Briefly, I would be hesitant to rely on

*This work was supported by Contract No. PH 43-65-594, Chemotherapy, National Cancer Institute, National Institutes of Health; by the Charles F. Kettering Foundation; by the Alfred P. Sloan Foundation; and by the American Cancer Society (Grant No. T 111).

27

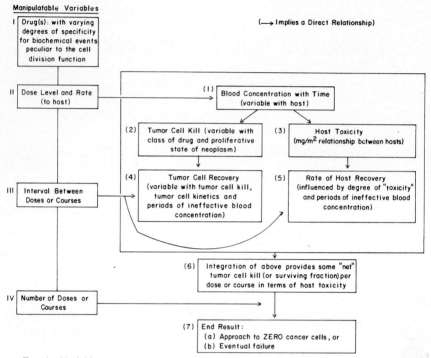

Manipulatable Variables

I | Drug(s): with varying degrees of specificity for biochemical events peculiar to the cell division function

(⟶ Implies a Direct Relationship)

II | Dose Level and Rate (to host)

(1) Blood Concentration with Time (variable with host)

(2) Tumor Cell Kill (variable with class of drug and proliferative state of neoplasm)

(3) Host Toxicity (mg/m^2 relationship between hosts)

III | Interval Between Doses or Courses

(4) Tumor Cell Recovery (variable with tumor cell kill, tumor cell kinetics and periods of ineffective blood concentration)

(5) Rate of Host Recovery (influenced by degree of "toxicity" and periods of ineffective blood concentration)

(6) Integration of above provides some "net" tumor cell kill (or surviving fraction) per dose or course in terms of host toxicity

IV | Number of Doses or Courses

(7) End Result: (a) Approach to ZERO cancer cells, or (b) Eventual failure

FIG. 1.—Variables and relationships worthy of consideration in design of any therapeutic trial.

approaches 1 and 2 alone because they might take too long if cancer is indeed "a hundred diseases." Personally, I suspect that the quantitative biochemical differences associated with the proliferative state of different types of cancer at different degrees of advancement may account for some or much of what has led us to describe cancer as a hundred diseases.

Table 1 is included to emphasize the fact that resting cells (cells not synthesizing deoxyribonucleic acid [DNA]) may be quite insensitive to certain anticancer agents (Pittillo, Schabel, and Skipper, in press). Similar differences have been observed between resting and dividing leukemic cells (Schabel, Skipper, Trader, and Wilcox, 1965) and between normal hematopoietic stem cells with a low growth fraction and transplanted lymphoma cell populations with a high growth fraction (Bruce, Meeker, and Valeriote, 1966).

The cycle-phase aspects of cell population kinetics which give a time parameter to DNA synthesis (albeit only a median) are relatable to classical knowledge of the mechanisms of action of certain anticancer agents (Table 2). Our problem would be much simpler conceptually if all cell populations

TABLE 1.—SENSITIVITY OF RESTING AND DIVIDING
BACTERIAL CELLS

	MINIMUM CONC. (μg/ml) TO KILL 90% (EQUAL EXPOSURES)		
	Resting Cells	Log Phase Cells	Ratio (Resting/Log Phase)
Amethopterin	>1,000	9.5	>105
6-MP	>1,000	112	>9
5-FU	>1,000	0.46	>2,174
Ara-C	>1,000	30	>33
Daunomycin	>1,000	23	>44
Porfiromycin	8.7	2.7	3
HN2	1.7	0.29	6
BCNU	215	16	13
Penicillin	>1,000 u.	72 u.	>14
Chlorotetracycline	>1,000	100	>10
Sulfonamide	>1,000	45	>22

Abbreviations: Ara-C, 1-β-D-arabinofuranosylcytosine · HCl; BCNU, urea, 1,3-bis(2-chloroethyl)-1-nitroso; 5-FU, 5-fluorouracil; HN2, nitrogen mustard; 6-MP, 6-mercaptopurine.

TABLE 2–DRUGS WITH VARYING DEGREES OF SPECIFICITY FOR
BIOCHEMICAL EVENTS PECULIAR TO THE CELL DIVISION FUNCTION

S (DNA, RNA, and Protein Synthesis)

G_1 + M + G_2 (RNA and Protein Synthesis)

Ⓐ only: S phase-specific re cell killing.

Ⓐ and Ⓑ simultaneously: S phase-specific with self-limitation.

AGENT	SITE(S) OF ACTION	END PRODUCT INHIBITION OR INACTIVATION	IMPLICATIONS RE CELL KILLING
Ara-C	DNA polymerase	DNA	S phase-specific
Hydroxyurea	Nucleotide reductase	DNA	S phase-specific
Methotrexate	Folic reductase	DNA, RNA, Prot.	S phase-specific with self-limit.
6-Mercaptopurine	De novo purine synth.	DNA, RNA	S phase-specific with self-limit.
Cytoxan	Reacts with DNA (others)	DNA (others)	Cycle phase-nonspecific
BCNU	?	?	Cycle phase-nonspecific
Actinomycin D	Complexes DNA	DNA, RNA	Cycle phase-nonspecific
Daunomycin	Complexes DNA	DNA, RNA	Cycle phase-nonspecific

NOTE: Some cycle phase nonspecific agents show marked selectivity for cell populations with a high growth fraction, possibly as a result of DNA repair in cells with a long sequestration in G_1 + M + G_2.

were homogeneous and all cells in a given tumor progressed in the cycle, from beginning G_1 to S to G_2 to M, at exactly the same rate. Quite obviously, they do not, even in long-transplanted murine leukemia systems. The median length of G_2 + M + G_1 in the early L1210 leukemia system is about 3.8 hours, but it takes about 24 hours for 99.999 per cent of an L1210 cell population to pass into S phase when, in the presence of an effective concentration of arabinosyl cytosine, they are rendered sterile. For S phase-specific drugs, it would appear that the fraction of neoplastic cells entering S phase per unit time underlies tumor sensitivity because effective blood concentrations cannot be maintained indefinitely. Agents which are S phase-specific with respect to cell killing but are self-limiting because they inhibit ribonucleic acid (RNA) and/or protein synthesis and passage of G_2 + M + G_1 cells into S phase have quite different optimal schedules than do S phase-specific agents (Table 4). The brilliant basic work of Cohen and Barner (1954) and, more recently, of Borsa and Whitmore (1969) on unbalanced growth, thymineless death, and "self-limitation" underlie some of these concepts.

In Figure 2, I have redrawn a chart which Dr. Gordon Zubrod and I devised some time ago. This chart may or may not help to communicate

FIG. 2.—Kinetic considerations and therapeutic implications. Note that Compartment B is not intended to represent a uniform static entity and may be considered simply as A cells with T_C's which are from longer to much longer than the median time. High growth fraction = high A/A + B + C. High growth fraction of viable cells = high A/A + B. Tumor growth = proliferation of A > loss to D. Tumor regression = loss to D > proliferation in A. "Normal" traffic sequence with advancement of disease may be A to B to C to D. "Cell cure" requires sterilization of A and B. Steady state in normal tissues = proliferation of A = loss to D. (Adapted from Skipper and Zubrod, 1968.)

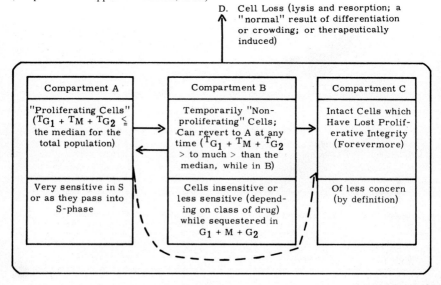

TABLE 3.—KINETIC PARAMETERS FOR MURINE LEUKEMIAS AND HUMAN ACUTE LEUKEMIAS

	Early L1210 Leukemia[a]	Advanced Spontaneous AK Leukemia[b]	Early 1st Passage AK Leukemia	Advanced ALL or AML[d]	Human Leuk. Cells in Log Phase Culture (Before "Crowding")[e]
Doubling Time (days)	0.5	ca 5	ca 1	ca 4 or >	ca 1
Median T_S (hrs)	9	ca 6		ca 20	12
Median T_{G_1} + T_M + T_{G_2} (hrs)	3.8	ca 14		ca 40	6
Median T_C (hrs)	12.8	ca 20		ca 60	18
T_S/T_C × 100	70%	ca 30%		ca 33%	67%
Pulse Thymidine Index	65%	5-37%		ca 5-15%	50%
24-Hour Thymidine Index	>99%			ca 25%	
Cell kill per day required to "stay even" (based on DT)	75%	ca 15%	50%	ca 18%	50%
Response to ara-C	"cures"	poor	"cures"	some remissions	
Response to Cytoxan	"cures"	increase in host lifespan	"cures"	some remissions (ALL)	

[a] References: Skipper, 1968; Simpson-Herren, unpublished data; Yankee, DeVita, and Perry, 1967; Wheeler, Bowdon, Wilkoff, and Dulmadge, 1967; Young, DeVita, and Perry, 1969.

[b] References: Schabel et al., in press; Skipper, Schabel, Trader, and Laster, in press; Metcalf and Wiadrowski, 1966.

[c] References: Schabel et al., in press; Skipper, Schabel, Trader, and Laster, in press.

[d] Reference: Killmann, S.-A., 1968.

[e] References: Todo, Fried, and Clarkson, 1969; Moore, Gerner and Minowada, 1968; Foley et al., 1968.

and avoid certain semantic problems. It helps me visualize kinetically heterogeneous cell populations, changing growth rates, growth fraction (Mendelsohn, 1965, in press), and cell loss (Steel, 1968) in terms of the problems and goals of therapy.

It would be difficult for me to overemphasize the fact that the kinetic behavior of cancer cell populations changes with increase in cell number and tumor mass, or "advancement of disease," in the following ways: (1) growth rates decrease (doubling times increase), (2) the fraction of viable cells passing through S phase per unit time decreases, and (3) cell loss by natural phenomena increases and accentuates the slowing of growth rate. I suspect that the slowing of the growth rate of the tumor is a reflection of increasing traffic between compartments, most often in the sequence A to B to C to D. I further suspect that early L1210 leukemia is a fair model for early acute lymphocytic leukemia (ALL) and acute myelocytic leukemia (AML), which clinicians rarely or never have the opportunity to confront, whereas advanced spontaneous AK leukemia or lymphoma in the mouse is a better model for advanced ALL or AML (Lin, Milley, and Bruce, 1969; Schabel et al., in press; Skipper, Schabel, Trader, and Laster, in press).

Table 3 shows some reported kinetic parameters for murine leukemias and advanced ALL and AML. It is of more than a little interest to us that early first-passage AK leukemia (about 10^6 cells) responds to therapy very much like long-passage AK or L1210 leukemia. Also, the kinetic behavior of uncrowded human leukemic cells (about 10^5/ml.) in culture is quite different from that of advanced ALL or AML. We have already pointed out that, although the median $T_G + T_M + T_{G_2}$ of early L1210 cell populations is 3.8 hours, the range is greater than 24 hours. From the reported median $T_{G_1} + T_M + T_{G_2}$ of about 40 hours for ALL or AML, we can imagine what the range might be. If agents like arabinosyl cytosine, amethopterin, or 6-mercaptopurine kill cells only in S phase, then such information is pertinent when attempting to translate optimal time schedules from the L1210 model to ALL or AML, when designing trials *de novo* against ALL or AML, or when interpreting available therapeutic trial data. The median length of S phase is also important information because, if blood concentrations of S phase-specific agents drop below effective levels for longer than T_s (minimum), some cells will pass through unharmed and divide. If the spacing of effective blood concentrations of arabinosyl cytosine is greater than 12 hours, we cannot kill L1210 leukemic cells (high growth fraction) faster than they are being replaced. Increase in survival time of the host may be achieved, but not "cell cures."

I do not have space to consider in detail the subject of drug concentration with time and cell kill in high growth fraction populations, but this is a very important subject. I will only comment that S phase-specific agents, or agents which are S phase-specific and self-limiting, are apt to be concentration independent above some effective blood concentration (Wilkoff *et al.*, 1967). In other words, concentrations of 10, 100, or 1,000 times higher than the effective blood concentration will not kill cells any faster, or the cells are quite insensitive to these agents until they initiate synthesis of DNA. Cell cycle phase-nonspecific drugs (which may be quite selective for high growth-fraction populations) are significantly concentration dependent with respect to rate of cell kill (concentration $\times$ time = constant for a given drug in a particular system [$C \times t = k$] for a given cell kill).

Relationships between mechanisms of action and schedule dependency of different agents against the high growth-fraction L1210 leukemia system are suggested by extensive data drastically summarized in Table 4 (Schabel, Skipper, Montgomery, and Brockman, unpublished data). The optimal schedule for S phase-specific agents was administration every three hours for eight doses, with three-day intervals for host recovery. This was not an optimal schedule for methotrexate, 6-mercaptopurine, or 5-fluorouracil, or for the cycle phase-nonspecific drugs. Based on either increase in host survival time or "cell cures," a chronic daily schedule is the worst schedule for Cytoxan or the nitrosoureas, presumably because the dose

TABLE 4.—SCHEDULE DEPENDENCE IN THE L1210 SYSTEM
(EARLY DISEASE BEFORE "CROWDING")

AGENT	POSSIBLE END PRODUCT INHIBITION OR INACTIVATION	"CURES" IN ANIMALS BEARING ABOUT 10^6 L1210 CELLS; HIGHEST NONLETHAL DOSE FOR EACH SCHEDULE (0.75-1.0 LD_{10})				
		Single Dose; Day 2	q^3hrs (x 8); Days 2, 6, 10 and 14	qd 2-16 Days	q^2d (x 8); 2-16 Days	q^4d (x 4); Days 2, 6, 10 and 14
1. Ara-C	DNA (only)	0/10	114/229	0/20	0/10	0/10
2. Hydroxyurea	DNA (only)	0/20	12/30	0/30	0/10	0/10
3. Guanazole	DNA (only)	0/10	7/20	0/10	0/10	0/10
4. Picolinaldehyde, 5-OH, T. S.	DNA (only)	0/10	14/30[a]	0/20	–	0/20
5. Methotrexate	DNA, RNA, Protein	0/60	0/40	0/120	0/30	0/80
6. 6-MP	DNA, RNA	0/20	0/20	0/80	0/10	0/10
7. 5-FU	DNA, RNA	0/10	0/30	0/20	0/20	0/10
8. Cytoxan	DNA (and others?)	44/99	0/10	0/40	0/10	0/10
9. BCNU	?	33/50	12/30 (10^7)	1/20	5/10	6/10
10. CCNU	?	357/425	6/60 (10^7)	0/10	5/10	18/40 (10^7)
11. Daunomycin	DNA, RNA (others?)	0/10	0/30	0/10	0/10	0/10
12. Actinomycin D	DNA, RNA (others?)	0/10	0/20	0/20	0/10	0/20

NOTE: [a]Three courses rather than four.
    Our goal is to kill leukemic cells faster than they are being replaced for long enough to reduce the viable number to ZERO—without ever over-dosing the host.
    Clearly (in this model before the leukemic cell population becomes "crowded") optimal scheduling can make the difference between success and failure. Also, it appears that the approach to optimal scheduling is quite different for agents which are: (1) cycle stage specific (e.g., S-phase specific); (2) cycle stage specific but self-limiting; (3) cycle stage nonspecific.
    Abbreviations: Ara-C, 1-β-D-arabinofuranosylcytosine · HCl; Picolinaldehyde, 5-OH, T. S., picolinaldehyde, 5-hydroxy-, thiosemicarbazone; 6-MP, 6-mercaptopurine; 5-FU, 5-fluorouracil; Cytoxan, cyclophosphamide; BCNU, urea, 1, 3-bis(2-chloroethyl)-1-nitroso; CCNU, urea, 1-(2-chloroethyl)-3-cyclohexyl-1-nitroso.

response is steep and the toxicity to the host is cumulative, unless longer host recovery periods are allowed.

I would like to be able to say that, with certain corrections based on relationships indicated in Figure 1 and Table 3, we can translate or alter the optimal schedules for different classes of agents for the L1210 system (with its high growth fraction) and apply them to ALL or AML. Unfortunately, we have not arrived at this point yet and may never get there. However, if we cannot learn to make such translations from high to lower growth-fraction leukemias, then we will try to do it with the spontaneous AK lymphoma system which appears a better kinetic counterpart for advanced ALL and AML. Work with this system is progressing very satisfactorily (Lin, Milley, and Bruce, 1969; Schabel *et al.,* in press; Skipper, Schabel, Trader, and Laster, in press).

Conclusions

Effort toward optimal scheduling is a worthwhile endeavor. It can make, and has made, the difference between success and failure in managing animal neoplasms and a few types of disseminated human cancer. The problem is how to arrive at optimal scheduling for different classes of agents, and their combinations, against a wide variety of human neoplasms with different kinetic behavior—without too many years of trial and error.

Can we gain some guidance from schedule-dependent trials in animal neoplasms having high, medium, and low growth fractions? Can we learn to make "translations," based on kinetic information so that we can reserve the really important, and necessarily long-term, clinical trials for the most important concepts and approaches?

An even better approach would be the development of techniques for sampling and quantitative assay of the fraction of human cancer cells surviving each dose or course of therapy. This does not seem an easy developmental chore at this point in time, but neither does it seem inconceivable.

Acknowledgments

The author wishes to acknowledge the contributions of ideas and data by many of his own associates, particularly Dr. Frank M. Schabel, Jr., and also the guidance received through continued collaboration with the scientific and clinical staffs of the National Cancer Institute, Sloan Kettering Institute for Cancer Research, The University of Texas M. D. Anderson Hospital and Tumor Institute at Houston, Roswell Park Memorial Institute, and other institutions.

Abbreviations

ALL—acute lymphocytic leukemia
AML—acute myelocytic leukemia
C—concentration
Cytoxan—cyclophosphamide
DNA—deoxyribonucleic acid
G_1—postmitotic phase of the cell cycle
G_2—postsynthetic phase of the cell cycle
k—constant for a given drug in a particular system
M—mitosis
RNA—ribonucleic acid
S—cell cycle phase during which the amount of DNA is duplicated while protein and RNA synthesis continue
t—time
T—time or length

REFERENCES

Borsa, J., and Whitmore, G. F.: Cell killing studies on the mode of action of methotrexate on L-cells in vitro. *Cancer Research,* 29:737-744, April 1969.
Bruce, W. R., Meeker, B. E., and Valeriote, F. A.: Comparison of the sensitivity of normal hematopoietic and transplanted lymphoma colony-forming cells to chemotherapeutic

agents administered in vivo. *Journal of the National Cancer Institute*, 37:233-245, August 1966.

Cohen, S. S., and Barner, H. D.: Studies on unbalanced growth in *Escherichia coli*. *Proceedings of the National Academy of Sciences of the U. S. A.*, 40:885-893, October 1954.

Foley, G. E., Lazarus, H., Farber S., Uzman, B. G., and Adams, R. A.: Studies on human leukemic cells in vitro. In *The Proliferation and Spread of Neoplastic Cells*, A Collection of Papers Presented at the 21st Annual Symposium on Fundamental Cancer Research, 1967, at The University of Texas M. D. Anderson Hospital and Tumor Institute at Houston. Baltimore, Maryland, The Williams and Wilkins Company, 1968, pp. 65-91.

Killmann, S.-A.: Acute leukemia: The kinetics of leukemic blast cells in man, an analytical review. *Series Haematologica*, 1(3):38-102, 1968.

Lin, H., Milley, G. I. A., and Bruce, W. R.: Effects of cyclophosphamide (CY), 1,3-bis(2-chloroethyl)-1-nitrosourea (BCNU), vinblastine (VLB) and cytosine arabinoside (ara-C) on lymphoma cells from the spontaneous lymphoma of AKR mice. (Abstract) *Proceedings of the American Association for Cancer Research*, 10:51, March 1969.

Mendelsohn, M. L.: Cell cycle kinetics and mitotically linked chemotherapy. *Cancer Research*. (In press.)

———: The kinetics of tumor cell proliferation. In *Cellular Radiation Biology*, A Collection of Papers Presented at the 18th Annual Symposium on Fundamental Cancer Research, 1964, at The University of Texas M. D. Anderson Hospital and Tumor Institute. Baltimore, Maryland, The Williams and Wilkins Company, 1965, pp. 498-513.

Metcalf, D., and Wiadrowski, M.: Autoradiographic analysis of lymphocyte proliferation in the thymus and in thymic lymphoma tissue. *Cancer Research*, 26:483-491, March 1966.

Moore, G. E., Gerner, R. E., and Minowada, J.: Studies of normal and neoplastic human hematopoietic cells in vitro. In *The Proliferation and Spread of Neoplastic Cells*, A Collection of Papers Presented at the 21st Annual Symposium on Fundamental Cancer Research, 1967, at The University of Texas M. D. Anderson Hospital and Tumor Institute at Houston. Baltimore, Maryland, The Williams and Wilkins Company, 1968, pp. 41-63.

Pittillo, R. F., Schabel, F. M., Jr., and Skipper, H. E.: On the sensitivity of resting and dividing cells. *Cancer Chemotherapy Reports*. (In press.)

Schabel, F. M., Jr., Skipper, H. E., Montgomery, J. A., and Brockman, R. W.: Unpublished data.

Schabel, F. M., Jr., Skipper, H. E., Trader, M. W., Laster, W. R., Jr., and Simpson-Herren, L.: Spontaneous AK leukemia (lymphoma) as a model system. *Cancer Chemotherapy Reports*, 53:329-344, December 1969.

Schabel, F. M., Jr., Skipper, H. E., Trader, M. W., and Wilcox, W. S.: Experimental evaluation of potential anticancer agents. XIX. Sensitivity of nondividing leukemic cell populations to certain classes of drugs in vitro. *Cancer Chemotherapy Reports*, 48:17-30, October 1965.

Simpson-Herren, L.: Unpublished data.

Skipper, H. E.: Cellular kinetics associated with "curability" of experimental leukemias. In Dameshek, W., and Dutcher, R. M., Eds.: *Perspectives in Leukemia*. New York, New York, Grune and Stratton, Inc., 1968, pp. 187-216.

Skipper, H. E., Schabel, F. M., Jr., Trader, M. W., and Laster, W. R., Jr.: Response to therapy of spontaneous, first passage, and long passage lines of AK leukemia. *Cancer Chemotherapy Reports*, 53:345-366, December 1969.

Skipper, H. E., and Zubrod, C. G.: Some thoughts concerning cancer and cancer therapy. *Medical Tribune and Medical News*, 9:11, 16, Oct. 10, 1968.

Steel, G. G.: Cell loss from experimental tumours. *Cell Tissue Kinetics*, 1:193-207, 1968.

Todo, A., Fried, J., and Clarkson, B.: Kinetics of proliferation of human hematopoietic cells in suspension culture. (Abstract) *Proceedings of the American Association for Cancer Research*, 10:93, March 1969.

Wheeler, G. P., Bowdon, B. J., Wilkoff, L. J., and Dulmadge, E. A.: The cell cycle of leukemia L1210 cells in vivo and in vitro. *Proceedings of the Society for Experimental Biology and Medicine*, 126:903-906, December 1967.

Wilkoff, L. J., Wilcox, W. S., Burdeshaw, J. A., Dixon, G. J., and Dulmadge, E. A.: Effects of antimetabolites on kinetic behavior of proliferating cultured L1210 leukemia cells. *Journal of the National Cancer Institute,* 39:965-975, November 1967.

Yankee, R. A., DeVita, V. T., and Perry, S.: The cell cycle of leukemia L1210 cells in vivo. *Cancer Research,* 27:2381-2385, December 1967.

Young, R. C., DeVita, V. T., and Perry, S.: The thymidine-^{14}C and -^{3}H double-labeling technic in the study of the cell cycle of L1210 leukemia ascites tumor in vivo. *Cancer Research,* 29:1581-1584, August 1969.

Current Status of the Relationship of Viruses to Leukemia, Lymphoma, and Solid Tumors*

LEON DMOCHOWSKI, M.D., Ph.D.

Department of Virology, The University of Texas
M. D. Anderson Hospital and Tumor Institute at Houston,
Houston, Texas

At The Ninth Annual Clinical Conference held in 1964, we reported some of the results of our electron microscope studies of human leukemia and lymphoma (Dmochowski *et al.*, 1966). At that time, we reported on the presence of virus particles in biopsy specimens from patients with different types of leukemia and malignant lymphoma. These virus particles were similar in size and structure, irrespective of the type of leukemia or lymphoma, and strikingly resembled in their mode of development and their relationship to cellular constituents the virus particles observed by us in different types of murine leukemia (Dmochowski, 1963). We pointed out that electron microscope studies of tumors from animals and human beings must be continued in association with immunological and biological studies to ascertain the tumor-inducing properties of these virus particles and their relationship to the disease (Dmochowski *et al.*, 1966). The results of our electron microscope studies on human leukemia have since been confirmed and extended by others (Dalton *et al.*, 1964).

In further electron microscope studies, we demonstrated the presence of the virus particles, now designated as type C murine leukemia virus particles (Dalton *et al.*, 1966), not only in tissues and organs of mice with leukemia but also in tissues and organs of mice with reticulum cell sarcoma

*This study was conducted under United States Public Health Service Contract No. PH43-65-604 within the Special Virus Cancer Program of the National Cancer Institute and supported in part by Grant No. CA-05831 from the National Cancer Institute, National Institutes of Health, United States Public Health Service.

37

resembling Hodgkin's disease, in mice with autoimmune disease, and in mice with various types of tumors induced by mouse sarcoma virus or viruses (Dmochowski, 1968a,b). We also reported the presence of similar particles in some specimens of lymph nodes, bone marrow, and plasma buffy coat from patients with different types of leukemia and lymphoma and in some specimens grown in tissue culture (Dmochowski, 1968-a,b).

Immunological methods have been helpful in the detection of known viruses. In connection with the electron microscope and tissue culture studies of cell lines obtained from patients with leukemia and lymphoma, immunological methods were applied by us three years ago in the search for the possible presence of viruses associated with human neoplasia. Some of the methods successfully applied for the detection of specific antigens associated with mouse leukemia antigens, such as mixed hemadsorption (Barth, Espmark, and Fagraeus, 1967) and immunofluorescence tests (Fink and Malmgren, 1963; Klein and Klein, 1964), have been applied to sera from patients with different types of leukemia and lymphoma and to sera from normal individuals. These tests were used in search for the possible presence of antibodies to viral agents or tumor antigens in sera of some patients and for the presence of viral or tumor antigens in some leukemia and lymphoma cells grown in tissue culture. Preliminary results obtained at that time (Dmochowski, 1968b) demonstrated a high degree of correlation between the results of the mixed hemadsorption and membrane immunofluorescence tests carried out with the same cell lines, except that in the mixed hemadsorption test normal sera did not react with leukemia or lymphoma cells, while some of the sera from normal donors gave positive immunofluorescence reactions with leukemia cells (Dmochowski, 1968b). These preliminary results indicated a high degree of reactivity in sera from leukemia patients against leukemia and lymphoma cells grown *in vitro* and low titer or no reaction with normal cell lines. Sera from apparently normal individuals gave negative reactions with leukemia, lymphoma, and normal cell lines. In view of these results, the positive immunological reactions required extension of immunological studies in an attempt to determine, if possible, the basis of these findings.

Before the results of these studies are presented, a brief summary of some of the findings in animal and human leukemia and solid tumors carried out by various investigators and ourselves will be given.

Both deoxyribonucleic acid (DNA) and ribonucleic acid (RNA) viruses have been shown to be the causative agents of neoplasia of animals of different species. However only the so-called cytoplasmic RNA viruses (Dalton *et al.*, 1966) involved in the origin of leukemia and solid tumors of animals and suspected to play a part in the etiology of similar types of neoplasia in man will be discussed in the present communication.

Cytoplasmic RNA viruses, described as type C particles (Dalton *et al.*,

1966), have now been shown to be the etiologic agent(s) in various types of murine leukemia such as lymphoid, myeloid, erythroid, and reticulum cell tumors (Dmochowski, in press). These viruses have recently been found to induce bone tumors of mice (Finkel, Biskis, and Jinkins, 1966) and bone tumors of rats and hamsters (Soehner and Dmochowski, 1969; Soehner, Fujinaga, and Dmochowski, in press). The RNA type C particles have been demonstrated in guinea pig leukemia (Opler, 1968) and in lymphoproliferative diseases of swine (Howard, Clarke, and Hackett, 1968). The RNA type C particles now have been demonstrated in spontaneous and induced neoplasms of cats and in specimens derived from these neoplasms grown in tissue culture. They have been shown to be the causative agents of leukemia and lymphosarcoma of cats (Jarrett, Crawford, Martin and Davie, 1964; Kawakami et al., 1967; Rickard et al., 1967; Rickard, Post, Noronha, and Barr, 1969). These particles have also been observed in dog lymphosarcoma (Seman, Proenca, Guillon, and Moraillon, 1967), in dog mammary tumors (Seman and Dmochowski unpublished data), and in cattle leukosis (Dutcher, 1968; Kawakami, Moore, and Theilen, in press; Olson, Miller, Miller, and Gillette, in press). It is of interest that these RNA type C particles also have been observed in mammary tumors of mice (Dmochowski and Maruyama, in press), rats (Chopra and Dutcher, in press), and women (Dmochowski, Seman, Myers, and Gallager, 1968). There exists an essential similarity in the ultrastructure and sites of replication of the C type particles in all types of leukemia, sarcoma, and mammary tumors of animals and, indeed, in those of man (Dmochowski, in press). These virus particles have been established to be causative in mouse, rat, and cat leukemia and solid tumors; however, this relationship remains to be ascertained in dog, cattle, and human neoplasia.

In animals, RNA type C virus particles have been found responsible not only for neoplastic lesions, but also for inflammatory and destructive lesions (Dmochowski, in press). It is imperative that we be aware of the possiblity of a similar part being played by these so-called type C virus particles in inflammatory, autoimmune, and neoplastic lesions of man. It should also be mentioned that murine sarcoma virus (Moloney strain) has been grown in human embryo cells (Boiron, Bernard, and Chuat, 1969). Murine type C (Rauscher leukemia) virus particles have also been grown successfully in human embryonic tissues (Wright, personal communication); cat leukemia type C virus has been grown in cat and human cell cultures (O'Connor and Fischinger, in press) and in human, canine, and porcine cells (Jarrett, in press).

In view of the morphological similarity of type C particles in leukemic tissues of animals of different species and their ability to replicate in tissues of animals of various species, the question of their antigenic relationship is an obvious one. Immunological studies on virus-induced animal tumors,

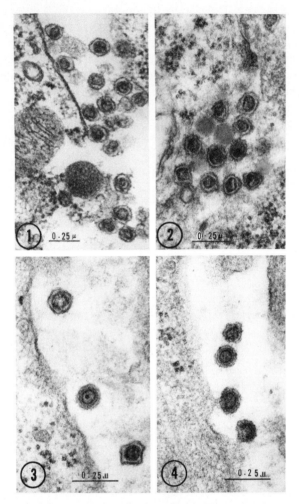

FIG. 1.—Bone marrow of a low-leukemia-strain (BALB/c) mouse with spontaneous leukemia. Appearance of type C virus particles. Reduced from × 67,500.

FIG. 2.—Spleen of a BALB/c strain mouse with induced reticulum cell sarcoma from an SJL/J strain mouse. Appearance of type C virus particles. Reduced from × 70,000.

FIG. 3.—Appearance of type C virus particles in bone tumor of an NZB (New Zealand Black) rat induced by Moloney murine sarcoma virus. Reduced from × 70,000.

FIG. 4.—Budding, immature, and mature type C virus particles in the same bone tumor as in Figure 3. Reduced from × 70,000.

including murine and feline leukemia, have demonstrated that tumors induced by the same oncogenic virus in animals of different species share specific antigens. Leukemia viruses of animals of different species also share common viral antigens, as demonstrated by different immunological techniques (Old, Boyse, and Stockert, 1964; Maruyama and Dmochowski, 1969; Maruyama, Dmochowski, and Rickard, in press; Hardy et al., in press). In spite of the difficulties of defining the nature and origin of the antigens of tumors induced by any one virus, there is no doubt that the antigens of various tumors induced by the same virus are serologically related, if not identical.

The appearance of the so-called type C virus particles (Dmochowski, 1968a,b) may be illustrated in a BALB/c strain mouse with spontaneous leukemia (Fig. 1) or with induced reticulum cell sarcoma (Fig. 2) and in a Moloney sarcoma virus-induced bone tumor in a rat (Figs. 3 and 4). The appearance of type C particles in human lymphosarcoma is shown in Fig-

FIG. 5.—Appearance of type C virus particles in lymph node from a patient with lymphosarcoma. Reduced from × 70,000.

FIG. 6.—Type C virus particle in human osteosarcoma. Reduced from × 70,000.

FIG. 7.—Type C virus particle in human rhabdomyosarcoma. Reduced from × 70,000.

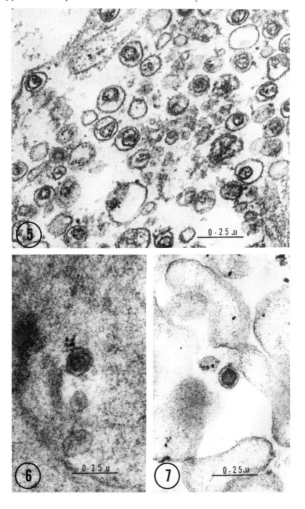

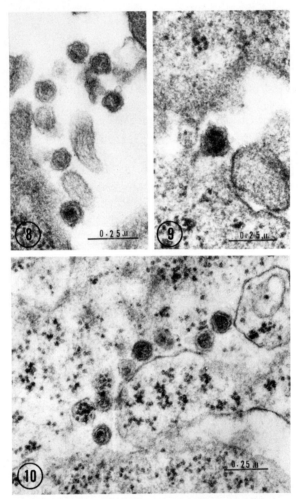

FIG. 8.—Appearance of type C virus particles in a mammary tumor of an RIII strain mouse. Tissue culture passage 45. Reduced from × 70,000.

FIG. 9.—Appearance of type C virus particle in human breast carcinoma. Reduced from × 70,000.

FIG. 10.—Appearance of type C virus particles in the thymus gland of a cat with spontaneous lymphoma. Reduced from × 66,000.

ure 5, and in human osteosarcoma and rhabdomyosarcoma in Figures 6 and 7. Type C virus particles in mouse mammary carcinoma are shown in Figure 8, and those in human breast cancer in Figure 9. These may be compared with type C particles in spontaneous lymphosarcoma of cat, shown in Figure 10.

During the past year, we have examined by electron microscopy specimens of various types from a total of 70 patients. The results of these studies are shown in Table 1. As may be seen, a number of patients with different types of leukemia, malignant lymphoma, and osteosarcoma showed the presence of small numbers of type C virus particles. These particles could be found only after prolonged examination of a considerable number of sections of the different specimens. An attempt was made to analyze the positive findings according to type of tissue examined and type of neoplasia affecting the patients (Table 2). Although judged from a small number of cases, it appears that the tumors or tissues involved in the neoplastic process are a better source of virus particles than other types of tissues. A further attempt was made to analyze the age distribution of cases positive for virus particles (Table 3). As may be seen, the greatest number of positive cases, at least in leukemia, were in the age group from nine to 15 years. In general, it appears that specimens from young untreated patients seem to be most promising in the search for virus particles. As far as tissue culture is concerned, the presence of occasional type C virus particles has

TABLE 1.—ELECTRON MICROSCOPE STUDIES OF TISSUE SECTIONS
PREPARED BY THE THIN-SECTIONING PROCEDURE*
(1968 to 1969)

TYPE OF NEOPLASIA	NO. OF PATIENTS EXAMINED	NO. OF PATIENTS WITH VP	NO. OF PATIENTS NEGATIVE FOR VP
Leukemia	48	11	37
Malignant lymphoma	14	3	11
Osteosarcoma	8	3	5
Totals	70	17	53

*Tissue sections were taken from lymph node biopsy and autopsy, blood plasma, buffy coat, tissue culture, spleen, bone marrow, and solid tumors.
Abbreviation: VP, particles resembling murine leukemia (type C) virus.

TABLE 2.—CASES POSITIVE FOR TYPE C VIRUS PARTICLES*
(ACCORDING TO TYPE OF TISSUE: THIN-SECTION ELECTRON MICROSCOPY)

TYPE OF NEOPLASIA	TOTAL POSITIVE SPECIMENS	TYPE OF TISSUE					
		Lymph Node	Spleen	Tumor	Buffy Coat	Bone Marrow	Tissue Culture
Leukemia	15	4	4	0	4	1	2
Malignant lymphoma	4	2	0	0	1	0	1
Osteosarcoma	3	0	0	3	0	0	0
Totals	22	6	4	3	5	1	3

*Particles resembling murine leukemia type C virus.

TABLE 3.—Cases Positive for Type C Virus Particles*
(According to Age: Thin-Section Electron Microscopy)

Type of Neoplasia	Total Positive Cases	Age (in Years)				
		0 to 8	9 to 15	16 to 29	30 to 59	60 and Above
Leukemia	11	1	6	2	0	2
Malignant lymphoma	3	1	0	0	1	1
Osteosarcoma	3	1	1	0	1	0
Totals	17	3	7	2	2	3

*Particles resembling murine leukemia type C virus.

been observed at irregular intervals during tissue culture passage. Ways and means have to be found to enrich the number of virus particles in tissue culture of specimens from patients with leukemia and solid tumors.

In an attempt to examine human leukemia and lymphoma cells for the possible presence of viral or tumor antigens and sera of patients with the diseases for antibodies to these antigens, a total of 437 sera were tested against 102 different specimens of fresh or cultured cells by mixed hemadsorption and indirect immunofluorescent antibody tests (Maruyama, Dmochowski, Bowen, and Hales, 1968). The results of these extensive tests may be summarized as follows:

Cells grown in tissue culture and derived from patients with different types of leukemia and lymphoma gave positive mixed hemadsorption and membrane immunofluorescence reactions with sera of some 30 per cent of patients with different types of leukemia and lymphoma (Tables 4 and 5). These reactions occur even in autologous serum-cell combinations. Normal cells also gave positive reactions with about 10 per cent of sera from leukemic patients, but not with normal donor sera (Tables 4 and 5). These results, at least with some sera, could not be attributed to isoantibodies or isoantigens (Maruyama, Dmochowski, Bowen, and Hales, 1968).

The mixed hemadsorption test has made it possible to demonstrate the presence of a common antigen or antigens not only in mouse leukemia cells induced by different murine leukemia viruses, but also in cells derived from mice, rats, hamsters, cats, and human embryos which had been infected with murine or feline leukemia viruses (Dmochowski and Maruyama, in press). It also has shown the presence of antibodies in sera of animals of different species immunized against different murine or cat leukemia viruses. These immune sera gave positive mixed hemadsorption reactions with cells infected with type C particles and derived from animals of different species, including cats and man (Tables 6 and 7).

TABLE 4.—SUMMARY OF RESULTS OF MIXED HEMADSORPTION TESTS

TYPE OF SERA	TYPE OF CELL CULTURES			
	Leukemia	Lymphoma	Other Neoplasms	Normal
Leukemia	14/46*	51/204	26/150	3/29
Lymphoma	7/42	30/235	44/179	3/76
Hodgkin's disease	17/71	29/189	41/160	0/53
Other neoplasms	4/14	10/81	22/109	2/19
Normal	0/7	5/42	5/77	0/10

*Numerator indicates number of sera positive. Denominator indicates number of sera tested.

TABLE 5.—SUMMARY OF RESULTS OF MEMBRANE IMMUNOFLUORESCENCE TESTS

TYPE OF SERA	TYPE OF CELL CULTURES			
	Leukemia	Lymphoma	Other Neoplasms	Normal
Leukemia	106/297*	19/75	18/49	7/75
Lymphoma	20/170	4/99	9/31	1/61
Hodgkin's disease	8/103	2/71	2/9	0/49
Other neoplasms	18/73	1/10	12/51	1/5
Normal	0/39	4/57	0/6	0/129

*Numerator indicates number of sera positive, showing 5 per cent or more of living cells with complete fluorescent ring. Denominator indicates number of sera tested.

TABLE 6.—MIXED HEMADSORPTION REACTION OF FELINE CELL CULTURES WITH ANTIMURINE LEUKEMIA VIRUS SERA

CULTURES	IMMUNE SERA					
	Anti-MLV* (Monkey)	Anti-RLV† (Monkey)	Anti-RLV‡ (Mouse)	Anti-RFLV§ (Rabbit)	Anti-FE-4# (Mouse)	TYPE C PARTICLES
F-491′	±	+	–	+ +	+ + +	+
F-503′	+	+ +	–	+ +	+ + +	+
FE-4	NT*	+ +	NT	+ +	+ + +	+
C-4¶	–	‥	–	–	+ + +	–
C-5¶	–	–	NT	NT	NT	NT
C-8¶	–	+	–	+	+ + +	+

*Anti-Moloney leukemia virus monkey serum.
†Anti-Rauscher leukemia virus monkey serum.
‡Anti-Rauscher leukemia virus mouse serum.
§Anti-rat adapted Friend leukemia virus rabbit serum.
#Anti-cat leukemia virus-infected feline embryo mouse serum.
′Bone marrow from cat with induced lymphosarcoma.
¶Normal young cat tissue.
Abbreviations: +, positive mixed hemadsorption reaction; –, negative mixed hemadsorption reaction; NT, not tested.

TABLE 7.—MIXED HEMADSORPTION REACTION OF RAUSCHER LEUKEMIA VIRUS-INFECTED
HUMAN EMBRYONIC KIDNEY CELL CULTURE
WITH IMMUNE SERA OF DIFFERENT TYPES

CULTURES	IMMUNE SERA					TYPE C PARTICLES
	Anti-RLV* (Monkey)	Anti-RLV† (Mouse)	Anti-RFLV‡ (Rabbit)	Anti-HeLa§ (Monkey)	Anti-FE-4≠ (Mouse)	
HEK-1-HRV′	+ + +	+ +	+ +	+ + + +	+ +	+
HEK-1 (control)	–	–	–	+ + + +	+	–

*Anti-Rauscher leukemia virus monkey serum.
†Anti-Rauscher leukemia virus mouse serum.
‡Anti-rat adapted Friend leukemia virus rabbit serum.
§Anti-HeLa cell monkey serum.
≠Anti-cat virus-infected feline embryo mouse serum.
′Human embryo kidney cells infected with Rauscher murine leukemia virus.
Abbreviations: +, positive mixed hemadsorption reaction; -, negative mixed hemadsorption reaction.

In an attempt to study the reaction of sera from patients with different types of neoplasia with cells from virus-induced animal tumors, 130 human sera were tested by mixed hemadsorption test with animal cell cultures containing type C virus particles. About 27 per cent of these sera gave titers of 16 or higher with Moloney sarcoma virus-induced hamster tumor cell cultures. These sera were all negative when tested with normal hamster embryo cultures (Table 8) (Maruyama, Dmochowski, and McGehee, 1969). Selected human sera which gave positive mixed hemadsorption reaction with the hamster tumor cell cultures were absorbed with sheep red blood cells, guinea pig erythrocytes, and guinea pig kidney tissue homogenates known to contain Forssman-like antigens. This reduced the titers of all sera, while guinea pig kidney homogenates completely removed activity of these sera, except for one serum specimen from a patient with malignant melanoma. There was no correlation between hemagglutination titer of these sera with sheep red blood cells and the mixed hemadsorption titer of the sera.

TABLE 8—MIXED HEMADSORPTION TITERS OF POSITIVE HUMAN SERA
AGAINST H(S)—MSV(M) CULTURES

SERA	NO. OF SERA TESTED	MHA TITERS					
		<16	16	32	64	128	256
Leukemia	16	6	6	2	1	1	0
Lymphoma	7	3	1	0	1	1	1
Hodgkin's disease	4	4	0	0	0	0	0
Other neoplasms	14	7	3	1	1	2	0
Normal	22	8	6	5	3	0	0

Abbreviation: H(S)—MSV(M), Moloney mouse sarcoma virus-induced tumor in Syrian hamster.

TABLE 9.—MIXED HEMADSORPTION (MHA) AND HEMAGGLUTINATION (HA)
TITERS OF SELECTED HUMAN SERA (UNABSORBED AND ABSORBED)
AGAINST H(S)-MSV(M) CULTURES

	MHA Titers				HA Titers	
SERA DIAGNOSIS	Unabs.	SRBC Abs.	GPRBC Abs.	GPKID Abs.	Unabs.	GPKID Abs.
1 Acute leukemia	128	8	16	<8	<4	NT
2 Reticulum cell sarcoma	256	32	32	<8	8	<8
3 Malignant melanoma	128	>32	16	16	<4	NT
4 Osteosarcoma	64	8	8	<8	4	NT
5 Polycythemia	128	16	16	<8	16	<8

Abbreviations: GPKID, guinea pig kidney cells; GPRBC, guinea pig red blood cells; H(S)-MSV(M), Moloney mouse sarcoma virus-induced tumor in Syrian hamster; SRBC, sheep red blood cells.

Both guinea pig kidney homogenates and guinea pig erythrocytes removed to a great extent the hemagglutinating activity of the sera (Table 9). The data indicate that Forssman and other heterophile-type antigens present in the hamster tumor cultures are responsible for a great part of the positive reaction of at least some human sera with Moloney sarcoma virus-induced hamster tumor cells (Maruyama, Dmochowski, and McGehee, 1969).

In a further attempt to examine the reactivity of human sera with cells derived from animal leukemia induced by type C virus particles, feline lymphoma cultures were tested with approximately 70 human sera. The results of mixed hemadsorption tests of feline cell cultures derived from leukemic (F-491, F-503, FE-4) and normal cats (C-4) with sera (diluted 1:64) obtained from patients with different types of neoplasia, normal relatives, and normal donors are summarized in Table 10. The incidence of

TABLE 10.—MIXED HEMADSORPTION REACTION OF FELINE CELL CULTURES
WITH HUMAN SERA OF DIFFERENT TYPES

	FELINE CELL CULTURES			
HUMAN SERA	F-491*	F-503*	FE-4†	C-4‡
Leukemia	5/20§	1/20	2/20	3/20
Lymphoma	3/10	3/10	0/2	1/2
Other neoplasms	3/8	4/13	NT	NT
Normal relatives	7/19	7/19	7/19	9/19
Normal donors	11/20	14/20	16/20	14/20

*Bone marrow from cat with induced lymphosarcoma.
†Cat embryo cells infected with cat leukemia virus.
‡Normal young cat tissues.
§Numerator indicates number of sera positive at the dilution of 1:64. Denominator indicates number of sera tested.
Abbreviation: NT, not tested.

positive tests with sera from apparently normal individuals was higher than that of sera from patients with leukemia, lymphoma, or other neoplastic diseases. However, no significant difference was observed between virus-infected cultures (F-491 and F-503) containing type C virus particles and a control uninfected feline culture (C-4) (Maruyama, Dmochowski, and McGehee, 1969). The data indicate that there is no apparent correlation between the presence of feline leukemia virus in test cells and the mixed hemadsorption reaction given by human sera. Further studies are needed to investigate the relationship of feline leukemia virus to human leukemia.

To investigate the nature of the antibodies involved, absorption experiments were carried out. Absorption with sheep red blood cells reduced the titer of the selected positive human sera, whereas absorption with guinea pig kidney homogenates removed the reaction. Absorption with purified Rauscher leukemia virus also reduced (two- or threefold) the titer of one of these positive human sera against all feline cell cultures tested. The data indicate that the antibodies in certain human sera which reacted with the feline cell cultures appear to be similar to Forssman and other heterophile antibodies. These data are in agreement with those obtained with cell cultures derived from Moloney sarcoma virus-induced hamster tumor. In view of the fact that absorption with purified Rauscher virus also reduced the titer of human sera tested, the possible relationship between viral coat antigens and the heterophile antigens remains to be clarified.

Recent studies using the immunofluorescence technique have revealed a high incidence of antibodies to osteosarcomas in the sera of patients with this disease and of their close associates which react with a common anti-

TABLE 11.—FIXED IMMUNOFLUORESCENCE OF SERA FROM PATIENTS WITH OSTEOSARCOMA

SERA PATIENT	CELLS FROM TISSUE CULTURE						
	OSTEOSARCOMA		Bone Marrow	OTHER TUMORS			
	Autologous	Homologous		Chondro-sarcoma	Giant Cell	Rhabdomyo-sarcoma	Ewing's
C	Neg.	1/5*	1/1§	NT	1/2	0/3	NT
D	+§	1/5	1/1	NT	1/2	1/3	0/1
H	Neg.	0/2	NT	NT	1/2	0/3	0/1
J	+	0/4	1/1	1/1	2/2	1/2	0/1
M	Neg.	0/4	0/1	0/1	1/2	0/2	0/1
O	NT	0/5	1/1	NT	1/2	0/3	0/1
R1	NT	0/3	0/1	0/1	1/2	1/3	0/1
R2	NT	0/3	1/1	1/1	1/2	0/3	0/1
S	NT	0/3	0/1	0/1	2/2	1/3	0/1
Z	NT	1/3	0/1	0/1	2/2	1/3	0/1

*Numerator indicates number of tissue cultures with positive fluorescence. Denominator indicates number of tissue cultures tested.

§Bone marrow was from patient D.

Abbreviation: NT, cells not available for testing.

gen (or antigens) in cells of human osteosarcomas (Morton and Malmgren, 1968).

In cooperation with Dr. E. S. Priori of the Department of Virology and Dr. Jordan R. Wilbur of the Department of Pediatrics, we recently have initiated studies using fixed immunofluorescence to explore the possible presence of antibodies in sera of patients with osteosarcomas. These studies have been extended to testing of sera from patients with osteosarcomas against cells of other tumors. The results of preliminary studies of 10 selected sera from patients with osteosarcomas are shown in Table 11 (Priori, Wilbur, and Dmochowski, in preparation).

In five autologous serum-sarcoma cell systems, cells of one of the five osteosarcomas showed positive perinuclear and cytoplasmic fluorescence by the indirect immunofluorescence method, both on frozen imprints of the tumor cells made at the time of surgical removal and on tissue culture cells derived from the osteosarcoma. Perinuclear fluorescence was observed in an autologous system in the case of a culture which had been derived from a bone marrow aspirate from an 11-year-old twin with osteosarcoma. In preliminary tests, the serum of the other twin was negative with the bone marrow of his twin.

In homologous systems, about 20 per cent of the sera from patients with osteosarcoma gave positive fluorescence.

The observation made with sera of the patients with osteosarcomas and cells derived from other tumors is of special interest. One of the six sera tested gave positive fluorescence with cells of a culture of chondrosarcoma. Every serum of the 10 tested gave a positive reaction with at least one of the two giant cell tumor cultures examined, and a number of sera gave positive fluorescence with cultures of rhabdomyosarcomas. It should be pointed out that 1 to 4 per cent of cells in positive cultures gave positive reactions. Cultures of Ewing's sarcoma, HeLa, or of normal human cells (WISH, or human embryonic cells) were negative when tested with the 10 sera of osteosarcoma patients (Priori, Wilbur, and Dmochowski, in preparation).

Recent studies on human osteosarcoma (Morton and Malmgren, 1968) and human liposarcoma (Morton, Hall, and Malmgren, 1969) suggest the presence of a viral agent with the morphological appearance of type C virus particles. Studies along these lines must be extended in both width and depth. Immunological studies reported by us on many serum-cell systems with autologous, homologous, and heterologous sera indicate that the antigenic changes observed appear to represent in part specific unmasking of normal host antigens shared by animals of different species and probably by human beings (Dmochowski and Maruyama, in press). These antigens may represent virus-specific cell surface antigens related to type C virus particle infection, which are, at least in part, immunologically similar in all the species so far examined.

Summary

Extensive electron microscope and immunological studies carried out by us and other investigators on animal leukemia and solid tumors have demonstrated an essential similarity of viruses involved in the origin of these diseases in animals of various species. Morphological evidence of similar virus particles in human leukemia and solid tumors and the results of immunological studies support further studies on the part played by RNA viruses in human neoplasia.

REFERENCES

Barth, R. F., Espmark, J. A., and Fagraeus, A.: Histocompatibility and tumor virus antigens identified on cells grown in tissue culture by means of the mixed hemadsorption reaction. *Journal of Immunology*, 98:888-892, May 1967.

Boiron, M., Bernard, C., and Chuat, J. C.: Replication of mouse sarcoma virus Moloney strain (MSV-M) in human cells. (Abstract) *Proceedings of the American Association for Cancer Research*, 10:8, March 1969.

Chopra, H. C., and Dutcher, R. M.: "C" type virus particles in rat tumors. In Dutcher, R. M., Ed.: *Proceedings of the 4th International Symposium on Comparative Leukemia Research*, Cherry Hill, New Jersey, 1969. Basel, Switzerland, and New York, New York, S. Karger. (In press.)

Dalton, A. J., de Harven, E., Dmochowski, L., Feldman, D., Haguenau, F., Harris, W. W., Howatson, A. F., Moore, D., Pitelka, D., Smith, K., Uzman, B., and Zeigel, R. (with suggestions from W. Bernhard and G. de-Thé): Suggestions for the classification of oncogenic RNA viruses. *Journal of the National Cancer Institute*, 37:395-397, September 1966.

Dalton, A. J., Moloney, J. B., Porter, G. H., Frei, E., and Mitchell, E.: Studies on murine and human leukemia. *Transactions of the Association of American Physicians*, 77:52-64, 1964.

Dmochowski, L.: Comparison of leukemogenic and sarcomagenic viruses at the ultrastructural level. In Dutcher, R. M., Ed.: *Proceedings of the 4th International Symposium on Comparative Leukemia Research*, Cherry Hill, New Jersey, 1969. Basel, Switzerland, and New York, New York, S. Karger. (In press.)

_____: The electron microscopic view of virus-host relationship in neoplasia. *Progress in Experimental Tumor Research*, 3:35-147, 1963.

_____: Recent studies on leukemia and solid tumors in mice and man. In Bendixen, H. J., Ed.: *Leukemia in Animals and Man*, Proceedings of the 3rd International Symposium on Comparative Leukemia Research, Paris, France, 1967. Basel, Switzerland, and New York, New York, S. Karger (Published as *Bibliotheca Haematologica* No. 30), 1968a, pp. 285-298.

_____: Viral studies in human leukemia and lymphoma. In Zarafonetis, C. J. D., Ed.: *Proceedings of the International Conference on Leukemia-Lymphoma*, The University of Michigan, Ann Arbor, Michigan, 1967. Philadelphia, Pennsylvania, Lea & Febiger, 1968b, pp. 97-113.

Dmochowski, L., Grey, C. E., Sykes, J. A., Dreyer, D. A., Mizuno, S., Langford, P., Rogers, T., Taylor, H. G., Shullenberger, C. C., and Howe, C. D.: Electron microscopy of human leukemia. In *Recent Advances in the Diagnosis of Cancer*, A Collection of Papers Presented at the 9th Annual Clinical Conference on Cancer, 1964, at The University of Texas M. D. Anderson Hospital and Tumor Institute. Chicago, Illinois. Year Book Medical Publishers, Inc., 1966, pp. 270-297.

Dmochowski, L., and Maruyama, K.: Immunological studies on leukemia and solid tumors of animals and man. In Severi, L., Ed.: Symposium on Immunity and Tolerance in Carcinogenesis, Perugia, 1969. (In press.)

Dmochowski, L., Seman, G., Myers, B., and Gallager, H. S.: Relationship of viruses to the origin of human breast cancer: An exploratory study of the submicroscopic appearance of human breast cancer. *Medical Record and Annals,* 61:384-387, 411, December 1968.

Dutcher, R. M.: Viral research on bovine leukosis. In Bendixen, H. J., Ed.: *Leukemia in Animals and Man,* Proceedings of the 3rd International Symposium on Comparative Leukemia Research, Paris, France, 1967. Basel, Switzerland, and New York, New York, S. Karger (Published as *Bibliotheca Haematologica* No. 30), 1968, pp. 116-135.

Fink, M. A., and Malmgren, R. A.: Fluorescent antibody studies of the viral antigen in a murine leukemia (Rauscher). *Journal of the National Cancer Institute,* 31:1111-1121, November 1963.

Finkel, M. P., Biskis, B. O., and Jinkins, P. B.: Virus induction of osteosarcomas in mice. *Science,* 151:698-701, February 11, 1966.

Hardy, W. D., Geering, G., Lloyd, L. J., deHarven, E., and Brodey, R. S.: Serological studies of feline leukemia virus. In Dutcher, R. M., Ed.: *Proceedings of the 4th International Symposium on Comparative Leukemia Research,* Cherry Hill, New Jersey, 1969. Basel Switzerland, and New York, New York, S. Karger. (In press.)

Howard, E. B., Clarke, W. J., and Hackett, P. L.: Experimental myeloproliferative and lymphoproliferative diseases of swine. In Bendixen, H. J., Ed.: *Leukemia in Animals and Man,* Proceedings of the 3rd International Symposium on Comparative Leukemia Research, Paris, France, 1967. Basel, Switzerland, and New York, New York, S. Karger (Published as *Bibliotheca Haematologica* No. 30), 1968, pp. 255-262.

Jarrett, O.: Growth of feline leukemia virus in human, canine, and porcine cells. In Dutcher, R. M., Ed.: *Proceedings of the 4th International Symposium on Comparative Leukemia Research,* Cherry Hill, New Jersey, 1969. Basel, Switzerland, and New York, New York, S. Karger. (In press.)

Jarrett, W. F. H., Crawford, E. M., Martin, W. B., and Davie, F.: A virus-like particle associated with leukemia (lymphosarcoma). *Nature,* 202:567-568, May 9, 1964.

Kawakami, T. G., Moore, A., and Theilen, G. H.: A comparative study of viral-like particles in plasma of cattle and of some known leukemogenic viruses. In Dutcher, R. M., Ed.: *Proceedings of the 4th International Symposium on Comparative Leukemia Research,* Cherry Hill, New Jersey, 1969. Basel, Switzerland, and New York, New York, S. Karger. (In press.)

Kawakami, T. G., Theilen, G. H., Dungworth, D. L., Munn, R. J., and Beall, S. G.: "C"-type viral particles in plasma of cats with feline leukemia. *Science,* 158:1049-1050, November 24, 1967.

Klein, E., and Klein, G.: Antigenic properties of lymphomas induced by the Moloney agent. *Journal of the National Cancer Institute,* 32:547-568, March 1964.

Maruyama, K., and Dmochowski, L.: Comparative studies of type C virus particle-containing cultures of different animal species by mixed hemadsorption reaction. *Texas Reports on Biology and Medicine,* 27:437-456, Summer 1969.

Maruyama, K., Dmochowski, L., Bowen, J. M., and Hales, R. L.: Studies of human leukemia and lymphoma cells by membrane immunofluorescence and mixed hemadsorption tests. *Texas Reports on Biology and Medicine,* 26:545-565, Winter 1968.

Maruyama, K., Dmochowski, L., and McGehee, M. P.: Comparative studies of leukemia and solid tumors of animals and man by mixed hemadsorption reaction. (Abstract) *Proceedings of the American Association for Cancer Research,* 10:55, March 1969.

Maruyama, K., Dmochowski, L., and Rickard, C. G.: Comparative studies of feline and human leukemia by mixed hemadsorption test. In Dutcher, R. M., Ed.: *Proceedings of the 4th International Symposium on Comparative Leukemia Research,* Cherry Hill, New Jersey, 1969. Basel, Switzerland, and New York, New York, S. Karger. (In press.)

Morton, D. L., Hall, W. T., and Malmgren, R. A.: Human liposarcomas: Tissue cultures containing foci of transformed cells with viral particles. *Science,* 165:813-815, August 22, 1969.

Morton, D. L., and Malmgren, R. A.: Human osteosarcomas: Immunologic evidence suggesting an associated infectious agent. *Science,* 162:1279-1281, December 13, 1968.

O'Connor, T. E., and Fischinger, P.: Physical alteration of a murine sarcoma-leukemia virus complex in mammalian cell cultures. In Dutcher, R. M., Ed.: *Proceedings of the 4th Inter-*

national Symposium on Comparative Leukemia Research, Cherry Hill, New Jersey, 1969. Basel, Switzerland, and New York, New York, S. Karger. (In press.)

Old, L. J., Boyse, E. A., and Stockert, E.: Typing of mouse leukemias by serological methods. *Nature,* 201:777-779, February 22, 1964.

Olson, C., Miller, L. D., Miller, J. M., and Gillette, K. G.: Studies on bovine lymphosarcoma. In Dutcher, R. M., Ed.: *Proceedings of the 4th International Symposium on Comparative Leukemia Research,* Cherry Hill, New Jersey, 1969. Basel, Switzerland, and New York, New York, S. Karger. (In press.)

Opler, S. R.: New oncogenic virus producing acute lymphatic leukemia in guinea pigs. In Bendixen, H. J., Ed.: *Leukemia in Animals and Man,* Proceedings of the 3rd International Symposium on Comparative Leukemia Research, Paris, France, 1967. Basel, Switzerland, and New York, New York, S. Karger (Published as *Bibliotheca Haematologica* No. 30), 1968, pp. 81-88.

Priori, E. S., Wilbur, J. R., and Dmochowski, L.: Studies of sera from patients with osteosarcoma by immunofluorescence test. *Proceedings of the American Association for Cancer Research.* (In press.)

Rickard, C. G., Barr, L. M., Noronha, F., Dougherty, E., III, and Post, J. E.: C-type virus particles in spontaneous lymphocytic leukemia in a cat. *Cornell Veterinarian,* 57:302-307, April 1967.

Rickard, C. G., Post, J. E., Noronha, F., and Barr, L. M.: A transmissible virus-induced lymphocytic leukemia of the cat. *Journal of the National Cancer Institute,* 42:987-1014, June 1969.

Seman, G. J., and Dmochowski, L.: Unpublished data.

Seman, G., Proenca, G., Guillon, J. C., and Moraillon, R.: Particules d'aspect viral dans les cellules du lymphosarcome du chien. *Bulletin de l'Academie Veterinaire de France,* 40(4): 211-214, 1967.

Soehner, R. L., and Dmochowski, L.: Induction of bone tumours in rats and hamsters with murine sarcoma virus and their cell-free transmission. *Nature,* 224:191-192, October 11, 1969.

Soehner, R. L., Fujinaga, S., and Dmochowski, L.: Neoplastic bone lesions induced in rats and hamsters by Moloney and Harvey murine sarcoma viruses. In Dutcher, R. M., Ed.: *Proceedings of the 4th International Symposium on Comparative Leukemia Research,* Cherry Hill, New Jersey, 1969. Basel, Switzerland, and New York, New York, S. Karger. (In press.)

Wright, B.: Personal communication.

Relationship Between Lymphoid Neoplasms and Immunologic Functions*

JOSEPH G. SINKOVICS, M.D.,
EIICHI SHIRATO, M.D., D.Sc.,
FERENC GYORKEY, M.D.,
JERRY R. CABINESS, B.S.,
AND CLIFTON D. HOWE, M.D.

Section of Clinical Tumor Virology and Immunology, Department of Medicine, The University of Texas M. D. Anderson Hospital and Tumor Institute at Houston, and Laboratory Service, Veterans Administration Hospital, Houston, Texas

IN ORDER TO INTRODUCE rational approaches to the immunotherapy for tumors of man, elementary basic studies are needed. The aim of such studies should be the documentation of the tumor-specific antigenicity of these neoplasms, the demonstration of immune reactions to these antigens, the recognition of means by which the tumor escapes these immune reactions, and a search for procedures that augment these immune reactions.

Compartmentalization of the Lymphoreticular System and an Immunological Concept of Malignant Lymphoma

Malignant transformation accompanies the development of the lymphoreticular system throughout its evolution from fish and reptiles to birds, mammals, and man (Cooper, Peterson, Gabrielsen, and Good, 1966; Good and Finstad, 1968). During the long process of evolution, the lymphoreticular system has undergone extensive compartmentalization. Not only thy-

*These studies were supported by United States Public Health Service Grants No. CA-6939 and No. CA-7923 and by Institutional Grant FR551-IN93. Dr. F. Gyorkey's work was supported by a Veterans Administration pathology research fund.

mus-dependent and gut-associated lymphatic tissues with functions as diverse as delayed hypersensitivity reactions and immune globulin production were formed, but within these two main faculties, numerous and as yet not fully recognized subdivisions have assumed existence (Good *et al.*, 1967). The gut-associated faculty operates by producing immunoglobulins (Ig) of the IgG, IgA, and IgE classes. Producers of 19S macroglobulins are large plasmacytoid lymphocytes occupying an intermediate position between the gut-associated and thymus-dependent faculties. The *modus operandi* of the thymus-dependent lymphoid faculty is not well understood, but it is known that cytotoxins are released by these cells during delayed hypersensitivity reactions (David, 1966; Ruddle and Waksman, 1968a, b; Williams and Granger, 1969). Lymphoid cells of the thymic faculty reach immunocompetence under the influence of thymic "hormones," the existence of which is postulated rather than proved (Stutman, Yunis, and Good, 1967; Law, Goldstein, and White, 1968).

The multiplicity of types of lymphoreticular neoplasia as recognized clinically and histologically in man suggests that this disorder takes its beginning in one of the highly specialized compartments of the lymphoreticular system. This compartment is either incapacitated by genetic or acquired factors and fails to resist an oncogenic agent, or the malignant transformation takes place during extraordinary immunogenic stimulation when intact immune compartments attempt to substitute for a defective or suppressed compartment, thus providing actively replicating cells for a potentially oncogenic agent. Presuming that malignantly transformed cells carry tumor-specific transplantation antigens, it may be expected that the intact faculties of the immune system will have attempted the rejection of the neoplastic cells. Histological evidence, particularly in Hodgkin's disease, supports this view (Lukes, 1964; Smithers, 1967; Crowther, Fairley, and Sewell, 1969). This conflict may result in the paradoxic histological and clinical features often termed as "autoimmune" complications of lymphoma.

Resemblances Between Lymphoma of Animals and Man
VIRAL ETIOLOGY

In the murine species, type C virus particles induce both thymic and extrathymic lymphoreticular neoplasms (Gross, 1961 a, b, c; Rich, 1968; Sinkovics, Gyorkey, and Shullenberger, in press). Type C virus particles usually reach full maturation in the malignantly transformed cells. The naturally occurring type C viruses represented by the Gross virus are ubiquitous in rodents and may exist without envelopes as strands of viral genes within neoplastic and nonneoplastic cells; it is assumed that the genome of the host suppresses the function of the viral genome. Should the host suffer a genetic insult, repression of host genes and derepression of viral genes takes place. Function of the viral genes results in the replication of viral genetic material, synthesis of viral envelopes and horizontal spread of infectious virus particles causing malignant transformation of newly invaded cells (Sinkovics, in press).

Type C virus particles are leukemogenic in the avian, feline, and canine species and probably also in cattle; although type C virus particles were seen in blood and lymph nodes of patients with leukemia and lymphoma (Dmochowski *et al.*, 1967), the etiologic role of this virus in neoplasia of man has not as yet been proved. The recent demonstration that malignant transformation (manifesting in cell-focus formation and in the appearance of new cellular antigens in cultures of human embryonic cells) takes place upon inoculation of fluid from osteosarcoma and liposarcoma cultures containing type C virus particles (Morton, Malmgren, Hall, and Shidlovsky, 1969; Morton, Hall, and Malmgren, 1969) offers a system by which the presence of an oncogenic virus in human lymphoma may be studied.

Accidental laboratory or intentional experimental infection with the Epstein-Barr (EB) virus results in the clinical picture of infectious mononucleosis (Henle, Henle, and Diehl, 1968; Grace, Blakeslee, and Jones, 1969). Antibodies to this virus or to lymphoid cells harboring this virus reach high titers in patients with Burkitt's lymphoma in remission or in patients recovering from infectious mononucleosis (Klein *et al.*, 1969). The EB virus causes or is associated with lymphoblastoid transformation of cultures deriving from patients with Hodgkin's disease, idiopathic thrombocytopenic purpura (Sinkovics, Sykes, Shullenberger, and Howe, 1967), nasopharyngeal carcinoma, or lymphoepithelioma (deThé, Ambrosioni, Ho, and Kwan, 1969). This virus also transforms normal lymphoid cells so that these cells establish themselves in culture and display chromosomal changes characteristic of lymphoid cell lines cultured from patients with Burkitt's lymphoma (Henle *et al.*, 1967; Gerber, 1969). Lymphoreticular neoplasia of animals, such as Marek's neurolymphomatosis of birds (Churchill, 1968; Nazerian, Solomon, Witter, and Burmester, 1968) and a fatal lymphoproliferative disease of squirrel and marmoset monkeys (Meléndez *et al.*, 1969) are reported to be caused by herpes viruses probably related to the EB virus of man. Since the EB virus occurs in lymphoid cells grown in suspension cultures from normal persons and from patients with infectious hepatitis and other pathological entities (Glade, Hirshaut, Douglas, and Hirschhorn, 1968), the possibility that this virus is not the initiator of the lymphoreticular cell proliferation in which it is found but a secondary invader taking advantage of rapidly proliferating lymphoid cells should be entertained seriously (Sinkovics, Gyorkey, and Shullenberger, in press; The cause of glandular fever, 1968).

PATHOGENESIS

Lymphoma in both rodents and man is characterized by profound immunological defects and autoimmune reactions. Mice infected with leukemia virus fail to produce antibodies or to mount homograft rejections or delayed sensitivity reactions (Peterson, Hendrickson, and Good, 1963; Dent, Peterson, and Good, 1965; Ceglowski and Friedman, 1968).

Conventional Swiss mice infected with cell-free extracts of a lymphoma developed runting and antibody-positive hemolytic anemia; survivors of this runt disease succumbed to lymphoma and recipients of lymphoma cells also showed either or both runt disease with autoimmune hemolytic anemia and lymphoma (Sinkovics 1962a, Sinkovics, Trujillo, Pienta, and Ahearn, in press). The NZB mice develop new germinal centers in the thymus, autoimmune hemolytic anemia, and immune-complex glomerulitis; these features are transferable with filtrate to Swiss mice (Mellors and Huang, 1967). Survivors of the autoimmune disease succumb to malignant lymphoma; extensive replication of type C virus particles takes place in these mice (East, Prosser, Holborow, and Jaquet, 1967; Mellors and Huang, 1967). Cell-induced chronic runt (homologous or allogeneic) disease often terminates in lymphoma in the recipient mice (Schwartz and André-Schwartz, 1968; Keast, 1968).

In man, lymphoreticular neoplasia is preceded by and associated with profound immunological defects (Miller, 1968), collagen diseases, and autoimmune complications such as antibody-positive hemolytic anemia, immune-complex glomerulitis, and preterminal wasting disease (Abbatt and Lea, 1958; Lea, 1964; Cammarata, Rodnan, and Jensen, 1963; Lee, Yamauchi, and Hopper, 1966; Dameshek, 1967; Talal, Sokoloff, and Barth, 1967; Brodovsky, Samuels, Migliore, and Howe, 1968; Bierman, 1968; Sinkovics, Trujillo, Pienta, and Ahearn, in press).

HISTOPATHOLOGY

Various types of malignant lymphoma resembling Hodgkin's disease, giant follicular lymphoma, and Burkitt's tumor of man have been found in mice (Dunn, 1954; Siegler, 1968; Butler, Szakacs, and Sinkovics, 1967).

In Hodgkin's disease of man, an extensive mesenchymal and lymphocytic defensive reaction takes place in response to neoplastic reticulum cells (Lukes, 1964; Smithers, 1967; Crowther, Fairley, and Sewell, 1969). In murine lymphoreticular neoplasia and soft tissue sarcoma, the mesenchymal defense reaction of the host may be so extensive that the neoplastic process resembles infectious granuloma (Siegler, 1968; Stanton, Law, and Ting, 1968).

The mere histological resemblance, for instance the display of the "starry-sky" histological pattern, does not necessarily endorse identical etiology of tumors of man and animals. However, these features are suggestive of similar pathogenesis, *i.e.* the establishment of lymphoreticular neoplasia in man and animals elicits defense reactions from the host that are directed to antigens specific for neoplastic cells and to viral agents harbored by the neoplastic cells.

Emergence of Immunoresistant Tetraploid Lymphoma Cells in Man and Mice

RECURRENCE OF BURKITT'S LYMPHOMA

The remission of Burkitt's lymphoma is associated with the appearance of high titers of antibodies directed against the EB virus and particularly against Burkitt's lymphoma cells (Klein *et al.*, 1969). Lymphocytes from patients with Burkitt's tumor destroy cells grown in vitro in primary monolayers from the autologous tumor (Chu, Stjernswärd, Clifford, and Klein, 1967). When Burkitt's lymphoma recurred in two patients after long remission, the tumors consisted of cells that were larger than usual. Chromosome analysis revealed that, in the primary Burkitt's tumor, the majority of the neoplastic cells possessed chromosomal sets in the diploid range, whereas in the recurrent tumor, the majority of the neoplastic lymphoid cells displayed karyotypes of the tetraploid range (Clifford *et al.*, 1968).

A distinction between neoplastic lymphoreticular cells with tetraploid karyotypes and normal diploid lymphoid cells representing the defense reaction of the host could be made in tissue cultures deriving from patients with Hodgkin's disease (Seif and Spriggs, 1967). Thus, it appears that tetraploid lymphoid cells emerge and by-pass immune defense mechanisms that are effective against diploid neoplastic cells.

A TETRAPLOID IMMUNORESISTANT MURINE LYMPHOMA

A situation reminiscent of that of Burkitt's lymphoma has recently been encountered in the mouse. A lymphoma consisting of neoplastic cells of diploid karyotype has been maintained by passages of cells in young adult Timco (Texas Inbred Mouse Company, Houston) Swiss mice. This lymphoma (protocol #620) exhibits the "starry-sky" histological pattern, produces mouse leukemia virus (Rauscher strain) particles, and is moderately sensitive to cytotoxic murine antisera, to immune murine lymphocytes, and to rejection mechanisms of the normal adult mouse (Sinkovics, Pienta, Trujillo, and Ahearn, 1969). When cultured, particularly in the presence of immune spleen cells, primary explants of this lymphoma released large lymphoid cells which grew as permanent cell lines. One cell line (protocol #818) derived from culture of lymphoma #620, without immune spleen

TABLE 1.—Comparisons of Two Lines of a Murine Lymphoma

Criteria	#620 (*in vivo*)	#818 (*in vitro*)
Histology	Lymphoma*	Lymphoma*
Growth	Slow, localized	Rapid, disseminated
Antigen	Rauscher virus	Rauscher virus
Rejection	Common†	Rare†
Reactions with		
immune lymphocytes	Sensitive	Resistant
antibodies	Cytotoxicity	Weak cytotoxicity
Electron microscopy	Type C, budding	Type C, budding malformed particles
Globulin production	Weak	Strong and virus-neutralizing
Chromosomes	Diploid range	Tetraploid range

*"Starry-sky" pattern. †Dose dependent.

cells added, was studied extensively. Cultured #818 cells possess chromosomal sets in the tetraploid range and display highly malignant features in young adult Timco Swiss mice (Table 1) (Sinkovics, Pienta, Trujillo, and Ahearn, 1969; Trujillo *et al.*, in press). A young adult Timco Swiss mouse is able to reject a tumor initiated by several million cells of #620 lymphoma, whereas 3,000 cells of the cultured tetraploid lymphoblasts of line #818 will grow invasively and kill the host. The tetraploid neoplastic lymphoblasts show immunoresistance when exposed to cytotoxic murine antibodies or lymphocytes (Sinkovics *et al.*, in press). These malignant cells continue to manufacture leukemia virus particles, but cell-free filtrates of the cultures fail to cause leukemia or lymphoma. These cells also produce gamma 1 and gamma 2a classes of immune globulins; the purified globulins neutralize the virulent mouse passage line (Rauscher strain) leukemia virus (Sinkovics, Pienta, Trujillo, and Ahearn, 1969; Trujillo *et al.*, in press). It has been proposed that the tetraploid cells acquired immunoresistance through the production of virus-neutralizing antibody. As immunoglobulins coat budding virus particles and viral neoantigenic sites on and within these cells, the cells may present themselves to the host as "self," *i.e.* coated by a film of self-type globulins. Although immune lymphocytes cannot, macrophages can react to such "opsonized" antigens; thus lymphocyte-mediated rejection of these neoplastic cells fails, but phagocytosis by mobile histiocytes continues to be operative.

In recent studies, the emergence of immunoresistant tetraploid lymphoma cells has been observed when #620 lymphoma cells were grown in vitro in the presence of spleen explants derived from Timco Swiss mice which previously rejected #620 lymphoma. Rejectors of this lymphoma were shown to produce antibodies that neutralize the leukemia virus and are cytotoxic to #620 lymphoma cells. The population of round lymphoid cells released from combined cultures of #620 lymphoma and immune spleen explants contained more larger cells (as measured in μ^3 in the Coulter Counter) than did the population of lymphoid cells released from cultures of #620 lymphoma alone, of #620 lymphoma and normal spleen explants, of normal spleen explants alone, and of immune spleen explants alone. Bioassays performed in the three-week-old Timco Swiss mice resulted in the development of progressive ascitic lymphosarcoma invading the liver in mice inoculated with lymphoid cells deriving from combined cultures of #620 tumor and immune spleen explants. Slow-growing solid lymphomas corresponding to the original #620 tumor developed in mice inoculated with lymphoid cells derived from cultures of #620 tumor alone or from cultures of #620 tumor and normal spleen explants. Preliminary karyotyping indicates a preponderance of tetraploid lymphoblasts in the invasive ascitic tumor (Fig. 1). No tumors developed in mice inoculated with lymphoid cells deriving from cultures of normal and immune spleen.

FIG. 1.—Foamy macrophage (M) with cell debris in its cytoplasm and lymphoid cells in the ascitic fluid of a mouse. In the center, a resting and a dividing lymphoid cell are visible; the dividing cell has a chromosomal set in the tetraploid range. This mouse was inoculated 2 weeks earlier with lymphoid cells floating in a combined culture of diploid lymphoma #620 and immune spleen explants. Wright's stain, × 70 objective, × 10 ocular.

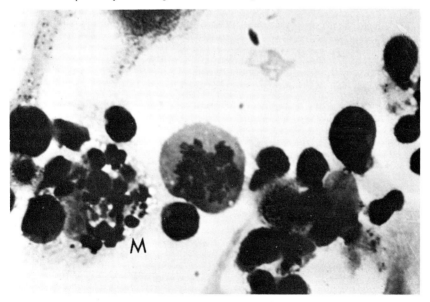

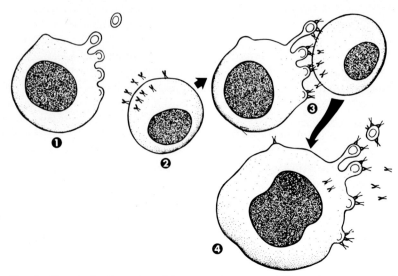

FIG. 2.—Hypothesis: Formation of immunoresistant tetraploid neoplastic lymphoid cells by fusion of the primary diploid neoplastic cell with plasma cell-producing virus-neutralizing antibody. The resulting tetraploid cell continues both genetically determined commitments: synthesis of leukemia virus and of virus-specific globulins; the globulin functions as "self-enhancing antibody." *1*, Virus-producing diploid immunosensitive lymphoma cell; *2*, Antibody (virus-neutralizing)-producing plasma cell; *3*, Juxtaposition of 1 and 2; *4*, Fusion of 1 and 2.

The hypothesis is proposed that immunoresistant tetraploid lympho-blasts emerge by fusion of diploid neoplastic lymphoblasts (#620 lymphoma cells) and antibody-producing plasma cells. The virion antigens on the membrane of the neoplastic cells attract the plasma cell by virtue of its virus-neutralizing antibody content (Fig. 2). The resulting tetraploid cell preserves its neoplastic features, loses its capacity to release virus free of antibody coat, and gains immunoresistance by being protected from lymphocyte-mediated rejection as the result of a self-type globulin coat covering the viral neoantigenic sites.

Immune Reactions of Patients with Lymphoma to Cultured "Neoplastic" Cells

ACTIVITIES OF LYMPHOCYTES IN PRIMARY TISSUE CULTURES

When lymphocytes destroy other cells in vitro, it is customary to postulate specific immunological activity. However, lymphocytes are known to utilize other, particularly fibroblast-like, cells as a feeder layer in culture; this association is very intimate, for groups of lymphocytes enter the cytoplasm of fibroblast-like cells where the lymphocytes may reside for several weeks and acquire coding material necessary for the synthesis of enzyme systems. A progeny of these lymphocytes will replicate first within, then also outside the fibroblast-like cells; the fibroblast-like cells slowly degenerate after harboring large colonies of lymphocytes (Sinkovics, Shullenberger, and Howe, 1966). Thus, cell destruction by lymphocytes occurs, but without an immunological principle involved. This type of association of lymphocytes with fibroblast-like cells was observed in primary cultures derived from patients with chronic lymphocytic leukemia and malignant lymphoma.

Another type of interaction between autologous lymphocytes and large elongated or epithelial cells occurs when the encounter of these cells results rapidly in cell death. Commonly, both lymphocytes and large cells succumb to a process of vacuolization and disintegration in this type of reaction. In addition to previously reported observations (Sinkovics, 1962b; Sinkovics, Sykes, Shullenberger, and Howe, 1967), this phenomenon has recently been observed in two cultures derived from Hodgkin's disease (cultures #1637

FIG. 3.—A large cell with multiple nucleoli is surrounded, invaded, and vacuolized by autologous lymphoid cells in primary culture of a lymph node from a patient (Mr. S.H.) with Hodgkin's disease. (*N*: nucleus of large target cell; *Ly*: lymphoid cells). Wright's stain, × 54 objective, × 10 ocular.

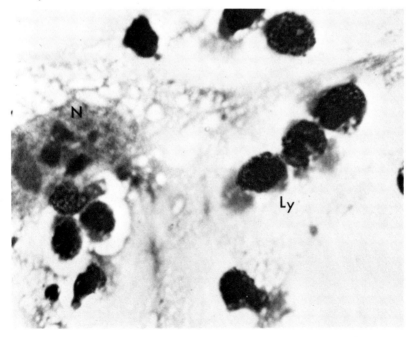

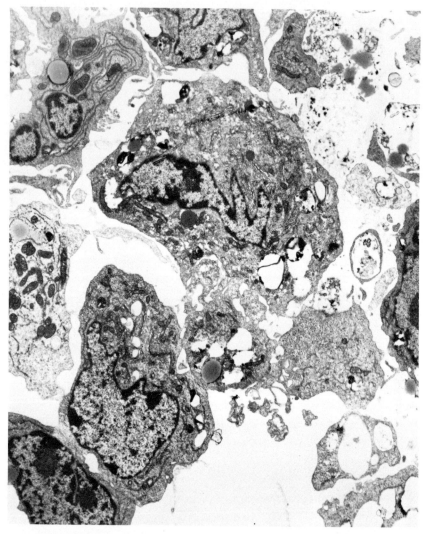

FIG. 4.—Lymphoid cells from culture # 1637. Electron microscopy, reduced from × 8,000.

and # 1711) and in one culture (culture # 1623) derived from lymphoepithelioma of the nasopharynx metastatic to the liver (Figs. 3, 4, and 5). Since
these patients may have received transfusions previously, it is not entirely
certain that the tissue cultures consisted of autologous cells only; it is

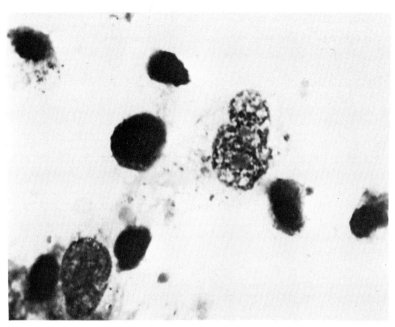

FIG. 5.—Degenerating cell with faint vacuolized cytoplasm and clumping of chromatin in the nucleus is surrounded by autologous lymphoid cells in primary culture of liver biopsy from a patient (Mr. J.B.) with lymphoepithelioma metastatic to the liver. Wright's stain, × 54 objective, × 10 ocular.

TABLE 2.—CULTURED "NEOPLASTIC" CELLS

CULTURE NO.	CLINICAL DIAGNOSIS*	MORPHOLOGIC CHARACTERISTICS OF CULTURE
# 778	Lymphocytic lymphoma (Mr. H.F.)	Large lymphoid cells, elongated cells, multinucleated cells
# 934	Reticulum cell sarcoma (Mr. L.F.S.)	Large lymphoid cells, epithelial and multinucleated cells
# 999	Infectious mononucleosis (Mrs. P.O.)	Large lymphoid cells, epithelial and multinucleated cells
# 1449	Embryonal rhabdomyosarcoma (Mrs. S.S.)	Multinucleated giant cells
# 1459	Chondrosarcoma (Mr. N.M.)	Multinucleated giant cells

*Of patient yielding culture.

possible that the cytotoxic lymphocytes derived from blood donors. It is known that one patient (Mr. S.H.) with Hodgkin's disease did not receive transfusion prior to the surgical lymph node biopsy from which the culture shown in Figure 3 was established.

REACTIONS OF PERIPHERAL LEUKOCYTES TO CULTURED
NEOPLASTIC CELLS

ESTABLISHED CULTURES OF PRESUMABLY NEOPLASTIC CELLS.—Salient features of the cultures utilized in this study are summarized in Table 2.

Culture #778 was grown from the lymph node of a patient (Mr. H.F.) with lymphocytic lymphoma; this culture has been in continuous growth since its initiation in 1966 (Sinkovics, Sykes, Shullenberger, and Howe, 1967; Sinkovics, 1968). The primary culture consisted of fibroblasts and scattered large round cells; the fibroblasts degenerated but the round cells began to grow in suspension in Bellco spinner bottles. After several months of growth in suspension, the cells showed an increased tendency to grow on the walls of the vessel, rather than in suspension. At the present time, the culture is being maintained in T flasks; it grows loosely adherent to glass.

FIG. 6.—Large lymphoid cells floating over a monolayer of fibroblasts in the primary culture (protocol #778) of a lymph node from a patient (Mr. H.F.) with lymphocytic lymphoma. Wright's stain, × 40 objective, × 10 ocular.

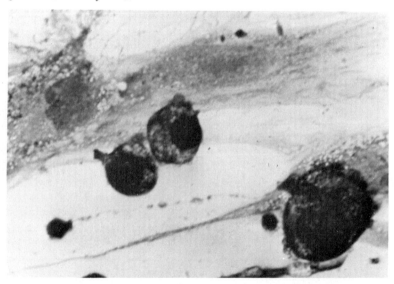

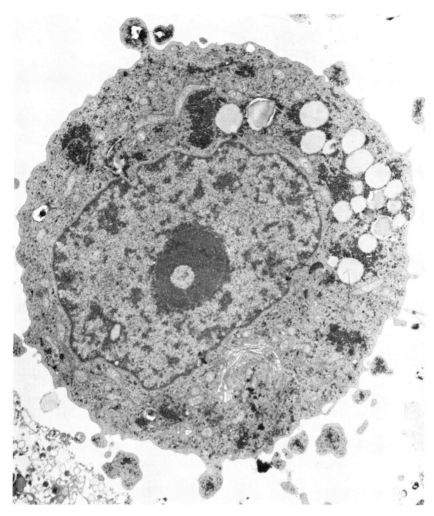

FIG. 7.—A round lymphoid cell grown in the suspended phase of culture #778. Electron microscope, original magnification × 16,000. (Courtesy of J. A. Sykes and L. Recher.)

No virus particles were seen in this culture (Recher, Sinkovics, Sykes, and Whitescarver, 1969), it could not be infected with the EB virus (Gerber, personal communication), and cell-free fluids derived from the culture failed to cause morphological transformation of human embryonic fibroblasts in our laboratory. EB viral or virus-coded antigens could not be found in this culture by fluorescent antibody staining (Vonka, personal communication). The

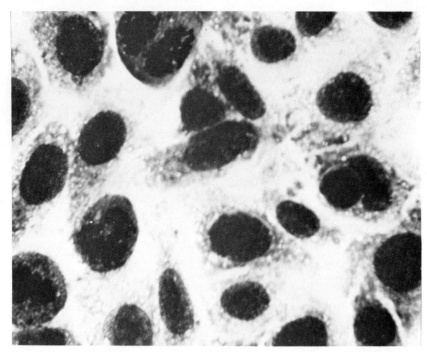

Fig. 8.—The appearance of culture #934 in passage 300. Wright's stain × 54 objective, × 10 ocular.

culture consists of slender cells with large nuclei, multinucleated giant cells, and large round cells growing into focus-like colonies (Figs. 6 and 7). The same patient (Mr. H.F.) yielded entirely similar cultures grown earlier in other laboratories; in these cultures, virus-like structures resembling type C particles and globulin production by the large round cells were demonstrated (Trujillo *et al.,* 1967).

Culture #934 derives from the lymph node of a patient (Mr. L.F.S.) with reticulum cell sarcoma (Dreyer, 1965). This culture has been maintained continuously in our laboratory since 1967. The culture consists of epithelial cells, multinucleated giant cells, and lymphoid cells in small numbers (Fig. 8). According to a former report (Dmochowski *et al.,* 1967), particles resembling type C virus were occasionally found in this culture. The presence of these particles could not be confirmed by other electron microscopists who examined the subline of the culture as maintained in our laboratory (Sykes and Recher, personal communication) and by two of us (P.G. and F.G.). Cell-free fluid from this culture did not cause morphological transformation of human embryonic fibroblasts in our laboratory. EB viral or virus-coded antigens could not be detected in this culture by fluorescent antibody staining (Vonka, personal communication).

Culture #999 derives from the bone marrow of a young woman (Mrs. P.O.) with lymphadenopathy and atypical Downey-type lymphocytes in the peripheral blood. The lymphadenopathy receded and the blood picture returned to normal; there was only equivocal rise of heterophile antibodies. This culture has been in continuous growth in our laboratory since 1967

FIG. 9.—Epithelial cells of culture #999 grown adherent to glass. Electron microscope, original magnification × 20,000. (Courtesy of J. A. Sykes and L. Recher.)

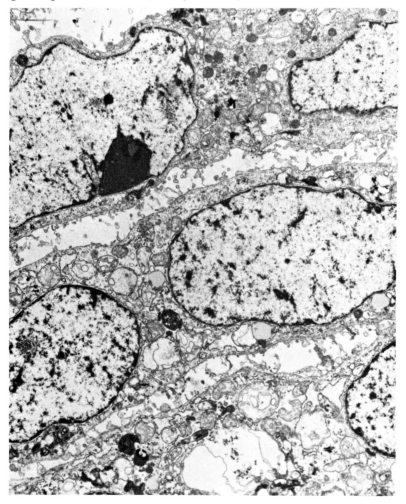

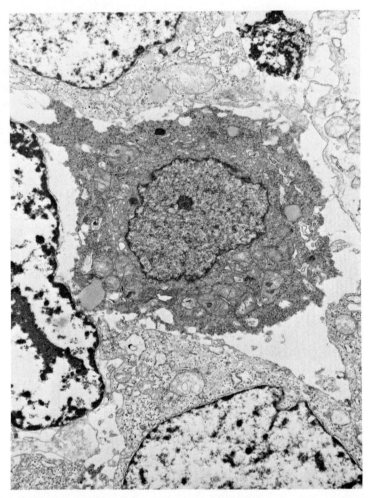

FIG. 10.—Culture #999, consisting of large pale epithelial and smaller dark, probably lymphoid, cells. Electron microscopy, original magnification × 16,000. (Courtesy of J. A. Sykes and L. Recher.)

(Sinkovics, 1968) and consists of epithelial cells, multinucleated giant cells, and lymphoid cells (Figs. 9 and 10). A former report described clusters of virus-like particles resembling type C virus in this culture (Sinkovics, Gyorkey, and Shullenberger, 1968), but repeated studies failed to confirm the continuous presence of these virus particles (Dmochowski, personal communication; Sykes and Recher, personal communication). Cell-free fluid from this culture did not cause morphological transformation of human embryonic fibroblasts in our laboratory. This culture could not be artificially infected with the EB virus (Gerber, personal communication); EB viral or virus-coded antigens could not be detected in this culture by fluorescent antibody staining (Vonka, personal communication).

Culture #1449 derives from a patient (Mrs. S.S.) with primary embryonal rhabdomyosarcoma of the breast. This culture has been in continuous growth in our laboratory since 1968. The culture consists of large elongated multinucleated cells (Fig. 11). Cell-free fluid of this culture did not cause malignant transformation in cultures of normal human embryonic fibroblasts. Filamentous structures resembling the ribonucleoprotein strands of myxoviruses were seen in the cultured cells (Fig. 12).

Culture #1459 derives from the right hip of a patient (Mr. N.M.) with chondrosarcoma. This culture has been in continuous growth in our laboratory since 1969. The culture consists of large cells with multilobulated large nuclei and of multinucleated giant cells (Figs. 13 and 14). Cell-free fluids from this culture failed to cause malignant transformation in cultures of normal human embryonic fibroblasts. Electron microscopic studies revealed cytoplasmic filamentous structures similar to those found in rhabdomyosarcoma also in this culture.

Patients.—Table 3 lists the patients involved in this study. Three authors of this paper (J.R.C., E.S., and J.G.S.) served as control donors of buffy coat white blood cells and sera.

EXPOSURE OF CULTURED CELLS TO PERIPHERAL WHITE BLOOD CELLS.—

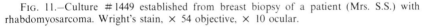

FIG. 11.—Culture #1449 established from breast biopsy of a patient (Mrs. S.S.) with rhabdomyosarcoma. Wright's stain, × 54 objective, × 10 ocular.

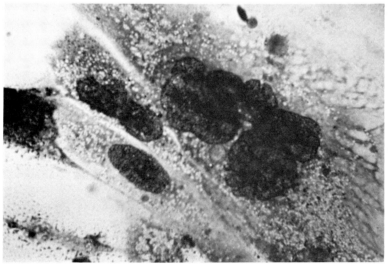

TABLE 3.—PATIENTS STUDIED

INITIALS	AGE	DIAGNOSIS AND STATUS	TYPE OF STUDY
Mrs. S.S.	42	Rhabdomyosarcoma, disseminated	Origin of culture #1449
Miss M.P.	18	Rhabdomyosarcoma, disseminated	Origin of culture #1517; reaction of WBC and plasma with cultures #1517 and #1449
Mrs. V.C.	24	Rhabdomyosarcoma, disseminated	Reaction of WBC with culture #1449
Mr. I.R.	47	Rhabdomyosarcoma, remission	Reaction of WBC and plasma with culture #1449
Mr. N.M.	59	Chondrosarcoma, regional	Origin of culture #1459; reaction of WBC and plasma with culture #1459
Mr. H.F.	64	Lymphocytic lymphoma, disseminated	Origin of culture #778; reaction of WBC and plasma with culture #778
Mr. L.S.	76	Reticulum cell sarcoma, disseminated	Origin of culture #934
Mrs. P.O.	23	Infectious mononucleosis	Origin of culture #999
Mr. S.H.	16	Hodgkin's disease, disseminated	Origin of culture #1637
Mr. E.K.	12	Hodgkin's disease, disseminated	Origin of culture #1711
Mr. J.B.	51	Lymphoepithelioma, disseminated	Origin of culture #1623
Mrs. E.G.	58	Reticulum cell sarcoma, disseminated	Reactions of WBC and plasma with culture #934
Mrs. P.V.	57	Reticulum cell sarcoma, disseminated	Reaction of WBC and plasma with culture #934
Mr. L.C.	57	Lymphocytic lymphosarcoma, disseminated	Reaction of WBC and plasma with cultures #778 and #934
Miss J.H.	23	Infectious mononucleosis; Hodgkin's disease, regional	Reaction of WBC with culture #999

Abbreviation: WBC, white blood cells (from buffy coat).

Heparinized blood was drawn from the patients and centrifuged. The plasma was stored frozen for antibody studies. The buffy coat was transferred into hematocrit tubes and centrifuged again. The buffy coat was pipetted off and mixed with presumably neoplastic cells, referred to thereon as target cells, which were obtained by trypsinization from established cultures. The cell mixtures contained white blood cells outnumbering target cells 100 to 200:1. The cell mixtures were seeded in Leighton tubes and grown in Ham's F10 medium containing 20 per cent heat-inactivated fetal calf serum. Cover slips from Leighton tube cultures were removed periodically and stained according to Wright's method. The target cells were counted in 10 to 15 fields on each slide using × 10 ocular and × 10 objective and the number of target cells in one field was arrived at by calculation; the results were plotted. The area of one cover slip was calculated to be $33,000,000\mu^2$. The area of one field seen through a special $\times$ 10 ocular and $\times$ 10 objective was calculated to be $80,000\mu^2$.

Leukocytes from the peripheral blood of a patient (Miss M.P.) with disseminated rhabdomyosarcoma were tested against the primary culture of her own tumor. Although no decrease of target cell growth was observed, leukocytes from a normal donor reduced the number of target cells by the

FIG. 12.–Cytoplasmic filamentous structures in a rhabdomyosarcoma cell of culture #1449. Electron microscopy, reduced from $\times$ 47,500.

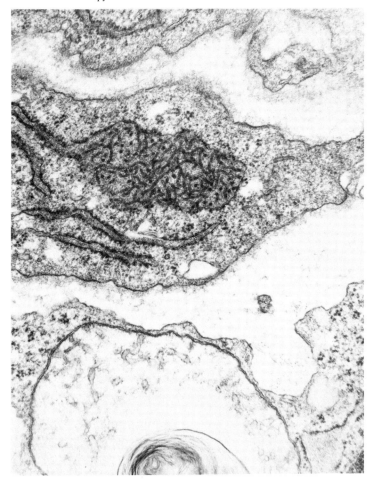

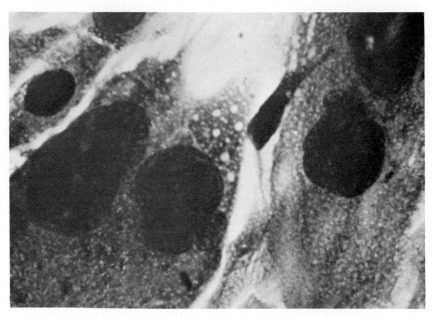

FIG. 13.—Culture #1459 established from surgical biopsy of the right hip from a patient (Mr. N.M.) with chondrosarcoma. Wright's stain, × 54 objective, × 10 ocular.

sixth day of incubation. Inspection of the cultures revealed that the primary culture (protocol #1517) of this tumor consisted of fibroblasts and of a few giant cells. The patient's lymphocytes spared the fibroblasts but damaged the giant cells. The leukocytes of the normal donor damaged the fibroblasts also, but the reaction was not immediate; it became evident only after several days of culturing. The leukocytes of this patient inhibited the growth of established allogeneic culture #1449 (Fig. 15). Repeated immunization of this patient with #1449 cells irradiated with 10,000 rads x-ray resulted in an augmented inhibitory effect of the patient's leukocytes on the target cells. The patient's lymphocytes surrounded and vacuolized #1449 cells in these cultures (Fig. 16). Two other patients with rhabdomyosarcoma (Mrs. V.C. and Mr. I.R.) were shown to circulate lymphocytes cytotoxic to #1449 cells. Leukocytes of normal donors also inhibited the growth of #1449 cells, but only after several days of co-culturing.

Leukocytes from the peripheral blood of a patient (Mr. N.M.) with locally growing chondrosarcoma of the right hip significantly inhibited the growth of presumably neoplastic cells established as a permanent culture from the autologous tumor (Fig. 17). Normal allogeneic leukocytes also inhibited the growth of this tumor, but the inhibition became evident only after several days of co-cultivation (Fig. 17). The heparinized plasma of this

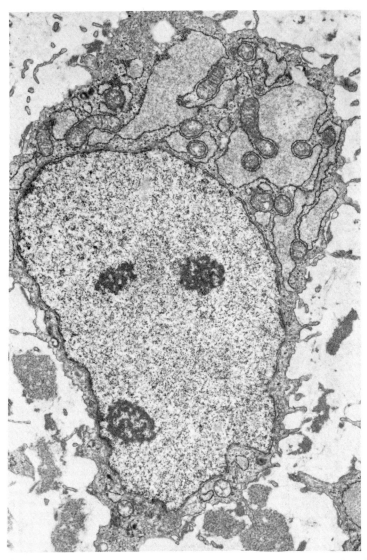

FIG. 14.–Chondrosarcoma cell in culture #1459. Electron microscopy, reduced from × 12,000.

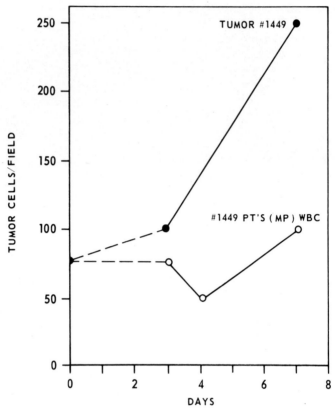

FIG. 15.—The growth of allogeneic rhabdomyosarcoma cells is inhibited by buffy coat lymphocytes of a patient (Miss M.P.). Interrupted line, calculated values; continuous line, actual cell counts on stained cover slips.

patient was "toxic" to the autologous cultured neoplastic cells (culture #1459). The patient's lymphocytes surrounded and vacuolized the autologous neoplastic target cells (Fig. 18), but autologous fibroblasts were not damaged.

Similar experiments were carried out with patients having malignant lymphomas. The leukocytes of a patient (Mr. H.F.) with lymphocytic lymphoma inhibited the growth of the presumably neoplastic autologous target cells (culture #778) and the plasma of the patient acted synergistically with the lymphocytes in suppressing the growth of the target cells (Fig. 19), however, the cytotoxic effect of the plasma may be due to its heparin content. Normal allogeneic lymphocytes exerted an inhibitory effect on these target cells, but only after several days of co-cultivation. The lymphocytes of this patient surrounded and invaded the target cells (Fig. 20); however, after

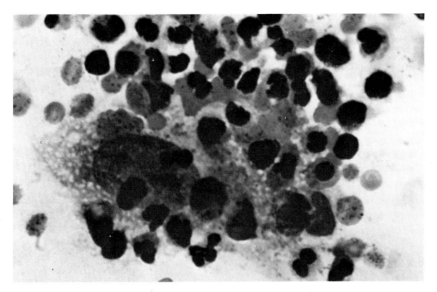

Fig. 16.—Allogeneic lymphoid cells (Miss M.P.) congregate on large cell of rhabdomyosarcoma culture #1449. Wright's stain, × 70 objective, × 10 ocular.

several days of co-cultivation, a symbiotic relationship between autologous lymphocytes and target cells had taken place. In this relationship, neither the target cells nor the lymphocytes seemed to suffer damage in spite of their close contact (Fig. 21).

Leukocytes from the peripheral blood of two patients (Mrs. E.G. and Mrs. P.V.) with reticulum cell sarcoma inhibited the growth of #934 cells before and after immunization with x-irradiated (10,000 to 12,000 rads) #934 cells (Figs. 22 and 23). These patients, in contrast to the patients previously studied, mobilized histiocytes (or macrophages) rather than lymphocytes to combat #934 cells (Figs. 24 and 25). However, leukocytes from a normal donor also vigorously inhibited #934 cells in culture, and the mediators of inhibition were macrophages rather than lymphocytes (Fig. 26); inhibition of #934 cells by normal macrophages was also immediate. Leukocytes from a patient with disseminated lymphocytic lymphosarcoma (Mr. L.C.) completely failed to inhibit the growth of #778 and #934 cells, and immunization with irradiated cells of cultures #778 and #934 did not result in the mobilization of cytotoxic lymphocytes or histiocytes. This patient was in the preterminal stage of his disease during these experiments.

A patient (Miss J.H.) developed sclerosing nodular type Hodgkin's disease in the cervical lymph nodes six months after recovering from infectious mononucleosis. Without actual proof, one may speculate that in this patient malignant transformation of some lymphoreticular cells occurred following

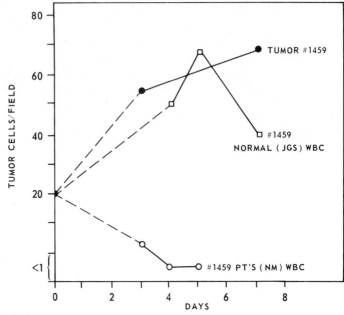

FIG. 17.—Immediate inhibition of growth of autologous tumor cells by buffy coat lymphocytes. Normal buffy coat lymphocytes undergo blastic transformation and begin to inhibit growth of tumor cells after five days of co-cultivation. Interrupted lines, calculated values; continuous lines, actual cell counts on stained cover slips.

FIG. 18.—Autologous lymphoid cells (Mr. N.M.) surround chondrosarcoma cell (culture # 1459); the target cell fails to spread out on the glass surface and eventually undergoes degeneration. Wright's stain, × 70 objective, × 10 ocular.

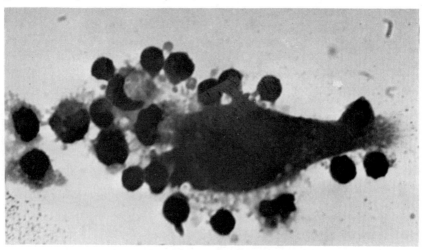

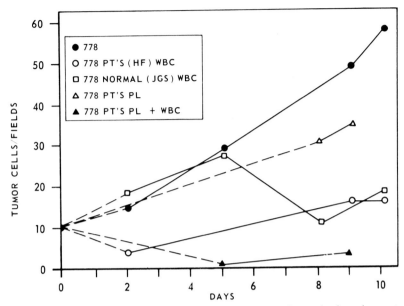

FIG. 19.—Immediate inhibition by buffy coat lymphocytes of growth of autologous target cells that are presumably neoplastic. Growth of target cells continues until the fifth day in the presence of normal buffy coat lymphocytes, and inhibition of growth occurs afterward. Patient's plasma is synergistic with growth-inhibitory autologous lymphocytes. Interrupted lines, calculated values; continuous lines, actual cell counts on stained cover slips.

a customarily benign virus infection. The leukocytes of this patient were tested against culture #999. Culture #999 may be regarded as a cell line deriving from infectious mononucleosis and subsequently undergoing malignant transformation in vitro (but without any trace of the EB virus). The leukocytes of this patient showed no immediate reaction with #999 cells; however, after co-cultivation for several days, suppression of growth occurred. Macrophages appeared to be the mediators rather than lymphocytes. Leukocytes of a normal donor suppressed #999 cells more effectively, and all white blood cell types seemed to participate in the reaction (Figs. 27 and 28).

PRODUCTION OF ANTIBODY TO NEOPLASTIC CELLS.—Recent reports indicate that patients with malignant melanoma, osteogenic sarcoma, liposarcoma, and Burkitt's lymphoma produce antibodies to autologous or allogeneic tumors of the corresponding histological types (Antigens in human sarcomas and melanomas, 1969; Klein et al., 1969). In the present study, culture #1449 was used as antigen against plasma of patients with rhabdomyosarcoma and cultures #934 and #778 were used as antigens

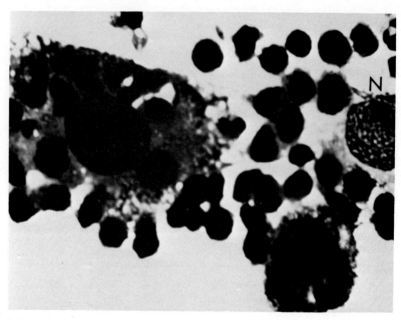

Fig. 20.—The large target cells (culture #778) are surrounded and vacuolized by autologous lymphocytes (Mr. H.F.); a bare target cell nucleus (*N*) with clumped chromatin is also visible. Wright's stain, × 70 objective, × 10 ocular.

Fig. 21.—Autologous lymphocytes (Mr. H.F.) and target cells (culture #778) co-exist after 12 days in culture. Wright's stain, × 54 objective, × 10 ocular.

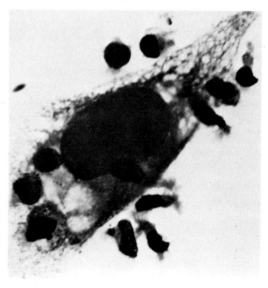

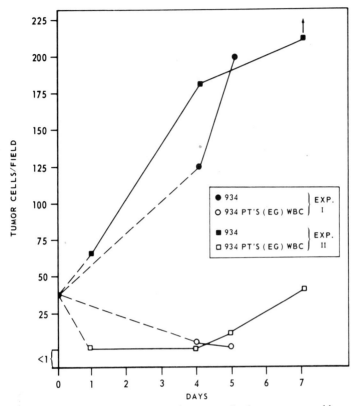

FIG. 22.—Inhibition of growth of allogeneic target cells that are presumably neoplastic by buffy coat cells of a patient with reticulum cell sarcoma. Interrupted lines, calculated values; continuous lines, actual cell counts on stained cover slips.

against plasma of patients with reticulum cell sarcoma and lymphoma. Questionable immunofluorescence (single resting cells fluorescing weakly in apple green color) was observed when acetone-fixed cultured cells were exposed to the plasma of patients with corresponding tumors and counter-stained with isothiocyanate-labeled antihuman gamma globulin rabbit serum (Figs. 29 and 30). Definitely positive immunofluorescence (numerous resting cells fluorescing strongly in bright apple green color) was observed in the indirect test when these cells were exposed to patients' plasma obtained after immunization with x-irradiated cultured cells of the corresponding type (Figs. 31 and 32). No fluorescence was observed with two normal sera. These preliminary studies do not permit a final conclusion; certain cells in cultures #934 and #778 may produce globulins of their

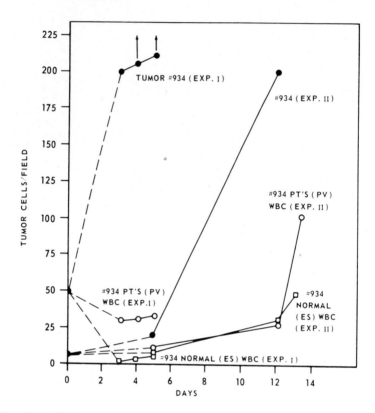

Fig. 23.—Inhibition of growth of allogeneic target cells that are presumably neoplastic by buffy coat cells of a patient with reticulum cell sarcoma and by buffy coat cells of a normal individual; inhibition is immediate in both cases. Regrowth of target cells occurs after twelfth day, when the patient's buffy coat white blood cells were exhausted. Interrupted lines, calculated values; continuous lines, actual cell counts on stained cover slips.

own. It is possible that there is a quantitative difference between the contents of antibodies directed to "common tumor-specific antigens" in plasma samples of patients obtained before and after immunization with the corresponding tumor cells.

CONCLUSION OF PRELIMINARY STUDIES.—Exposure of cultured allogeneic target cells, either presumably neoplastic or normal fibroblastic, to normal peripheral leukocytes resulted in suppressed growth of target cells. Inhibition of growth was not immediate, but became evident after several days of co-culturing. During co-cultivation, blastic transformation of normal lymphoid cells occurred. Thus, the probability of an immune reaction acquired in vitro should be considered. The mediators of this reaction were lymphocytes when fibroblastic, rhabdomyosarcoma, or chondrosarcoma

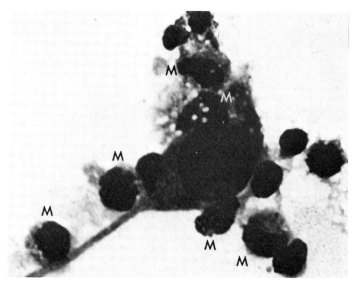

FIG. 24.–The large target cell of culture #934 is surrounded by allogeneic macrophages *(M)* and lymphocytes (Mrs. E.G.). Wright's stain, × 70 objective, × 10 ocular.

FIG. 25.–Allogeneic macrophages *(M)* (Mrs. P.V.) surround target cells of culture #934. Wright's stain, × 54 objective, × 10 ocular.

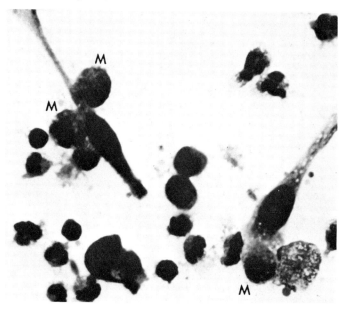

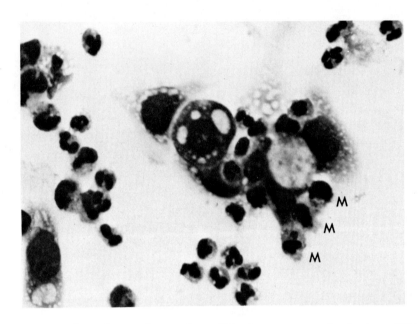

FIG. 26.—Allogeneic normal macrophages (*M*) adhere to target cells of culture #934; the target cells undergo vacuolization. Polymorphonuclear leukocytes do not participate in this reaction. Wright's stain, × 54 objective, × 10 ocular.

FIG. 27.—Several allogeneic lymphoid cells (*Ly*) and macrophages (*M*) (Miss J.H.) adhere to a vacuolized large target cell of culture #999. Wright's stain, × 54 objective, × 10 ocular.

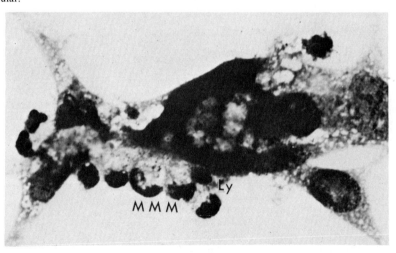

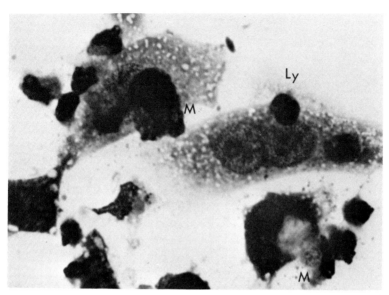

FIG. 28.—Normal allogeneic lymphoid cells (*Ly*) and macrophages (*M*) adhere to target cells of culture #999. Wright's stain, × 70 objective, × 10 ocular.

FIG. 29.—Indirect fluorescent antibody stain using acetone-fixed cells of culture #1449 exposed to plasma of a patient (Miss M.P.) with rhabdomyosarcoma and counter-stained with fluorescein isothiocyanate-labeled antihuman globulin. Cytoplasmic fluorescence of occasional cell groups was observed. Fluorescence microscopy, × 25 objective, × 10 ocular.

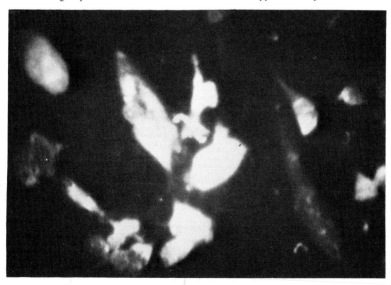

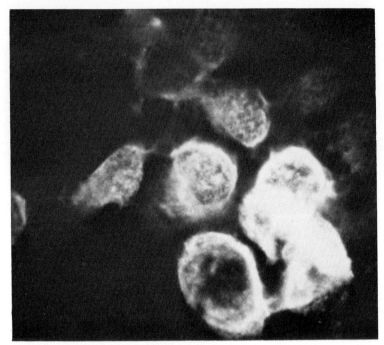

FIG. 30.—Indirect fluorescent antibody stain using acetone-fixed cells of culture #934 exposed to plasma of a patient (Mrs. E.G.) with reticulum cell sarcoma and counter-stained with fluorescein isothiocyanate-labeled antihuman globulin. Cytoplasmic fluorescence of occasional cell groups was observed. Fluorescence microscopy, × 54 objective, × 10 ocular.

cells were used as targets. Against a culture (#934) derived from reticulum cell sarcoma, macrophages were mobilized. Presumably, the target cells are globulin producers, thus attracting macrophages which preferably engulf "opsonized" antigens.

Patients with rhabdomyosarcoma or chondrosarcoma circulated lymphoid cells which reacted immediately with allogeneic (#1449) cultured tumor cells or with autologous (#1459) cultured tumor cells. Destruction of target cells by lymphoid cells was seen. The distinction between the immediate reaction of these patients as opposed by the delayed reaction of the normal individuals to these target cells requires more precise studies to be carried out in quadruplicate so that statistical analysis may be applied. The immediate reaction suggests that these patients circulate lymphoid cells presensitized to autologous tumor-specific antigens and that the same antigens occur on allogeneic neoplastic cells of the same histological type.

If fibroblastic and neoplastic cells are not clearly distinguished in primary cultures of tumors exposed to autologous leukocytes, a false-negative reading of the results may occur. A mere count of target cells, or colony-count of these cells would not reveal suppression of growth if the majority of the target cells were normal fibroblasts; however, lymphocytes of the patient may still display cytotoxicity to a few neoplastic cells lying in the network of fibroblastic cells. Another possible interpretation of the reaction between lymphocytes and target cells as falsely negative may take place when the results are read too late. In certain instances, lymphocytes severely inhibit the target cells at the beginning, but after an initial suppression of growth, the target cells, adapted well to in vitro conditions, exhaust and outgrow the supply of lymphocytes that are not as yet adapted to growing in vitro.

False-positive reactions are possible, too, especially when the lymphocytes of patients are tested against allogeneic tumors. Cytotoxic activity may be acquired in vitro so rapidly that it may appear as a reaction between presensitized lymphocytes and target cells. Cytotoxins released from presensitized lymphocytes reacting with a specific antigen may nonspecifically

FIG. 31.—Indirect fluorescent antibody stain using acetone-fixed cells of culture #1449 exposed to plasma of a patient (Miss M.P.) after immunization of the patient with x-irradiated #1449 cells. The preparation was counter-stained with fluorescein isothiocyanate-labeled antihuman globulin. Cytoplasmic fluorescence of cell groups was frequently observed. Fluorescent microscopy, × 25 objective. × 10 ocular.

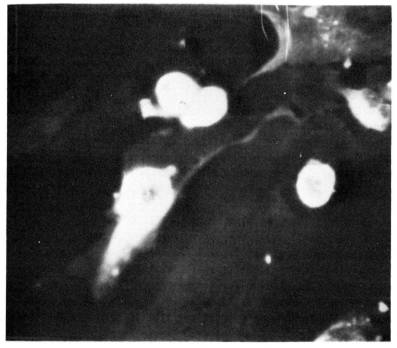

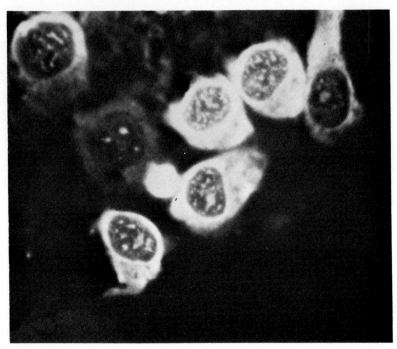

FIG. 32.—Indirect fluorescent antibody stain using acetone-fixed cells of culture #934 exposed to plasma of a patient (Mrs. E.G.) after immunization of the patient with x-irradiated #934 cells. The preparation was counter-stained with fluorescein isothiocyanate-labeled antihuman globulin. Cytoplasmic fluorescence of cell groups was frequently observed. Fluorescent microscopy, × 54 objective, × 10 ocular.

damage normal fibroblasts lying nearby (Ruddle and Waksman, 1968a, b). Lymphoid cells may utilize target cells as a feeder layer in vitro and afflict protracted damage to the target cells, but without an immunological principle involved (Sinkovics, Shullenberger, and Howe, 1966). Also, the reaction between macrophages and certain target cells, whether the macrophages were derived from patients or from normal individuals, was also of the immediate type.

The filamentous structures found in cultured cells of rhabdomyosarcoma and chondrosarcoma are possibly ribonucleoprotein strands of an as yet unidentified myxovirus. These structures endow the cells with virion-type neoantigenicity as well as with transplantation-type neoantigens coded for by these structures. Type C viruses closely resemble myxoviruses; thus, it is well within the range of justifiable conjectures to regard these strands as possible defective type C viruses with oncogenic potency, until proved otherwise.

Prospects of Immunization Against Malignant Lymphoma

Virus-induced tumors of experimental animals yield to immunotherapy. It was possible to prevent viral leukemia in the mouse by active immunization using live attenuated virus, killed virus, or subliminal doses of neoplastic cells (Sinkovics, in press). Neoplastic cells of this type carry both virion-associated and virus-coded but not virion-associated tumor-specific transplantation antigens. The process of oncogenesis by SV40 virus in hamsters could be intercepted by applying active immunization with properly incapacitated tumor cells (Hilleman, 1968). Passive immunization has been shown to be effective against neoplastic cells growing in a disseminated fashion, such as leukemia (Old, Stockert, Boyse, and Geering, 1967), but solid tumors often respond with enhanced growth to attempts at passive immunization (Kaliss, 1962; Hutchin, 1968). Adoptive immunization, when runt (homologous or allogeneic) disease was not fatal, resulted in both prevention and effective treatment of murine leukemia or lymphoma (Sinkovics, Bertin, and Howe, 1965; Spärck and Volkert, 1965). A strong synergistic action between chemo- and radiotherapy and immunotherapy has been demonstrated in certain types of experimental tumors (Haddow and Alexander, 1964; Mihich, 1969).

Although not proved, the viral etiology of leukemias, sarcomas, and malignant lymphomas of man is most probable. Tumors of man induced by related viruses would possess related tumor-specific transplantation antigens. The existence of common tumor antigens and the probability of a viral etiological agent have recently been suggested in neuroblastoma (Hellström, Hellström, Pierce, and Bill, 1968) and in osteogenic sarcoma and liposarcoma of man (Morton, Malmgren, Hall, and Shidlovsky, 1969; Morton, Hall, and Malmgren, 1969). Thus, active immunization with autologous or allogeneic tumor cells, properly incapacitated by x-ray irradiation, may result in an augmented immune reaction to the common tumor-specific antigens. While in experimental animals antitumor activity of splenic lymphocytes was demonstrable only several days or weeks after the removal of the bulk of the tumor (Mikulska, Smith, and Alexander, 1966), it is most encouraging that circulating leukocytes of patients with advanced malignant disease still displayed the capacity for destroying target cells in vitro and that macrophages of patients with reticulum cell sarcoma retained similar activity.

The selective cytotoxicity of lymphocytes in autologous cultures deriving from Hodgkin's disease and lymphoepithelioma offers an avenue to adoptive immunotherapy. If these lymphocytes represent the clone committed to react to tumor-specific antigens in these neoplasms, established cultures of these lymphocytes may be used for immunotherapy. The risks involved in this approach are the possible malignant growth potential of these lymphocytes and the possibility that activated EB virus will be reinduced into the patients with the lymphocytes.

Summary

In a murine lymphoma consisting of immunosensitive diploid cells, immunoresistant tetraploid cells emerged. The immunoresistant cells produced both leukemia virus particles and virus-neutralizing globulins. It is suggested that the globulins act as "self-enhancing" antibody by coating neoantigenic sites of the neoplastic cells. The neoplastic cells thus escape lymphocyte-mediated rejection. Tetraploid immunoresistant cells emerge when diploid lymphoma cells and antibody-producing immune spleen cells are brought together. It is proposed that tetraploid immunoresistant cells are formed by the fusion of diploid lymphoma cells and antibody-producing plasma cells. Analogy between the remission of diploid primary and the appearance of tetraploid recurrent Burkitt's lymphoma and the above-described murine lymphoma is quite evident.

Lymphoblastoid reconversion of tissue cultures deriving from patients with Hodgkin's disease and lymphoepithelioma was observed. The lymphoid cells were cytotoxic to large autochthonous cells resembling Reed-Sternberg cells and to epithelial cells, respectively.

Lymphocytes and macrophages of patients with sarcomas and malignant lymphomas were capable of suppressing the growth and damaging cells of established cultures derived from rhabdomyosarcoma, chondrosarcoma, reticulum cell sarcoma, lymphocytic lymphoma, and infectious mononucleosis.

Immunization of patients with irradiated sarcoma cells resulted in the production of antibodies and cytotoxic lymphoid cells.

Filamentous structures resembling ribonucleoprotein strands of a myxovirus were seen in cultured cells of chondro- and rhabdomyosarcoma.

Acknowledgments

The authors thank Dr. C. C. Shullenberger for his clinical contributions to this presentation and Drs. J. A. Sykes and L. Recher of The Southern California Cancer Center, Los Angeles, California, for the preparation of Figures 7, 9, and 10 and many other electron microscopic pictures related to this work but not shown in this paper. The participation of Drs. M. J. Ahearn, B. Drewinko, and J. M. Trujillo in these studies is greatly appreciated. The authors are obliged for outstanding assistance to Mesdames Phyllis Gyorkey, Elaine Thornell, and Barbara Click and to Miss Ann Cork.

REFERENCES

Abbatt, J. D., and Lea, A. J.: Leukaemogens. *Lancet*, 2:880-883, October 25, 1958.

Antigens in human sarcomas and melanomas. (Editorial) *British Medical Journal*, 3:543, September 6, 1969.

Bierman, S. M.: The role of immunologic aberrations in the pathogenesis of lymphomas. *Archives of Dermatology*, 97:699-711, June 1968.

Brodovsky, H. S., Samuels, M. L., Migliore, P. J., and Howe, C. D.: Chronic lymphocytic leukemia, Hodgkin's disease, and the nephrotic syndrome. *Archives of Internal Medicine*, 121:71-75, January 1968.

Butler, J. J., Szakacs, A., and Sinkovics, J. G.: Virus-induced murine lymphoma resembling Burkitt's tumor. *American Journal of Pathology*, 51:629-637, October 1967.

Cammarata, R. J., Rodnan, G. P., and Jensen, W. N.: Systemic rheumatic disease and malignant lymphoma. *Archives of Internal Medicine*, 111:330-337, March 1963.

The cause of glandular fever. (Editorial) *Lancet*, 1:576-577, March 16, 1968.

Ceglowski, W. S., and Friedman, H.: Immunosuppressive effects of Friend and Rauscher leukemia disease viruses on cellular and humoral antibody formation. *Journal of the National Cancer Institute*, 40:983-995, May 1968.

Chu, E. H. Y., Stjernswärd, J., Clifford, P., and Klein, G.: Reactivity of human lymphocytes against autochthonous and allogeneic normal and tumor cells in vitro. *Journal of the National Cancer Institute*, 39:595-617, October 1967.

Churchill, A. E.: Herpes-type virus isolated in cell culture from tumors of chickens with Marek's disease. I. Studies in cell culture. *Journal of the National Cancer Institute*, 41: 939-950, October 1968.

Clifford, P., Gripenberg, U., Klein, E., Fenyo, E. M., and Manolov, G.: Treatment of Burkitt's lymphoma. *Lancet*, 2:517-518, August 31, 1968.

Cooper, M. D., Peterson, R. D. A., Gabrielsen, A. E., and Good, R. A.: Lymphoid malignancy and development, differentiation, and function of the lymphoreticular system. *Cancer Research*, 26:1165-1169, June 1966.

Crowther, D., Fairley, G. H., and Sewell, R. L.: Significance of the changes in the circulating lymphoid cells in Hodgkin's disease. *British Medical Journal*, 2:473-477, May 24, 1969.

Dameshek, W.: Certain forms of leukemia as immunoproliferative disorders. In *Carcinogenesis: A Broad Critique*, A Collection of Papers Presented at the 20th Annual Symposium on Fundamental Cancer Research, 1966, at The University of Texas M. D. Anderson Hospital and Tumor Institute at Houston. Baltimore, Maryland, The Williams and Wilkins Company, 1967, pp. 141-155.

David, J. R.: Delayed hypersensitivity in vitro: Its mediation by cell-free substances formed by lymphoid cell-antigen interaction. *Proceedings of the National Academy of Sciences of the U.S.A.*, 56:72-77, July 15, 1966.

Dent, P. B., Peterson, R. D. A., and Good, R. A.: A defect in cellular immunity during the incubation period of passage A leukemia in C3H mice. *Proceedings of the Society for Experimental Biology and Medicine*, 119:869-871, July 1965.

DeThé, G., Ambrosioni, J. C., Ho, H. C., and Kwan, H. C.: Lymphoblastoid transformation and presence of herpes-type viral particles in a Chinese nasopharyngeal tumour cultured in vitro. *Nature*, 221:770-771, February 22, 1969.

Dmochowski, L.: Personal communication.

Dmochowski, L., Yumoto, T., Grey, C. E., Hales, R. L., Langford, P. L., Taylor, H. G., Freireich, E. J, Shullenberger, C. C., Shively, J. H., and Howe, C. D.: Electron microscopic studies of human leukemia and lymphoma. *Cancer*, 20:760-777, May 1967.

Dreyer, D. A.: Development of a cell line from a transformed tissue culture of human lymph node cells. (Abstract) *Abstract of Papers Presented at the 16th Annual Meeting of the Tissue Culture Association*, 1965, p. 81.

Dunn, T. B.: Normal and pathologic anatomy of the reticular tissue in laboratory mice, with a classification and discussion of neoplasms. *Journal of the National Cancer Institute*, 14: 1281-1433, June 1954.

East, J., Prosser, P. R., Holborow, E. J., and Jaquet, H.: Autoimmune reactions and virus-like particles in germ-free NZB mice. *Lancet*, 1:755-757, April 8, 1967.

Gerber, P.: Lymphocytes altered by Epstein-Barr virus. (Interview) *Medical Tribune*, 10:1 20, September 25, 1969.

Gerber, P.: Personal communication.

Glade, P. R., Hirshaut, Y., Douglas, S. D., and Hirschhorn, K.: Lymphoid suspension cultures from patients with viral hepatitis. *Lancet*, 2:1273-1275, December 14, 1968.

Good, R. A., and Finstad, J.: The association of lymphoid malignancy and immunologic functions. In Zarafonetis, C. J. D., Ed.: *Proceedings of the International Conference on Leukemia-Lymphoma*, The University of Michigan, Ann Arbor, Michigan, 1967. Philadelphia, Pennsylvania, Lea & Febiger, 1968, pp. 175-197.

Good, R. A., Finstad, J., Gewurz, H., Cooper, M. D., and Pollara, B.: The development of immunological capacity in phylogenetic perspective. *American Journal of Diseases of Children*, 114:477-497, November 1967.

Grace, J. T., Jr., Blakeslee, J., Jr., and Jones, R., Jr.: Induction of infectious mononucleosis in man by the herpes type virus (HTV) in Burkitt lymphoma cells in tissue culture. (Abstract) *Proceedings of the American Association for Cancer Research*, 10:31, March 1969.

Gross, L.: Induction of leukemia in mice following inoculation of filtrates from mouse tumors. In Gross, L.: *Oncogenic Viruses*. New York, New York, Oxford and London, England, and Paris, France, Pergamon Press, 1961a, pp. 252-280.

_____: Mouse leukemia. In Gross, L.: *Oncogenic Viruses*. New York, New York, Oxford and London, England, and Paris, France, Pergamon Press, 1961b, pp. 153-231.

_____: Radiation-induced leukemia in mice. In Gross, L.: *Oncogenic Viruses*, New York, New York, Oxford and London, England, and Paris, France, Pergamon Press, 1961c, pp. 232-251.

Haddow, A., and Alexander, P.: An immunological method of increasing the sensitivity of primary sarcomas to local irradiation with x-rays. *Lancet*, 1:452-457, February 29, 1964.

Hellström, I. E., Hellström, K. E., Pierce, G. E., and Bill, A. H.: Demonstration of cell-bound and humoral immunity against neuroblastoma cells. *Proceedings of the National Academy of Sciences of the U.S.A.*, 60:1231-1238, August 1968.

Henle, W., Diehl, V., Kohn, G., zur Hausen, H., and Henle, G.: Herpes-type virus and chromosome marker in normal leukocytes after growth with irradiated Burkitt cells. *Science*, 157:1064-1065, September 1, 1967.

Henle, G., Henle, W., and Diehl, V.: Relation of Burkitt's tumor-associated herpes-type virus to infectious mononucleosis. *Proceedings of the National Academy of Sciences of the U.S.A.*, 59:94-101, January 1968.

Hilleman, M. R.: Approaches to prevention of leukemia in man. In Dameshek, W., Ed.: *Perspectives in Leukemia*. New York, New York, Grune & Stratton, 1968, pp. 272-292.

Hutchin, P.: Mechanisms and functions of immunologic enhancement. *Surgery, Gynecology and Obstetrics*, 126:1331-1356, June 1968.

Kaliss, N.: The elements of immunological enhancement. A consideration of mechanisms. *Annals of the New York Academy of Sciences*, 101:64-79, November 20, 1962.

Keast, D.: Runting syndromes, autoimmunity, and neoplasia. *Advances in Cancer Research*, 43-71, 1968.

Klein, G., Clifford, P., Henle, G., Henle, W., Geering, G., and Old, L. J.: EBV-associated serological patterns in a Burkitt lymphoma patient during regression and recurrence. *International Journal of Cancer*, 4:416-421, July 15, 1969.

Law, L. W., Goldstein, A. L., and White, A.: Influence of thymosin on immunological competence of lymphoid cells from thymectomized mice. *Nature*, 219:1391-1392, September 28, 1968.

Lea, A. J.: An association between the rheumatic diseases and the reticuloses. *Annals of Rheumatic Disease*, 23:480-484, November 1964.

Lee, J. C., Yamauchi, H., and Hopper, J., Jr.: The association of cancer and the nephrotic syndrome. *Annals of Internal Medicine*, 64:41-51, January 1966.

Lukes, R. J.: Prognosis and relationship of histological features to clinical stage. *Journal of the American Medical Association*, 190:914-915, December 7, 1964.

Meléndez, L. V., Hunt, R. D., Daniel, M. D., Garcia, F. G., and Fraser, C. E. O.: Herpes-virus saimiri. II. Experimentally induced malignant lymphoma in primates. *Laboratory Animal Care,* 19:378-386, June 1969.

Mellors, R. C., and Huang, C. Y.: Immunopathology of NZB/BL mice. VI. Virus separable from spleen and pathogenic for Swiss mice. *Journal of Experimental Medicine,* 126:53-62, July 1, 1967.

Mihich, E.: Combined effects of chemotherapy and immunity against leukemia L1210 in DBA/2 mice. *Cancer Research,* 29:848-854, April 1969.

Mikulska, Z. B., Smith, C., and Alexander, P.: Evidence for an immunological reaction of the host directed against its own actively growing primary tumor. *Journal of the National Cancer Institute,* 36:29-35, January 1966.

Miller, D. G.: The immunologic capability of patients with lymphoma. *Cancer Research,* 28: 1441-1448, July 1968.

Morton, D. L., Hall, W. T., and Malmgren, R. A.: Human liposarcomas: Tissue cultures containing foci of transformed cells with viral particles. *Science,* 165:813-815, August 22, 1969.

Morton, D. L., Malmgren, R. A., Hall, W. T., and Shidlovsky, G.: Immunologic and virus studies with human sarcomas. *Surgery,* 66:152-161, July 1969.

Nazerian, K., Solomon, J. J., Witter, R. L., and Burmester, B. R.: Studies on the etiology of Marek's disease. II. Finding of a herpesvirus in cell culture. *Proceedings of the Society of Experimental Biology and Medicine,* 127:177-182, January 1968.

Old, L. J., Stockert, E., Boyse, E. A., and Geering, G.: A study of passive immunization against a transplanted G+ leukemia with specific antiserum. *Proceedings of the Society of Experimental Biology and Medicine,* 124:63-68, January 1967.

Peterson, R. D. A., Hendrickson, R., and Good, R. A.: Reduced antibody forming capacity during the incubation period of passage A leukemia in C_3H mice. *Proceedings of the Society of Experimental Biology and Medicine,* 114:517-520, November 1963.

Recher, L., Sinkovics, J. G., Sykes, J. A., and Whitescarver, J.: Electron microscopic studies of suspension cultures derived from human leukemic and nonleukemic sources. *Cancer Research,* 29:271-285, February 1969.

Rich, M. A.: Virus-induced murine leukemia. In Rich, M. A., Ed.: *Experimental Leukemia.* New York, New York, Appleton-Century-Crofts, 1968, pp. 15-49.

Ruddle, N. H., and Waksman, B. H.: Cytotoxicity mediated by soluble antigen and lympho-cytes in delayed hypersensitivity. I. Characterization of the phenomenon. *Journal of Experimental Medicine,* 128:1237-1254, December 1, 1968a.

_____: Cytotoxicity mediated by soluble antigen and lymphocytes in delayed hypersen-sitivity. III. Analysis of mechanism. *Journal of Experimental Medicine,* 128:1267-1279, December 1, 1968b.

Schwartz, R. S., and André-Schwartz, J.: Malignant lymphoproliferative diseases: Interactions between immunological abnormalities and oncogenic viruses. *Annual Review of Medicine,* 19: 269-282, 1968.

Seif, G. S. F., and Spriggs, A. I.: Chromosome changes in Hodgkin's disease. *Journal of the National Cancer Institute,* 39:557-570, September 1967.

Siegler, R.: Pathology of murine leukemias. In Rich, M. A., Ed: *Experimental Leukemia.* New York, New York, Appleton-Century-Crofts, 1968, pp. 51-95.

Sinkovics, J. G.: Abnormal immune and other complicating phenomena associated with a viral mouse leukemia. *Journal of Infectious Diseases,* 110:282-296, May-June 1962a.

_____: Intracellular lymphocytes in leukaemia. *Nature,* 196:80-81, October 6, 1962b.

_____: Lymphoid cells in long-term cultures. *Medical Record and Annals,* 61:50-56, Feb-ruary 1968.

_____: Immunology of neoplasia: Experimental tumors. In Harris, J. E., and Sinkovics, J. G.: *Immunology of Malignant Disease.* St. Louis, Missouri, C. V. Mosby Company. (In press.)

Sinkovics, J. G., Bertin, B. A., and Howe, C. D.: Some properties of the photodynamically inactivated Rauscher mouse leukemia virus. *Cancer Research,* 25:624-627, June 1965.

Sinkovics, J. G., Gyorkey, F., and Shullenberger, C. C.: A comparison of murine and human leukemia. In Clarke, W. J., and Howard, E. B., Eds.: *Myeloproliferative Disorders of Ani-*

mals and Man. Amsterdam, The Netherlands, Excerpta Medica (U.S. Atomic Energy Commission, Washington, D. C.). (In press.)
: Infectious mononucleosis. Lancet, 1:476-477, March 2, 1968.
Sinkovics, J. G., Pienta, R. J., Ahearn, M. J., Trujillo, J. M., and Mikulik, F. M.: Activities of immune lymphoid cells against leukemia virus-carrier murine neoplastic cells. Bibliotheca Haemotologica. (In press.)
Sinkovics, J. G., Pienta, R. J., Trujillo, J. M., and Ahearn, M. J.: An immunological explanation for the starry sky histological pattern of a malignant lymphoma. Journal of Infectious Diseases, 120:250-254, August 1969.
Sinkovics, J. G., Shullenberger, C. C., and Howe, C. D.: Cell destruction by lymphocytes. Lancet, 1:1215-1216, May 28, 1966.
Sinkovics, J. G., Sykes, J. A., Shullenberger, C. C., and Howe, C. D.: Patterns of growth in cultures deriving from human leukemic sources. Texas Reports on Biology and Medicine, 25:446-467, Fall 1967.
Sinkovics, J. G., Trujillo, J. M., Pienta, R. J., and Ahearn, M. J.: Leukemogenesis stemming from autoimmune disease. In Genetic Concepts and Neoplasia, A Collection of Papers Presented at the 23rd Annual Symposium on Fundamental Cancer Research, 1969, at The University of Texas M. D. Anderson Hospital and Tumor Institute at Houston. Baltimore, Maryland, The Williams & Wilkins Company. (In press.)
Smithers, D. W.: Hodgkin's disease—II. British Medical Journal, 2:337-341, May 6, 1967.
Spärck, J. V., and Volkert, M.: Effect of adoptive immunity on experimentally induced leukaemia in mice. Nature, 206:578-579, May 8, 1965.
Stanton, M. F., Law, L. W., and Ting, R. C.: Some biologic, immunogenic, and morphologic effects in mice after infection with a murine sarcoma virus. II. Morphologic studies. Journal of the National Cancer Institute, 40:1113-1129, May 1968.
Stutman, O., Yunis, E. J., and Good, R. A.: Functional activity of a chemically induced thymic sarcoma. Lancet, 1:1120-1123, May 27, 1967.
Sykes, J. A., and Recher, L.: Personal communication.
Talal, N., Sokoloff, L., and Barth, W. F.: Extrasalivary lymphoid abnormalities in Sjögren's syndrome (reticulum cell sarcoma, "pseudolymphoma," macroglobulinemia). American Journal of Medicine, 43:50-65, July 1967.
Trujillo, J. M., Ahearn, M. J., Pienta, R. J., Gott, C., and Sinkovics, J. G.: Immunocompetence of leukemic murine lymphoblasts. I. Ultrastructure, virus and globulin production. Cancer Research. (In press.)
Trujillo, J. M., Butler, J. J., Ahearn, M. J., Shullenberger, C. C., List-Young, B., Gott, C., Anstall, H. B., and Shively, J. A.: Long-term culture of lymph node tissue from a patient with lymphocytic lymphoma. II. Preliminary ultrastructural, immunofluorescence and cytogenetic studies. Cancer, 20:215-224, February 1967.
Vonka, V.: Personal communication.
Williams, T. W., and Granger, G. A.: Lymphocyte in vitro cytotoxicity: Mechanism of lymphotoxin-induced target cell destruction. Journal of Immunology, 102:911-918, April 1969.

Features Suggesting Curability in Leukemia and Lymphoma*

JOSEPH H. BURCHENAL, M.D.

Division of Applied Therapy, Sloan-Kettering Institute for Cancer Research, and the Department of Medicine, Memorial Hospital for Cancer and Allied Diseases, New York, New York

IN THE MANAGEMENT of infectious disease, many different agents, both antimetabolites and antibiotics, are available which through either bacteriostatic or bacteriocidal action will control the disease and allow the patient to return to normal health. Most of these agents have a high specific toxicity for the organism involved as compared to the human host and thus are much more specific than most of the agents we have for the management of leukemias and lymphomas. Despite this great specificity, however, it is extremely difficult to completely eradicate infections in patients who have diminished host defenses, such as those with agammaglobulinemia or acute leukemia in relapse. Thus, it would appear that, for the successful management of infectious disease, one needs both chemotherapeutic specificity and adequate host defense.

In the management of the leukemias and lymphomas, we began with agents with relatively little specificity (Farber *et al.,* 1948), but now, because of more appropriate and exact dosage schedules and the use of simultaneous or sequential combinations, this specific activity has been increased considerably. By analogy with the therapeutic situation in patients with infectious disease, however, it seems unlikely that cures could be achieved in patients with leukemia and lymphoma without the benefit of host defenses (Burchenal, 1966).

In searching for features suggesting curability in patients with leukemias and lymphomas, it might be well to review the status of certain other

*These studies were supported in part by National Cancer Institute Grants No. CA-08748 and No. CA-05826, American Cancer Society Grant No. T-45, and a grant from the Hearst Foundation.

disseminated tumors which have a high degree of curability. As seen in Table 1, perhaps 95 per cent of the patients with choriocarcinoma of the uterus can achieve initial complete remission, as shown by the disappearance of all evidence of disease, including return of the chorionic gonadotropin level to normal (Hertz et al., 1958; Lewis, 1967; Li, Hertz, and Spenser, 1956). With the present forms of treatment consisting of repeated intensive short courses of methotrexate followed by actinomycin D in those who demonstrate resistance to methotrexate, approximately 75 per cent of patients can achieve long-term remissions (Lewis, 1967). In these cases, long-term remission (defined as more than one year without evidence of disease) is essentially synonymous with cure since less than 1 per cent of the 75 per cent have relapsed after a remission lasting one year. Choriocarcinoma of the uterus has the highest rate of spontaneous regression of any known metastatic tumor, and there are two reports in the literature (Rider and Cinader, 1966; Robinson and Ratzkowsky, 1965) in which apparent cures have been achieved by immunologic methods alone. It is probable, however, that the most important factors in the curability of patients with choriocarcinoma are (1) the great sensitivity of the tumor to chemotherapy and (2) the availability of an extremely precise technique for measuring the levels of chorionic gonadotropin in the urine to detect the presence of a minute amount of tumor.

The curability of up to half of the patients with metastatic Wilms' tumor, as shown by Farber (1966) and others (Tan, personal communication) (Table 1), also appears to be related to the tumor's sensitivity to actinomycin D and the fact that most metastases are pulmonary and therefore can be

TABLE 1.—INCIDENCE OF INITIAL AND LONG-TERM REMISSIONS

TYPE OF CANCER	No. OF PATIENTS	No. of Initial Remissions	% of Initial Remissions*	% of Long-Term Remissions†		
Choriocarcinoma of the uterus (1955-1966)	279		95	57		
Choriocarcinoma of the uterus (1965-1966)	58		95	75		
Wilms' tumor (Farber, 1966, Group A)	31		–	58 (2-9 years)		
Wilms' tumor (Farber, 1966, Group B)	55		–	24 (2+ years)		
Wilms' tumor (1956-1964) (Tan, personal communication)	23		–	35 (6-12 years)		
Testicular tumors	154		15	8 (1-10 years)		
Burkitt's tumor (Burkitt, 1967; Ngu, 1967; Clifford, 1967; and Burchenal, 1967)	245		–	15		
Burkitt's tumor stages I and II (Ziegler et al., in press)	12	12	100	92	still in remission at time of report	Preliminary data suggest 50% surviving 1-2 years
Burkitt's tumor stage III (Ziegler et al., in press)	38	28	74	66		
Burkitt's tumor stage IV (Ziegler et al., in press)	7	2	29	0		
Burkitt's tumor, U.S. (Carbone et al., 1969)	12			50 (1-2 years)		
Hodgkin's disease stages III and IV (DeVita, Serpick, and Carbone, 1969)	43		81	28 (more than 2 years)‡		

*Of those patients surviving 30 days of therapy.
†Almost all patients with choriocarcinoma or Burkitt's tumor in unmaintained remission for over one year do not relapse.
‡At time of report, 20 of 35 patients (57 per cent) were still in remission.

followed precisely by radiography. It would appear that, for both these diseases, the availability of a precise method of determining the residual tumor allows the chemotherapist to continue therapy until all evidence of the disease is destroyed. Without such techniques, he might discontinue therapy when the patient was apparently without disease but when a few functional neoplastic cells actually remained. It is also probable that there are host defenses against the neoplastic cells in patients with both these conditions, although such evidence has not been developed yet.

Patients with testicular tumors are much less curable than those with choriocarcinoma of the uterus, which again suggests that the more complete remissions of trophoblastic tumors may be partially the result of greater antigenic differences between the host and a tumor of fetal origin in contrast to the differences between the host and a spontaneous autochthonous tumor. However, even in patients with this spontaneous disease, occasionally one can achieve long-term remissions which in all probability could be considered cures. The group at Memorial Hospital (Li, 1961; Li, Whitmore, and Golbey, 1959; Li, Whitmore, Golbey, and Grabstald, 1960; Mackenzie, 1966) studied 154 patients treated either with triple combination therapy consisting of repeated intensive courses of methotrexate, actinomycin D, and an alkylating agent or with actinomycin D alone; they found 15 per cent complete remissions, of which roughly half appeared to be permanent cures.

For the leukemias and lymphomas, the features suggesting curability are most evident in patients with Burkitt's tumor (Burkitt, 1958). Individuals with this disease were first treated successfully by Burkitt (Oettgen, Burkitt, and Burchenal, 1963), who used intensive short courses of methotrexate; some of the patients treated at that time are still alive with no evidence of disease (Burkitt, 1967). At a meeting in 1967, the results reported by Ngu (1967), Burkitt (1967), and Clifford (1967) were collected. Of 245 patients, 38 (15 per cent) had long-term regressions (Burchenal, 1967), which may be defined as no evidence of disease for more than one year after discontinuing therapy. A follow-up on these 38 patients shows that only two have relapsed in the ensuing two years. Both of these were in the series reported by Clifford, and both relapsed after approximately four years without evidence of disease (Clifford et al., 1968). It is possible that these two cases may not represent relapses, but may be reinduction of a new disease in the patients, particularly in view of the chromosomal changes reported (Clifford et al., 1968). These 38 long-term survivors were treated primarily with alkylating agents such as Cytoxan, nitrogen mustard, and Orthomerphalan, and a few were treated with the antimetabolite, methotrexate. When the patients treated at Kampala were studied by Morrow, Pike, and Kisuule (1967), it was shown that a much higher incidence of long-term remissions was seen in those with stages I and II disease than in those with stages III or IV dis-

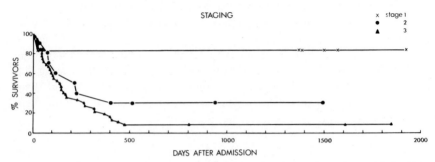

FIG. 1.—Effect of stage on percentage of long-term remissions in patients with Burkitt's tumor. (Redrawn from Morrow, Pike, and Kisuule, 1967.)

ease, and it appeared that the curability might be as high as 80 per cent in patients with stage I disease (Fig. 1).

More recently, Ziegler *et al.* have reported a series of 57 consecutive cases from the Lymphoma Treatment Center; these patients were treated with 40 mg./kg. Cytoxan intravenously either as a single dose or repeated every three weeks for a total of six doses (Ziegler *et al.*, in press; Ziegler, personal communication). As seen in Table 1, there were 100 per cent initial complete responses in the patients with stages I and II disease, 74 per cent initial complete remissions in those with stage III disease, and 29 per cent in those with stage IV disease. Eleven of 12 patients with stages I and II disease were still in remission, 25 of 38 patients with stage III disease were still in remission, but all patients with stage IV disease had died at 34 weeks. It is too early to ascertain the percentage of long-term remissions which will be achieved in these various groups in Ziegler's series, but it appears that the results in the patients with stages I and II disease, and even in those with stage III disease, will be considerably better than results achieved elsewhere. It is interesting to speculate why the results should be so much better in patients with stages I and II disease than in those with stages III or IV disease. There usually is less actual volume of disease in stages I and II than in stage III. Also, the tumor in stages I and II, being limited to the jaw, can be observed much more carefully than the intra-abdominal stage III disease. Patients with localized jaw disease also may be less likely to be immunologically deficient than those with far-advanced disease.

It was originally thought that the excellent results in Africa perhaps were caused by a possible nonspecific stimulation of the reticuloendothelial system by constant exposure to malaria and infectious disease. It is of interest, however, that Carbone *et al.* (1969), in treating 12 nonmalarial American patients with Burkitt's tumor by using multiple-dose Cytoxan therapy, showed that six of the 12 had no evidence of disease for periods of from 50 to 112 weeks.

The recent studies of DeVita, Serpick, and Carbone (1969) on a combined treatment of patients with stages III and IV Hodgkin's disease is of great interest. Thirty-five of 43 patients given six two-week cycles of therapy consisting of 1.4 mg./m² vincristine and 6 mg./m² nitrogen mustard on days 1 and 8, 100 mg./m² procarbazine per os daily for 14 days of each cycle, and 40 mg./m² prednisone per os daily for 14 days of cycles 1 and 4 achieved complete remissions. Twenty of these 35 were still in remission at the time of the report, and 12 had been without evidence of disease for more than 24 months after discontinuation of therapy (Table 1).

If the differences in the incidence of long-term complete remissions between stages I and II as contrasted to stages III and IV of Burkitt's tumor could be extrapolated to Hodgkin's disease, even better results might be expected in patients with stages I and II Hodgkin's disease than the already stated excellent results achieved in those with advanced disease. This particular combination presently is being studied in patients with all stages of Hodgkin's disease by Ziegler (personal communication) at the Lymphoma Treatment Center in Uganda, where radiotherapy is not available. The results in patients with stages I and II disease will be of tremendous interest to all investigators in the field of chemotherapy.

Both Klein and Ziegler have conducted interesting immunologic studies on patients with Burkitt's tumor. Klein, Clifford, Klein, and Stjernswärd (1967) first demonstrated by indirect immunofluorescence the presence of an antibody against living Burkitt's tumor cells in the sera of patients with this tumor. They observed a higher titer in those patients who later achieved a complete remission than in those who had less satisfactory responses.

The Henles (Henle and Henle, 1965, 1966), using a fixed-cell indirect immunofluorescence technique, noted in the sera of patients with Burkitt's tumor antibodies against Epstein-Barr (EB) virus particles in the Burkitt's tumor cells. Old et al. (1966) demonstrated the presence of an antibody against a soluble antigen from the Jijoye line of Burkitt's tumor cells in the sera of patients with Burkitt's tumor and postnasal space carcinoma, but did not study differences in titers between responders and nonresponders to therapy.

Ziegler (Fass, Herberman, and Ziegler, in preparation), using a preparation consisting mainly of membranes of autochthonous Burkitt's tumor cells, found a much higher incidence of positive skin tests among patients with Burkitt's tumor after chemotherapy than before. He also noted that those with a positive test generally remained in long-term complete remission, whereas those who had a negative skin test tended to relapse rapidly. This supports the contention that both sensitivity to the particular chemotherapeutic agent and an immunologic response on the part of the host are necessary to achieve an enduring remission.

Morton (personal communication) accumulated somewhat similar data on cancer patients undergoing definitive surgical treatment. By using delayed hypersensitivity to dinitrochlorobenzene (DNCB) as an indication of immunologic competence, he correlated positive skin tests with good operative results and negative tests with early recurrence. Various authors (Lewis *et al.*, 1969; Morton, Malmgren, Holmes, and Ketchum, 1968; Oettgen *et al.*, 1968), using immunofluorescence or cytotoxicity techniques, have shown that patients with localized melanoma have an antibody against their own or allogeneic tumor cells, whereas patients with disseminated disease or normal volunteers do not possess this antibody. Whether the positive skin tests described by Ziegler (Fass, Herberman, and Ziegler, in preparation) represent specific immunity against the patients's tumor or whether they are a general indication of immunologic competence remains to be ascertained.

Mathé and his colleagues (1967, 1969) recently have reported on the use of immunotherapy in patients with acute leukemia in remission. In this series, all control patients had relapsed by 130 days, whereas eight of 20 treated with repeated injections of Bacille Calmette Guerin (BCG) and/or pooled irradiated allogeneic leukemic cells were still surviving with no evidence of disease from one to almost four years after discontinuation of chemotherapy. Skurkovich, Kisljak, Machonova, and Begunenko (1969) recently have reported on the use of active and adoptive immunotherapy in patients with acute leukemia in relapse. Although these results are of great interest and indicate the possibility of increasing host resistance, it seems probable that even better and more lasting results could be achieved by using such techniques in patients in complete remission resulting from previous chemotherapy.

Prior to 1947, there was no specific therapy for acute leukemia, and the disease was generally regarded as hopeless. After the discovery of the ability of the folic acid antagonists to produce remissions in children with acute leukemia by Farber *et al.* (1948), followed in a few years by discovery of the therapeutic effects of corticosteroids (Farber *et al.*, 1950; Pearson and Eliel, 1950) and the purine antagonists (Burchenal *et al.*, 1953), it became possible to achieve palliative results in a high percentage of patients and to increase the median survival time. A small number of patients treated with one or all of these drugs alone or in combination survived more than five years from diagnosis. The collection of such cases from hematologists from many parts of the world definitely proved that such long-term remissions could be achieved occasionally in true cases of acute leukemia, even with therapy which was only palliative in the great majority of patients (Burchenal and Murphy, 1965; Burchenal, 1967; Burchenal, in press a). By 1967, 159 such cases had been collected, and preliminary studies of the relapse rate after five years could be made. These studies led to the prediction that at least half of those patients with acute leukemia surviving five years from the diagnosis would survive indefinitely (Burchenal, 1967). In reviewing these same patients in 1969, we found only 10 who had relapsed in the ensuing two years. These relapses occurred between five and 12 years after diagnosis (Fig. 2). A repeat study of the relapse rate (defined as the number of patients who relapsed per number of patients at risk) for each year again showed that most relapses occur in the sixth, seventh, and eighth year after diagnosis and that more than half the patients surviving five years may be expected to remain free of the disease indefinitely.

The original studies proved that long-term survivals in acute leukemia do occur, and it was no longer necessary to collect more cases at random to prove this point; however, these initial studies gave no indication of the rate. The first reported five-year survival rate was that by Zuelzer (1968), who treated 229 consecutive children with acute lymphoblastic leukemia by a cyclic regimen using prednisone, 6-mercaptopurine, and methotrexate; 4.3 per cent of these children were alive at five years. Various forms of intensive therapy have been used by many groups since 1963, and the median survival time has increased rapidly (Acute Leukemia Group B, 1965; Freireich, Karon, and Frei, 1964; Henderson, Freireich, Karon, and Rossee, 1966; Henderson, in press; Selawry, personal communication). The figures from Acute Leukemia Group B, as reported recently by Holland (1969) (Fig. 3), are indicative of the continuing progress. In the 227 patients treated by members of the group in 1960 and 1961, approximately 2 per cent survived five years; for patients treated in 1962 and 1963, the five-year survival rate was 5 per cent; and for those treated in 1964 and 1965, it was

FIG. 2.—Survival of 159 patients with acute leukemia who are living more than five years after diagnosis.

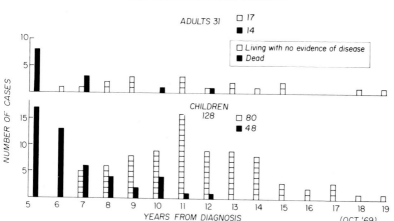

SURVIVAL OF 159 PATIENTS WITH ACUTE LEUKEMIA
LIVING MORE THAN 5 YEARS FROM DIAGNOSIS

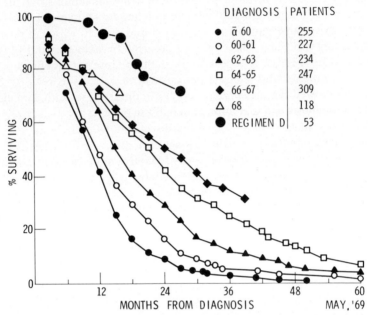

FIG. 3.—Survival curves of various groups of patients treated by members of Acute Leukemia Group B from 1960 to 1968. (Courtesy of Holland, 1969.)

10 per cent. In certain other series of intensively treated patients, the five-year mark also has been reached. Bernard (personal communication) has reported that 12 of 52 patients (23 per cent) given intensive combination therapy during 1964 and 1965 have survived over 4.5 years. If the increasing rate of survival at two years in the more recently treated series of patients (Regimen D) (Fig. 3) continues, one also might expect at least as high a percentage of five-year survivors in these groups.

It is possible that the addition of L-asparaginase (Broome, 1961; Clarkson *et al.,* in press; Hill *et al.,* 1967; Kidd, 1953; Oettgen *et al.,* 1967; Tallal *et al.,* in press) to various forms of intensive therapy also may increase this percentage. The long-term unmaintained remissions occasionally obtained with this drug in combination with cytosine arabinoside and vincristine suggest that this possibility may indeed be the case (Burchenal, in press b, c, d) (Fig. 4).

In summary, the features suggesting curability in patients with leukemia and lymphoma are: (1) the curability of patients with certain other types of disseminated neoplastic disease such as trophoblastic tumors and Wilms' tumor, (2) the evidence in man of host resistance against certain tumors such as Burkitt's tumor and localized melanoma, (3) the exciting suggestion of the possible value of active specific or nonspecific immunotherapy in

R.V. 16 YRS ♂ ACUTE LYMPHOBLASTIC LEUKEMIA

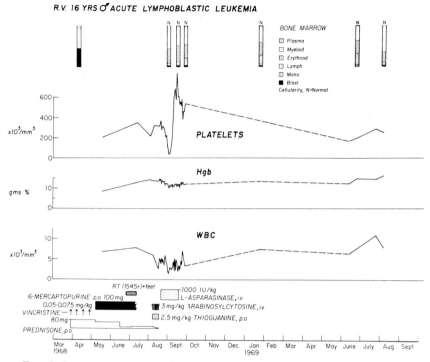

FIG. 4.—Long-term unmaintained remissions after sequential therapy with vincristine, prednisone, 6-mercaptopurine, cytosine arabinoside, thioguanine, and L-asparaginase.

patients with acute leukemia, (4) the significant although small five-year survival rate in patients with acute leukemia and Burkitt's tumor, and (5) the evidence of a much higher wave of long-term remissions following new and more intensive combination therapy in patients with both Burkitt's tumor and acute leukemia. It would be surprising indeed, if these series of patients now under treatment with both chemotherapy and immunotherapy did not produce significantly higher five-year and indefinite survival figures than those at present.

REFERENCES

Acute Leukemia Group B (Selawry, O. S., Hananian, J., Wolman, I. J., Abir, E., Chevalier, L., Gourdeau, R., Denton, R., Gussoff, B. D., Levy, R., and Burgert, O., Jr.): New treatment schedule with improved survival in childhood leukemia. Intermittent parental vs daily oral administration of methotrexate for maintenance of induced remission. *Journal of the American Medical Association,* 194:75-81, October 4, 1965.

Bernard, J.: Personal communication.

Broome, J. D.: Evidence that the L-asparaginase activity of guinea pig serum is responsible for its antilymphoma effects. *Nature,* 191:1114-1115, September 9, 1961.

Burchenal, J. H.: Analysis of long-term survival in acute leukemia and Burkitt's tumor—effects to be expected from intensive therapy and asparaginase. *Proceedings of the Sixth National Cancer Conference, Denver, 1968.* Philadelphia, Pennsylvania, J. B. Lippincott Co. (In press a.)

————: Clinical evaluation and future prospects of asparaginase. In Mathé, G.: *Proceedings of the Plenary Session of the European Organization for Research on Treatment of Cancer, Paris, 1969.* (In press b.)

————: Experimental studies with L-asparaginase in mouse leukemias. Proceedings of the Symposium on Experimental and Clinical Effects of L-Asparaginase. In Oettgen, H. F.: *Recent Results in Cancer Research.* Berlin and Heidelberg, West Germany, and New York, New York, Springer-Verlag. (In press c.)

————: Formal discussion: Long-term survival in Burkitt's tumor and acute leukemia. *Cancer Research,* 27:2616-2618. December 1967.

————: Geographic chemotherapy—Burkitt's tumor as a stalking horse for leukemia: Presidential address. *Cancer Research,* 26:2393-2405, December 1966.

————: Success and failure in present chemotherapy and the implications of asparaginase. *Cancer Research.* (In press d.)

Burchenal, J. H., and Murphy, M. L.: Long-term survivors in acute leukemia. *Cancer Research,* 25:1491-1494, October 1965.

Burchenal, J. H., Murphy, M. L., Ellison, R. R., Sykes, M. P., Tan, T. C., Leone, L. A., Karnofsky, D. A., Craver, L. F., Dargeon, H. W., and Rhoads, C. P.: Clinical evaluation of a new antimetabolite, 6-mercaptopurine, in the treatment of leukemia and allied diseases. *Blood, The Journal of Hematology,* 8:965-999, November 1953.

Burkitt, D.: Chemotherapy of jaw tumours. In Burchenal, J. H., and Burkitt, D. P., Eds.: *Treatment of Burkitt's Tumour* (UICC Monograph Series, Vol. 8). Berlin and Heidelberg, West Germany, and New York, New York, Springer-Verlag, 1967, pp. 94-101.

————: A sarcoma involving the jaw in African children. *British Journal of Surgery,* 46:218-223, November 1958.

Carbone, P. P., Berard, C. W., Bennett, J. M., Ziegler, J. L., Cohen, M. H., and Gerber, P.: National Institutes of Health Clinical Staff Conference. *Annals of Internal Medicine,* 70:817-832, April 1969.

Clarkson, B. D., Krakoff, I., Burchenal, J. H., Karnofsky, D., Golbey, R., Dowling, M., Oettgen, H., and Lipton, A.: Clinical results of treatment with *E. Coli* L-asparaginase in adults with leukemia, lymphoma and solid tumors. *Cancer.* (In press.)

Clifford, P.: Observations on the treatment of Burkitt's lymphoma. In Burchenal, J. H., and Burkitt, D. P., Eds.: *Treatment of Burkitt's Tumour* (UICC Monograph Series, Vol. 8). Berlin and Heidelberg, West Germany, and New York, New York, Springer-Verlag, 1967, pp. 77-93.

Clifford, P., Gripenberg, U., Klein, E., Fenyö, E. M., and Manolov, G.: Treatment of Burkitt's lymphoma. *Lancet,* 2:517-518, August 31, 1968.

DeVita, V. T., Serpick, A., and Carbone, P. P.: Combination chemotherapy of advanced Hodgkin's disease (HD): The NCI program, a progress report. (Abstract) *Proceedings of the American Association for Cancer Research,* 10:19, March 1969.

Farber, S.: Chemotherapy in the treatment of leukemia and Wilms' tumor. *Journal of the American Medical Association,* 198:826-836, November 21, 1966.

Farber, S., Diamond, L. K., Mercer, R. D., Sylvester, R. F., Jr., and Wolff, J. A.: Temporary remissions in acute leukemia in children prolonged by folic acid antagonist, 4-aminopteroyl-glutamic acid (aminopterin). *New England Journal of Medicine,* 238:787-793, June 3, 1948.

Farber, S., Shwachman, H., Toch, R., Downing, V. O., Kennedy, B. H., and Hyde, J.: The effect of ACTH in acute leukemia in childhood. In Mote, J. R., Ed.: *Proceedings of the First Clinical ACTH Conference.* New York, New York, Blakiston Co., 1950, p. 328.

Fass, L., Herberman, R., and Ziegler, J. L.: Cutaneous hypersensitivity to Burkitt lymphoma cell extracts. (In preparation.)

Freireich E. J, Karon M., and Frei, E., III: Quadruple combination therapy (VAMP) for acute lymphocytic leukemia of childhood. (Abstract) *Proceedings of the American Association for Cancer Research,* 5:20, March 1964.

Henderson, E. S.: Evidence that drugs in multiple combinations have materially advanced the treatment of human malignancies. *Cancer Research.* (In press.)

Henderson, E. S., Freireich, E. J, Karon, M., and Rossee, W.: High dose combination chemotherapy in acute lymphocytic leukemia of childhood. (Abstract) *Proceedings of the American Association for Cancer Research,* 7:30, April 1966.

Henle, G., and Henle, W.: Evidence for a persistent viral infection in a cell line derived from Burkitt's lymphoma. *Journal of Bacteriology,* 89:252-258, January 1965.

———: Immunofluorescence in cells derived from Burkitt's lymphoma. *Journal of Bacteriology,* 91:1248-1256, March 1966.

Hertz, R., Bergenstal, D. M., Lipsett, M. B., Price, E. B., and Hilbish, T. F.: Chemotherapy of choriocarcinoma and related trophoblastic tumors in women. *Journal of the American Medical Association,* 168:845-854, October 18, 1958.

Hill, J. M., Roberts, J., Loeb, E., Khan, A., MacLellan, A., and Hill, R. W.: L-Asparaginase therapy for leukemia and other malignant neoplasms. *Journal of the American Medical Association,* 202:882-888, November 27, 1967.

Holland, J. F.: Who should treat acute leukemia? *Journal of the American Medical Association,* 209:1511-1513, September 8, 1969.

Kidd, J. G.: Regression of transplanted lymphomas induced in vivo by means of normal guinea pig serum. I. Course of transplanted cancers of various kinds in mice and rats given guinea pig serum, horse serum, or rabbit serum. *Journal of Experimental Medicine,* 98:565-582, December 1, 1953.

Klein, G., Clifford, P., Klein, E., and Stjernswärd, J.: Search for tumor specific immune reactions in Burkitt lymphoma patients by the membrane immunofluorescence reaction. In Burchenal, J. H., and Burkitt, D. P., Eds.: *Treatment of Burkitt's Tumour* (UICC Monograph Series, Vol. 8). Berlin and Heidelberg, West Germany, and New York, New York, Springer-Verlag, 1967, pp. 209-232.

Lewis, J., Jr.: Chemotherapy for metastatic gestational trophoblastic neoplasms. *Clinical Obstetrics and Gynecology,* 10:330-341, June 1967.

Lewis, M. G., Ikonopisov, R. L., Nairn, R. C., Phillips, T. M., Hamilton Fairley, G., Bodenham, D. C., and Alexander, P.: Tumour-specific antibodies in human malignant melanoma and their relationship to the extent of the disease. *British Medical Journal,* 3:547-552, September 6, 1969.

Li, M. C.: Management of choriocarcinoma and related tumors of uterus and testis. *Medical Clinics of North America,* 45:661-676, May 1961.

Li, M. C., Hertz, R., and Spenser, D. B.: Effect of methotrexate therapy upon choriocarcinoma and chorioadenoma. *Proceedings of the Society for Experimental Biology and Medicine,* 93:361-366, November 1956.

Li, M. C., Whitmore, W., and Golbey, R.: Effect of combined drug therapy upon metastatic choriocarcinoma. (Abstract) *Proceedings of the American Association for Cancer Research,* 3:37, March 1959.

Li, M. C., Whitmore, W. F., Jr., Golbey, R., and Grabstald, H.: Effects of combined drug therapy on metastatic cancer of the testis. *Journal of the American Medical Association,* 174:1291-1299, November 5, 1960.

Mackenzie, A. R.: Chemotherapy of metastatic testis cancer: Results in 154 patients. *Cancer,* 19:1369-1376, October 1966.

Mathé, G.: Personal communication.

Mathé, G., Amiel, J. L., Schwarzenberg, L., Schneider, M., Cattan, A., Schlumberger, J. R., Hayat, M., and de Vassal, F.: Active immunotherapy for acute lymphoblastic leukaemia. *Lancet,* 1:697-699, April 5, 1969.

Mathé, G., Turpin, F., Schlumberger, J. R., Amiel, J. L., Schwarzenberg, L., Schneider, M., and Cattan, A.: Some observations on lymphoblastic neoplasias. In Burchenal, J. H., and Burkitt, D. P., Eds.: *Treatment of Burkitt's Tumour* (UICC Monograph Series, Vol. 8). Berlin and Heidelberg, West Germany, and New York, New York, Springer-Verlag, 1967, pp. 71-76.

Morrow, R. H., Pike, M. C., and Kisuule, A.: Survival of Burkitt's lymphoma patients in Mulago Hospital, Uganda. *British Medical Journal,* 4:323-327, November 11, 1967.

Morton, D. L.: Personal communication.

Morton, D. L., Malmgren, R. A., Holmes, E. C., and Ketchum, A. S.: Demonstration of antibodies against human malignant melanoma by immunofluorescence. *Surgery,* 64:233-240, July 1968.

Ngu, V. A.: Clinical experience in the therapy of Burkitt tumour. In Burchenal, J. H., and Burkitt, D. P., Eds.: *Treatment of Burkitt's Tumour* (UICC Monograph Series, Vol. 8). Berlin and Heidelberg, West Germany, and New York, New York, Springer-Verlag, 1967, pp. 71-76.

Oettgen, H. F., Aoki, T., Old, L. J., Boyse, E. A., de Harven, E., and Mills, G. M.: Suspension culture of a pigment-producing cell line derived from a human malignant melanoma. *Journal of the National Cancer Institute,* 41:827-843, October 1968.

Oettgen, H. F., Burkitt, D., and Burchenal, J. H.: Malignant lymphoma involving the jaw in African children: Treatment with methotrexate. *Cancer,* 16:616-623, May 1963.

Oettgen, H. F., Old, L. J., Boyse, E. A. Tallal, L., Leeper, R. D., Schwartz, M. K., and Kim, J. H.: Inhibition of leukemias in man by L-asparaginase. *Cancer Research,* 27:2619-2631, December 1967.

Old, L. J., Boyse, E. A., Oettgen, H. F., de Harven, E., Geering, G., Williamson, B., and Clifford, P.: Precipitating antibody in human serum to an antigen present in cultured Burkitt's lymphoma cells. *Proceedings of the National Academy of Sciences of the U.S.A.,* 56:1699-1704, December 1966.

Pearson, O. H., and Eliel, L. P.: Use of pituitary adrenocorticotropic hormone (ACTH) and cortisone in lymphomas and leukemias. *Journal of the American Medical Association,* 144:1349-1353, December 16, 1950.

Rider, W. D., and Cinader, B.: Immunotherapy for trophoblastic disease. (Abstract) *Ninth International Cancer Congress: Abstracts of Papers,* Tokyo, Japan, October 23-29, 1966, p. 599.

Robinson, E., and Ratzkowski, E.: Chemotherapy and immunotherapy of a patient with choriocarcinoma. *Gynaecologia,* 160 (2):87-93, 1965.

Selawry, O.: Personal communication.

Skurkovich, S. V., Kisljak, N. S., Machonova, L. A., and Begunenko, S. A.: Active immunization of children suffering from acute leukaemia in acute phase with "live" allogeneic leukaemic cells. *Nature,* 223:509-511, August 2, 1969.

Tallal, L., Tan, C., Oettgen, H., Wollner, N., McCarthy, M., Helson, L., Burchenal, J., Karnofsky, D., and Murphy, M. L.: *E. coli* L-asparaginase in the treatment of leukemia and solid tumors in 131 children. *Cancer.* (In press.)

Tan, C. T. C.: Personal communication.

Ziegler, J. L.: Personal communication.

Ziegler, J. L., Morrow, R. H., Jr., Fass, L., Kyalwazi, S. K., and Carbone, P. P.: Treatment of Burkitt's lymphoma with cyclophosphamide. *Cancer.* (In press.)

Zuelzer, W. W.: Therapy of acute leukemia in childhood. In Zarafonetis, C. J. D., Ed.: *Proceedings of the International Conference on Leukemia-Lymphoma,* The University of Michigan, Ann Arbor, Michigan, 1967. Philadelphia, Pennsylvania, Lea & Febiger, 1968, pp. 451-461.

Cytogenetic Contributions to the Study of Human Leukemias*

JOSE M. TRUJILLO, M.D.,
MANUEL N. FERNANDEZ, M.D.,†
C. C. SHULLENBERGER, M.D.,
LUIS H. RODRIGUEZ, M.D., AND
ANN CORK, M.A.

*Departments of Medicine and Pathology, The University of Texas
M. D. Anderson Hospital and Tumor Institute at Houston, Houston, Texas*

A SERIES OF TECHNICAL IMPROVEMENTS in the handling of mammalian chromosomes during the latter part of the 1950's facilitated the cytogenetic study of neoplastic cells. The improved cytological techniques were initially applied to suitable material such as transplantable ascites tumor, which contains free single cells suspended in fluid and often has a high mitotic index. Since 1960, however, the method has been used extensively in the investigation of the chromosomal constitution of human leukemic cells (Levan, 1967). A retrospective examination of the numerous publications which have crowded the literature during the last 10 years enables one to distinguish two main and, to a certain extent, successive research trends. The initial one mainly involves the basic cancer researcher, and the second originated primarily with the clinician or, to be more specific, the hematologist. Certainly, we do not wish to imply that a line of separation has existed between these two approaches timewise or in any other way. This obviously would be impossible because of the mere fact that we are dealing with a disease of human beings. However, the fact remains that the initial cytogenetic studies of human leukemia were centered around the then exciting possibility that a straightforward confirmation of the Boveri ideas

---

*This work was supported by Grant No. CA 06939-05 from the National Cancer Institute, National Institutes of Health, United States Public Health Service.

†Present address: Chief of Hematology Clinic, Puerta de Hierro, Madrid, Spain.

would be found, whereas later, the emphasis was changed to the use of chromosomal parameters for clinical characterization (Court Brown and Tough, 1963; Hungerford, 1961; Hauschka, 1961; Tjio, Carbone, Whang, and Frei, 1966; Whang-Peng, Canellos, Carbone, and Tjio, 1968). To be perfectly truthful, a group of dedicated investigators, with the help of data obtained from experimental models and with the use of newer and more sophisticated methods, are assiduously looking for a meaningful answer to the basic question created by the wide range of chromosomal variations found in neoplastic cells (Baikie, 1966; Kato, 1968a, b; Levan, 1967; Sandberg, Takagi, Sofuni, and Crosswhite, 1968).

In the light of what has been said, cytogenetic contributions to the study of human leukemia can be considered in two categories: those which have added significantly to a better clinical characterization of the various pathological processes encompassed by the term *leukemia* and those which have increased our basic knowledge of the disease and broadened our understanding of the neoplastic process in general. We will elaborate now on the first category and, later, briefly touch upon the second one. Throughout the entire paper, the established lines of classification of the neoplasias of the hematological system will be followed although, for the more chronic disorders, we will utilize primarily the categories set forward by the late William Dameshek.

Chronic Myeloproliferative Diseases

The group of chronic myeloproliferative diseases, as defined by Dameshek (Dameshek and Gunz, 1964), includes the following entities: (1) chronic granulocytic leukemia, (2) polycythemia vera, (3) myelosclerosis with myeloid metaplasia, and (4) thrombocythemia.

CHRONIC GRANULOCYTIC LEUKEMIA

Without any doubt, one of the most significant advances in the knowledge of this interrelated group of neoplastic disorders of the hematopoietic tissue was the discovery by Nowell and Hungerford (1961) of a defective, small chromosome known as the Philadelphia (Ph^1) chromosome. This finding served as a major stimulus for the cytogenetic investigation of human leukemia. Almost a decade has elapsed since the initial report by investigators of the Ph^1 chromosome, and several hundred patients have had chromosomal studies done at various periods during the course of their disease. Analysis of the pertinent data accumulated so far in the cytogenetic laboratory of The University of Texas M. D. Anderson Hospital and Tumor Institute at Houston in conjunction with the results emanating from other centers in this country and abroad permits us, at this time, to draw some

TABLE 1.—Presence of the Ph[1] Chromosome in Patients
Diagnosed as Having Chronic Granulocytic
Leukemia (CGL) on Admission to Anderson Hospital
Between 1961 and 1967

Total No. of CGL Cases	With Ph[1] Study	Ph[1] Present (+)	Ph[1] Not Found With Adequate Study	With Incomplete Study
68	58	52	4	2

TABLE 2.—Leukocyte Alkaline Phosphatase Determinations
in 32 Chronic Granulocytic Leukemia Patients Before
Treatment

Marker Chromosome	Total No.	Score 0	Score Low	Score High
Ph[1](+)	28	15	8	2
Ph[1](−)	4	0	3	1

definite conclusions, the majority of which have significant clinical relevance.

Conclusion 1.—The Ph[1] chromosome marker was present in 90 to 95 per cent of the typical cases of chronic granulocytic leukemia (Table 1) (Fitzgerald, Adams, and Gunz, 1963; Krauss, Sokal, and Sandberg, 1964; Nowell and Hungerford, 1964; Sandberg, Ishihara, Crosswhite, and Hauschka, 1962; Tjio, Carbone, Whang, and Frei, 1966; Whang-Peng, Canellos, Carbone, and Tijo, 1968). On this basis alone, it can be stated that the Ph[1] chromosome, when compared with other parameters such as the level of alkaline phosphatase in the peripheral blood, is the most reliable diagnostic tool available (Table 2) (Rosen and Teplitz, 1965; Winkelstein, Goldberg, Tishkoff, and Sparkes, 1967). In addition, such a high incidence of association draws a sharp line of distinction between the typical cases of chronic granulocytic leukemia, which are almost invariably Ph[1]-positive, and the other disorders grouped under chronic myeloproliferative conditions.

Conclusion 2.—Discussion of the so-called Ph[1]-negative chronic granulocytic leukemia patients requires separate consideration of the childhood and the adult cases. Cytogenetic studies of the former group were initially done by us in Los Angeles during 1962 (Reisman and Trujillo, 1963). Although chronic granulocytic leukemia is extremely rare in infancy, we were able to study nine affected children; in four of the nine, no Ph[1] chromosome was found. Clinical and hematological analysis of these patients demonstrated that the Ph[1]-negative group differed in certain respects from the others, *i.e.,* they frequently had early thrombocytopenia with bleeding tendencies, they were less responsive to the usual forms of therapy (Myleran), and their disease ran a shorter course. The poorer prognosis of some of these patients had been previously noted by others who had, therefore, made a distinction between the juvenile and the adult types of leukemia in children, since the latter resembled the disease seen in the older age group. Confirmation of the absence of the Ph^1 chromosome in the children with the juvenile type of chronic granulocytic leukemia was soon obtained and reported by Hardisty, Speed, and Till (1964). With four cases of their own, they were able to report: "Our findings lead to the conclusion that the presence or absence of the Ph^1 chromosome provides the surest means of distinguishing between the adult and juvenile types of granulocytic leukemia, and the strongest reason for regarding them as two different entities."

The adult group of Ph^1-negative patients showing clinical and hematological chronic granulocytic leukemia, although apparently more heterogenous, also seems to present a few statistically significant hematological differences from the Ph^1-positive patients, as emphasized by Tjio, Carbone, Whang, and Frei (1966). According to their report, the median white blood cell count and the median platelet count were 41,500 and 180,000/mm^3, respectively, in 13 Ph^1-negative patients, compared with median white blood cell and platelet counts of 133,700 and 388,000 in 60 Ph^1-positive individuals. More important, the Ph^1-negative patient seems to respond poorly to therapy and has, as a whole, a poorer prognosis than the Ph^1-positive patient, as demonstrated again by the workers of the National Institutes of Health who found the median duration of survival from the time of diagnosis to be 18 months for the former and 45 months for the latter (Tjio, Carbone, Whang, and Frei, 1966). To date, in our laboratory, we have encountered only a small number of adult individuals who could be categorized as Ph^1-negative cases of chronic granulocytic leukemia, and they seem to follow the general clinical pattern already described. The question whether the above-mentioned differences between the Ph^1-positive and the Ph^1-negative patients are indicative of the existence of two separate diseases, as some investigators believe, cannot be settled here, but the fact remains that the presence or absence of the Ph^1 chromosome in a clinical condition otherwise indistinguishable from chronic granulocytic leukemia has therapeutic and prognostic implications.

Conclusion 3.—Adequate hematological identification of the hematopoietic cells carrying a particular type of chromosomal aberration was an early aim in several laboratories. By comparing results obtained from parallel hematological and cytogenetic characterizations of bone marrow samples from patients with chronic granulocytic leukemia, we, in Los Angeles, were able to postulate as early as 1962 that both the myeloid and the erythroid cells carry the Ph[1] chromosome (Trujillo and Ohno, 1963). Confirmatory evidence was soon afterwards provided (Whang *et al.*, 1963) which, in addition, included the presence of the same chromosome marker in octoploid bone marrow cells, most likely representing elements of the megakaryocytic line. Later, Clein and Flemans (1966), with the help of special staining procedures for demonstrating the presence of iron, and, more recently, Rastrick (1969), utilizing ^{59}Fe uptake with modified fixation methods, have been able to prove almost beyond any doubt that the mitotic erythroid cells contain the Ph[1] chromosome.

This finding has a dual significance. First, it is strong evidence in favor of the existence of a common precursor cell for the erythrocytic, myelocytic, and megakaryocytic elements in clear distinction from the lymphocytic cells which appear uninvolved (Fig. 1). Second, the widespread presence of this marker chromosome in the bone marrow significantly broadens the scope of the disease. Therefore, what is now known as chronic granulocytic leukemia should actually be considered as a condition affecting not only the myeloid tissue, as the name implies, but also the entire hematopoietic system.

Conclusion 4.—For some time, it has been known that chemotherapy or splenic x-irradiation could produce excellent remission in the clinical and hematological abnormalities of the majority of patients with chronic granulocytic leukemia. In those cases in which the therapeutic response is especially good, most of the clinical and hematological parameters (*i.e.,* palpable spleen high white blood cell count, low hemoglobin level, and increased myeloid erythroid ratio) all return to normal. Under these circumstances, simple microscopic examination of a bone marrow smear fails to demonstrate any residual evidence of disease. Serial chromosomal studies in these

FIG. 1.—A schematic representation of the sequence of events which probably resulted in the appearance of the Ph[1] chromosome in the myeloid as well as erythroid elements. (Redrawn from Trujillo and Ohno, 1963.)

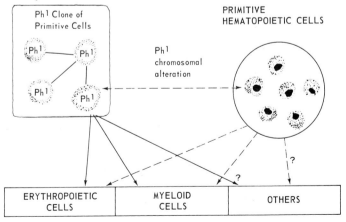

TABLE 3.—CAUSES OF DEATH IN CHRONIC GRANULOCYTIC LEUKEMIA

TOTAL No.	ACUTE PHASE (BLASTIC CRISIS)	BONE MARROW FAILURE	MYELOFIBROSIS AND MYELOID METAPLASIA	OTHER	UNKNOWN
34	23(67.6%)	6(17.6%)	0	3(8.8%)	2(5.8%)

patients undergoing therapy have shown a decrease in the number of Ph^1-positive cells in the peripheral blood (which coincides with the gradual disappearance of immature myelocytic cells from the circulation) and thus marks the initial effect of the treatment (Carbone *et al.*, 1963; Sandberg, Ishihara, Crosswhite, and Hauschka, 1962; Sandberg, Kikuchi, and Crosswhite, 1964; Tough *et al.*, 1962). During periods of complete remission when no immature hematopoietic elements are found in the peripheral blood, no Ph^1-positive cells can be recovered from the blood cultures. However, as Tough and associates (1962) in Edinburgh, and Sandberg, Ishihara, Crosswhite, and Hauschka (1962) in this country demonstrated, the Ph^1 chromosome persists in the bone marrow at the initial level of incidence even during the most complete and perfect remission. The clinical implications of these cytogenetic findings are of great importance and, as has been previously stated by Carbone and associates (1963), suggest that present approaches to the treatment of patients with chronic granulocytic leukemia are only palliative. In other words, the persistence of the Ph^1 chromosome in hematologically normal marrows during remission can, in all probability, be equated to survival of cells carrying the cytogenetic mark of chronic granulocytic leukemia. It follows that no new form of therapy can be considered as a definite cure for the disease unless serial chromosomal analyses demonstrate permanent eradication of the Ph^1-positive clone of cells from the bone marrow.

Conclusion 5.—The most common cause of death from chronic granulocytic leukemia is a transformation to a more acute phase, often called blastic crisis (Table 3). Chromosomal studies during the acute phase demonstrate a high incidence of karyotypic abnormalities other than the Ph^1 chromosome (Fitzgerald, 1966; Goh, 1967; Kemp, Stafford, and Tanner, 1964; Spiers and Baikie, 1968). Quite often, these aberrations are manifested by the presence of multiple clones of aneuploid cells in which the Ph^1 chromosome and, at times, other markers are invariably present, suggesting that clonal evolution is the underlying mechanism (Fitzgerald, 1966; Spiers and Baikie, 1968). The presence of identical markers in several aberrant clones means that multiple lines of cells, karyotypically different but interrelated, are evolving one from another through successive steps of misdivision, thus creating an evolutionary trend for the appearance of more successful and, probably, therapy-resistant clones. Bent Pedersen (1967a, b, 1968) has lately added emphasis to this evolutionary trend of aneuploid cells resulting in the appearance of hyperdiploid Ph^1-positive clones by suggesting that these cells are more resistant to cytostatic agents. In one patient who had received toxic doses of Myleran for several weeks, we obtained cytogenetic evidence highly suggestive of increased drug resistance, demonstrated by the fact that peripheral blood cultures of this person yielded two basic types of metaphases: Ph^1-negative cells showing a high incidence of chromosomal damage and Ph^1-positive pseudodiploid and aneuploid cells with all chromosomes intact (Fig. 2A and B).

In summary, it can be stated that, although blastic crisis is not always accompanied by karyotypic aberrations other than the Ph^1 chromosome, the late appearance of additional chromosomal abnormalities in Ph^1-positive patients almost invariably signals the development of the acute or terminal phase of the disease. In accordance with the present evidence, it is likely that these late-developing aneuploid clones are resistant to previous types of drug therapy.

Conclusion 6.—In 1962, a group of workers in Edinburgh studied six patients with chronic granulocytic leukemia who had been treated by splenic irradiation; they showed that, soon after the treatment, there was a fall to almost zero in the number of Ph^1-positive cells in peripheral blood (Tough *et al.*, 1962). As mentioned previously, this decrease coincides with a lowering in the number of circulating immature hematopoietic cells and can be considered part of the usual response of the disease to this form of therapy. We have had the opportunity to study a few similar cases, but the most remarkable one showed the appearance of a new Ph^1-positive aneuploid clone after splenic irradiation, both in the peripheral blood and in the bone marrow cells (Fig. 3). Later, splenectomy was performed in this patient, and direct chromosomal studies of a small portion of the spleen after short-term incubation demonstrated the same type of aneuploid cell. The data obtained by the Edinburgh group plus our own observations indicate that the spleen plays a significant role in maintaining the Ph^1-positive cells in circulation. Moreover, the case we have just described demonstrates that a new clone originating in the spleen, probably as a result of the irradiation, is able not only to circulate in the blood but also to seed the bone marrow, thus raising the possibility that a significant proportion of stem cells could circulate in the vascular system and travel between the spleen and the bone marrow and vice versa. Whether the mobilization of stem cells is actually accelerated in patients with chronic granulocytic leukemia and whether the spleen plays a more active role in the development or evolution of the disease than merely serving as a reservoir are matters for future investigation. However, it appears that the use of the chromosomal tool can contrib-

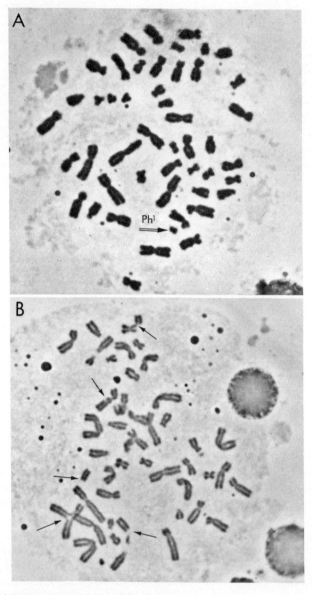

FIG. 2.—Metaphases from peripheral blood cultures of a patient with chronic granulocytic leukemia in blastic crisis after receiving toxic doses of Myleran (approximately 20 mg. per day) for several weeks. *A*, Ph[1]-positive hyperdiploid metaphase with 48 chromosomes. The chromosomes appear intact (double arrow: Ph[1] chromosome). *B*, Ph[1]-negative diploid metaphase from phytohemagglutinin-stimulated blood cultures showing a great deal of chromosomal damage (arrows).

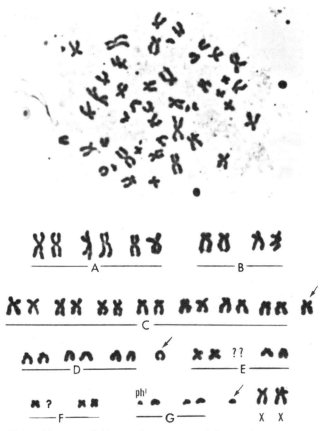

FIG. 3.—Ph¹-positive aneuploid metaphase recovered from a bone marrow culture of a patient with chronic granulocytic leukemia in blastic crisis. The patient had received heavy x-irradiation to the spleen.

ute significantly to the clarification of the mechanism of action of splenic irradiation in patients with chronic granulocytic leukemia.

Cytogenetic studies of the other disorders in the chronic myeloproliferative group have not produced such a straightforward picture to date. The mixed results can be attributed to several factors: (1) The disorders, including some atypical cases of chronic granulocytic leukemia, constitute an ill-defined group with overlapping clinical and hematological aspects. (2) Frequent transitions are found between the various forms, and mixed or borderline cases do exist. (3) The use of different clinical and hematological criteria for the classification of the disorders is widespread. In general, however, the typical cases easily can be distinguished, as observed in patients with chronic granulocytic leukemia. A major problem exists, however, for cases of myelofibrosis. Quite often, polycythemia vera terminates with the same clinical and histological picture as myelofibrosis and more rarely, a few patients with chronic granulocytic leukemia have been known to develop marked fibrosis of the bone marrow. Results of chromosomal studies on these conditions are summarized in the following sections.

POLYCYTHEMIA VERA

The best cytogenetic investigation of polycythemia vera that we are aware of was conducted by Kay, Lawler, and Millard (1966) and includes a group of 43 patients. Of 11 untreated patients, there was aneuploidy of some cells in four, and of all cells in three, with partial reversion to euploidy in the latter group after ^{32}P treatment. Of the remaining 32 patients who had already been treated with ^{32}P, different types of chromosomal abnormalities were present in at least two thirds. Notable preponderance of aneuploid clones was found in a few patients who had developed leukemia. Although many of these chromosomal aberrations could have resulted from the ^{32}P therapy, the finding of aneuploid clones in some patients long after therapy, especially in those who had developed leukemia, is of definite significance. This is especially true since it has been postulated that the incidence of acute leukemia in patients with polycythemia vera is much higher after ^{32}P treatment. In contrast to the results obtained by H. E. M. Kay and associates (Kay, Lawler, and Millard, 1966), results of cytogenetic studies of polycythemia vera in our laboratory and in other centers have, in general, been negative. It is obvious, therefore, that further work in this area is warranted.

MYELOFIBROSIS

A few reports of chromosomal abnormalities involving the C group in patients with myelofibrosis are in the literature (Cohen, 1967; Forrester and Louro, 1966; Kiossoglou, Mitus, and Dameshek, 1966); the most significant is the one by Kiossoglou and associates. The majority of the typical cases, however, show no chromosomal abnormalities. As had been noticed by others (Jackson and Higgins, 1967; Kiossoglou, Mitus, and Dameshek, 1966; Mitus, Coleman, and Kiossoglou, 1969), we, too, have seen atypical disorders which present aneuploidy with involvement of the C group. It is our considered opinion that most of these patients actually belong to another category closer to, if not identical with, acute leukemia.

THROMBOCYTHEMIA

Basically, the karotypes of patients with thrombocythemia have been found to be diploid.

Acute Leukemia

The result of chromosomal studies in patients with acute leukemia show that approximately 50 per cent of the cases are associated with the presence of aneuploidy in the bone marrow cells, whereas in the remaining 50 per cent, only diploid karotypes are found (Fitzgerald, Adams, and Gunz, 1964; Sandberg, Takagi, Sofuni, and Crosswhite, 1968; Trujillo et al., unpublished data). Earlier studies on acute leukemia in children show a higher incidence of chromosomal abnormalities (Norwell, 1968; Reisman, Zuelzer, and Thompson, 1964). In accordance with Sandberg, Takagi, Sofuni, and Crosswhite (1968), the aneuploidy associated with the acute leukemias shows a great deal of variability from case to case; in their recent publication, these investigators presented chromosomal data on 219 cases of acute leukemia. Among their more significant observations are: (1) general stability of the initial karyotype during the phases of remission and relapse and (2) the apparent lack of hypodiploidy in patients with acute lymphoblastic leukemia compared to that in those with acute myeloblastic leukemia, in whom hyper- and hypodiploidy can be present. They also stress the apparent randomness of the chromosomal changes found in patients with acute leukemia. We will present here, on a preliminary basis, data obtained so far in our laboratory, some of which appear to contradict a few of the points raised by Sandberg and his associates.

As shown in Table 4, up to the present time, we have adequately studied 59 adult patients with acute leukemia (Trujillo et al., unpublished data). About 50 per cent of them present definite aneuploid clones in the bone marrow. The individual karyotypic changes noted in these clones are presented in Table 5. A significant proportion of these aberrations reveal pseudodiploidy, a type of alteration which has not been emphasized before, probably because of the difficulties involved in the meticulous analysis required for proper identification (Fig. 4). In contrast to what has been stated by Sandberg and associates (Sandberg, Takagi, Sofuni, and Cross-

TABLE 4.—COMPARATIVE INCIDENCE OF CHROMOSOMAL ALTERATIONS IN PATIENTS WITH ACUTE LEUKEMIA

INVESTIGATORS	No. of CASES	No. with ANEUPLOIDY	No. with DIPLOIDY	% ANEUPLOIDY
Reisman, Zuelzer, and Thompson, 1964	13 (Children)	13	0	100%
Sandberg, Takagi, Sofuni, and Crosswhite, 1968	219 (Adults and children)	108	111	50%
Trujillo et al., unpublished data	59 (Adults)	27	32	46%

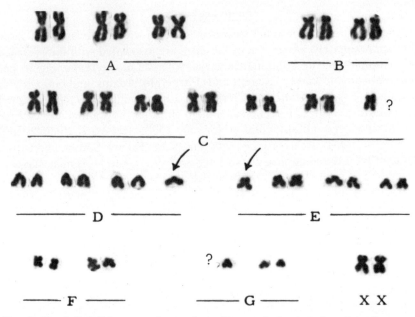

FIG. 4.—Pseudodiploid karyotype in a patient with acute leukemia before chemotherapy.

white, 1968), preliminary examination of our data shows a tendency to repetition of certain specific cytogenetic profiles (Table 5). A more critical analysis will be done at a later date when more material has been accumulated. Perhaps the most significant finding, which is also in contrast to what Sandberg and associates have described, is the fact that, during remission, the aneuploid clones disappear completely from the bone marrow and are totally replaced by diploid cells (Table 6). During relapse, these aneuploid clones, showing the same karyotypic changes, reappear. This is of great clinical significance and agrees with what Reisman, Zuelzer, and Thompson (1964) have found in children with acute lymphatic leukemia.

In summary, from cytogenetic studies of acute leukemia, the following conclusions can be drawn: (1) Although the presence of an occasional aneuploid cell in the bone marrow is probably without major significance, especially in older individuals, the existence of a significant proportion of well-established pseudodiploid and aneuploid clones of cells in the hematopoietic tissue is highly indicative of a neoplastic process. (2) Even if only 50 per cent of the cases of adult acute leukemia are diploid, whenever pseudodiploidy or aneuploidy is encountered, the chromosomal changes define specifically the leukemic cells and, as such, can be utilized by the clinician to determine the response to therapy. (3) From the data presented in this paper, it seems that disappearance of the pseudodiploid or aneuploid cells precedes as well as accompanies clinical and hematological remission. Conversely, reappearance of the abnormal clones is a sure indication of relapse.

Other Leukemic Conditions

We will present a few remarks concerning other disorders intimately related to leukemia on which cytogenetic studies have been reported. Our experience in this area is small, but a few points are pertinent.

TABLE 5.—CYTOGENETIC PROFILES IN PATIENTS WITH ACUTE LEUKEMIA

PATIENT	KARYOTYPE
C.C.	46,XX,C-,D+,E+,G-
	46,XX,D+,G-
D.W.	45,XY,C-,D+,E+,2G-
B.W.	45,XY,C-,D+,E+,2G-
R.G.	46,XY,C-,D+,E+,G-
	47,XY,C-,2D+,E+,G-
W.T.	45,XY,C-,D+,E+,2G-
D.Mc.	44,XY,B-,E+,2G-
E.D.	46,XY,D+,E+,2G-
C.F.	46,X,Y-?,C-,2E+
O.W.	45,X,Y-,D+,G-
	44,X,Y-,B-,D+,G-
L.G.	47,XX,B+,C-,D(q+),E+
B.L.	46,XY,C+,D+(q+),E-,G-
R.S.	45,XX,C-,D-,G+
	45,XX,C-
L.W.	46,XY,B(q+)
D.V.	47,XY,C+
R.R.	47,XY,C+
J.F.	47,XX,C+
C.B.	47,XX,C+
C.H.	48,XX,2C+
	47,XX,2C+,D-
J.V.	45,XY,C-
M.P.	45,XX,C-
K.D.	45,XX,E-
O.F.	47,XY,G+
G.T.	48,XY,E+,G+
N.W.	49,XY,A2(q+),C+,D+,F+
	50,XY,A2(q+),C+,D+,2F+
	51,XY,A2(q+),3C+,D+,F+

TABLE 6.—CYTOGENETIC PROFILES OF SEVERAL ANEUPLOID PATIENTS
RESPONDING TO THERAPY AND WITH DISEASE CURRENTLY IN REMISSION

PATIENT	BEFORE TREATMENT	DURING REMISSION	DURATION OF REMISSION
C.C.	46,XX,C-,D+,E+,G- 46,XX,D+,G-	46,XX	First—6 months Second—since Nov. 1968
E.D.	46,XY,D+,E+,2G-	46,XY	Since Nov. 1968
L.G.	47,XX,B+,C-,D(q+),E+	46,XX	Since Dec. 1968
D.W.	45,XY,C-,D+,E+,2G-	46,XY	Since May 1969
B.W.	45,XY,C-,D+,E+,2G-	46,XY	Since May 1968
O.F.	47,XY,G+	46,XY	Since Apr. 1969

Last year, Nowell (1968) reported the presence of aneuploid clones in a number of patients with "preleukemia." A significant proportion of these individuals developed true leukemia and died within three months, whereas only a small number of preleukemia patients without chromosomal changes in the marrow at the time of the study actually developed leukemia. Therefore, according to Nowell (1968), a preleukemic patient with an abnormal cell clone in his marrow is more prone to develop true leukemia within a short time than the patient in whom no chromosomal abnormality is detectable. Additional studies to determine the practical prognostic value of chromosomal analysis in this area are needed.

The apparent association between familial chronic lymphocytic leukemia and a specific inherited chromosomal abnormality in the G group has been reported, but has not been sustained by further studies (Gunz, Fitzgerald, and Adams, 1962). Chromosomal studies of chronic lymphocytic leukemia have failed so far to show any definite alteration (Nowell, 1968).

Cytogenetic studies of multiple myeloma and Waldenström's macroglobulinemia have shown the presence of a marker chromosome in a number of cases. However, since many other apparently identical cases have failed to present any chromosomal changes, the significance of this finding cannot be assessed (Nowell, 1968).

Conclusions

A few words should be added concerning the possible significance of chromosomal aberrations in human leukemic cells in particular and in neoplastic cells in general. The pertinence of the changes observed so far to the basic cancer researcher is obvious although, because of their protean nature, these alterations are difficult to assess. Repeating Baikie (1966), I shall re-emphasize that "initial chromosomal studies have, of course, failed to solve any of the major problems of etiology, prevention or cure of human leukemias." However, the British investigator further states, and rightly so: "To deny importance to chromosomal changes in leukemic cells is to deny the central role of the chromosomes in the organization of the cells."

It is obvious by this time that chromosomal changes are not necessary for the development and maintenance of the leukemic state since, as mentioned above, a significant proportion of patients with leukemia are devoid of any chromosomal abnormalities. However, the specificity of the Ph[1] chromosome in patients with chronic granulocytic leukemia, which is definitely not an inherited anomaly (Dougan, Scott, and Woodliff, 1966; Jacobs, Luce, and Cailleau, 1966), and the high incidence of chromosomal abnormalities in patients with acute leukemia pose a basic question. Recent experiments on viral and chemical carcinogenesis, both in vivo and in vitro, show that the transition from normal to neoplastic cells is often preceded by a phase of karyotypic alterations until an abnormal clone with a deviating karyotype finally becomes established (Levan, 1967). In man it has been found that individuals with a few inherited conditions, such as the Bloom and the Fanconi syndromes, have an increased liability to acute leukemia (Bloom, 1966; German, Archibald, and Bloom, 1965). In patients with both conditions, a variety of chromosomal aberrations have been found in both peripheral blood and fibroblast cultures. In addition, it is known that individuals with inherited chromosomal anomalies, such as Down's syndrome, etc., are also more prone to develop leukemia and other neoplasias. Todaro and Martin (1967) recently demonstrated that cultured fibroblasts from these individuals are also more susceptible to in vitro viral neoplastic transformation. It appears, therefore, that, although aneuploidy is not a precondition to neoplasia, whenever it is present, it confers an additional advantage to the tumoral growth by significantly extending the freedom or autonomy of the neoplastic cells.

Since the normal mitotic process, diploidy included, is genetically controlled, disturbance in the constancy of this mechanism may be the microscopic reflection of deep alterations in the genome. According to Levan (1967), it is logical to assume that "the swarm of chromosomal disturbances following in the wake of carcinogenesis are [sic] symptoms of a 'mutative noise' on a sub-microscopic level." A model of carcinogenesis, therefore, can be conceived in which the initial and more transcendental event takes place at a genic level. Depending, perhaps, on several factors (the type of carcinogenic agent, the metabolic state of the cell, the stage of cell differentiation, cell age, etc.), this primary event may or may not alter the genes involved in regulating the mechanism of chromosomal replication and the stability of the mitotic process. Whenever these genes become involved in the changes induced by carinogenesis, real mutations in these areas are probably established and a chromosomal alteration takes place, thus inducing karyotypic changes and creating new ground for cell evolution at the chromosomal level. Hopefully, by further concentrated effort, we will be able to clarify this confused field.

Acknowledgments

We would like to mention that the cytogenetic data utilized in the latter part of this work is part of a long-term collaborative study of acute leukemias undertaken jointly by the staffs of the cytogenetic laboratory of the Department of Clinical Pathology and the hematology section of the Department of Developmental Therapeutics. Special acknowledgment is given to Doctors E. Frei, E. J Freireich, and J. Hart for their cooperation.

REFERENCES

Baikie, A. G.: Chromosomal aspects of leukaemia. In *The XI Congress of the International Society of Haematology, Plenary Sessions,* the University of Sydney, Australia, 1966. Sydney, Australia, Victor C. N. Blight, Government Printer, 1966, pp. 198-210.

Bloom, D.: The syndrome of congenital telangiectatic erythema and stunted growth. *Journal of Pediatrics,* 68:103-113, January 1966.

Carbone, P. P., Tjio, J. H., Whang, J., Block, J. B., Kremer, W. B., and Frei, E., III: The effect of treatment in patients with chronic myelogenous leukemia: Hematologic and cytogenetic studies. *Annals of Internal Medicine,* 59:622-628, November 1963.

Clein, G. P., and Flemans, R. J.: Involvement of the erythroid series in blastic crisis of chronic myeloid leukaemia: Further evidence for the presence of Philadelphia chromosome in erythroblasts. *British Journal of Haematology,* 12:754-758, November 1966.

Cohen, S. M.: Chronic myelogenous leukemia with myelofibrosis: Four years after autoimmune hemolytic anemia. *Archives of Internal Medicine,* 119:620-625, June 1967.

Court Brown, W. M., and Tough, I. M.: Cytogenetic studies in chronic myeloid leukemia. *Advances in Cancer Research,* 7:351-381, 1963.

Dameshek, W., and Gunz, F.: Leukemia and the myeloproliferative disorders. In Dameshek, W., and Gunz, F.: *Leukemia.* 2nd edition. New York, N. Y., and London, England, Grune & Stratton, 1964, pp. 356-402.

Dougan, L., Scott, I. D., and Woodliff, H. J.: A pair of twins, one of whom has chronic granulocytic leukaemia. *Journal of Medical Genetics,* 3:217-219, September 1966.

Fitzgerald, P. H.: A complex pattern of chromosome abnormalities in the acute phase of chronic granulocytic leukaemia. *Journal of Medical Genetics,* 3:258-264, December 1966.

Fitzgerald, P. H., Adams, A., and Gunz, F. W.: Chromosome studies in adult acute leukemia. *Journal of the National Cancer Institute,* 32:395-417, February 1964.

———: Chronic granulocytic leukemia and the Philadelphia chromosome. *Blood, The Journal of Hematology,* 21:183-196, February 1963.

Forrester, R. H., and Louro, J. M.: Philadelphia chromosome abnormality in agnogenic myeloid metaplasia. *Annals of Internal Medicine,* 64:622-627, March 1966.

German, J., Archibald, R., and Bloom, D.: Chromosomal breakage in a rare and probably genetically determined syndrome of man. *Science,* 148:506, April 23, 1965.

Goh, K.: Cytogenetic studies in blastic crises of chronic myelocytic leukemia. *Archives of Internal Medicine,* 120:315-320, September 1967.

Gunz, F. W., Fitzgerald, P. H., and Adams, A.: An abnormal chromosome in chronic lymphocytic leukaemia. *British Medical Journal,* 2:1097-1099, October 27, 1962.

Hardisty, R. M., Speed, D. E., and Till, M.: Granulocytic leukaemia in childhood. *British Journal of Haematology,* 10:551-566, October 1964.

Hauschka, T. S.: The chromosomes in ontogeny and oncogeny. *Cancer Research,* 21:957-974, September 1961.

Hungerford, D. A.: Chromosome studies in human leukemia. I. Acute leukemia in children. *Journal of the National Cancer Institute,* 27:983-1011, November 1961.

Jackson, J. F., and Higgins, L. C.: Group C monosomy in myelofibrosis with myeloid metaplasia. *Archives of Internal Medicine,* 119:403-406, April 1967.

Jacobs, E. M., Luce, J. K., and Cailleau, R.: Chromosome abnormalities in human cancer: Report of a patient with chronic myelocytic leukemia and his nonleukemic monozygotic twin. *Cancer,* 19:869-876, June 1966.

Kato, R.: *Chromosomal studies on Carcinogenesis in the Chinese Hamster,* Ph.D. Dissertation. University of Lund, Lund, Sweden, 1968a, 15 pp.

———: Chromosome breakage induced by a carcinogenic hydrocarbon in Chinese hamster cells and human leukocytes in vitro. *Hereditas,* 59(1):120-141, 1968b.

Kay, H. E. M., Lawler, S. D., and Millard, R. E.: The chromosomes in polycythaemia vera. *British Journal of Haematology,* 12:507-528, September 1966.

Kemp, N. H., Stafford, J. L., and Tanner, R.: Chromosome studies during early and terminal chronic myeloid leukaemia. *British Medical Journal,* 1:1010-1014, April 18, 1964.

Kiossoglou, K. A., Mitus, W. J., and Dameshek, W.: Cytogenetic studies in the chronic myeloproliferative syndrome. *Blood, The Journal of Hematology,* 28:241-252, August 1966.

Krauss, S., Sokal, J. E., and Sandberg, A. A.: Comparison of Philadelphia chromosome-positive and -negative patients with chronic myelocytic leukemia. *Annals of Internal Medicine,* 61:625-635, October 1964.

Levan, A.: Some current problems of cancer cytogenetics. *Hereditas,* 57(3):343-355, 1967.

Mitus, W. J., Coleman, N., and Kiossoglou, K. A.: Abnormal (marker) chromosomes in two patients with acute myelofibrosis. *Archives of Internal Medicine,* 123:192-197, February 1969.

Nowell, P. C.: Chromosome abnormalities in human leukemia and lymphoma. In Zarafonetis, C. J. D.: Ed.: *Proceedings of the International Conference on Leukemia-Lymphoma,* The University of Michigan, Ann Arbor, Michigan, 1967. Philadelphia, Pennsylvania, Lea & Febiger, 1968, pp. 47-53.

Nowell, P. C., and Hungerford, D. A.: Chromosome changes in human leukemia and a tentative assessment of their significance. *Annals of the New York Academy of Sciences,* 113:654-662, February 28, 1964.

———: Chromosome studies in human leukemia. II. Chronic granulocytic leukemia. *Journal of the National Cancer Institute,* 27:1013-1035, November 1961.

Pedersen, B.: Cytogenetic structure of aneuploid blood culture cell populations during progression and treatment of chronic myelogenous leukaemia. *Acta pathologica et microbiologica scandinavica,* 69(2):192-204, 1967a.

———: Evolutionary trends of aneuploid blood culture cell populations during progression and treatment of chronic myelogenous leukaemia. *Acta pathologica et microbiologica scandinavica,* 69(2):185-191, 1967b.

———: Influence of hyperdiploidy on Ph^1 prevalence response to therapy in chronic myelogenous leukaemia. *British Journal of Haematology,* 14:507-512, May 1968.

Rastrick, J. M.: A method for the positive identification of erythropoietic cells in chromosome preparations of bone marrow. *British Journal of Haematology,* 16:185-191, January-February 1969.

Reisman, L. E., and Trujillo, J. M.: Chronic granulocytic leukemia of childhood: Clinical and cytogenetic studies. *Journal of Pediatrics,* 62:710-723, May 1963.

Reisman, L. E., Zuelzer, W. W., and Thompson, R. I.: Further observation on the role of aneuploidy in acute leukemia. *Cancer Research,* 24:1448-1455, September 1964.

Rosen, R. B., and Teplitz, R. L.: Chronic granulocytic leukemia complicated by ulcerative colitis: Elevated leukocyte alkaline phosphatase and possible modifier gene deletion. *Blood, The Journal of Hematology,* 26:148-156, August 1965.

Sandberg, A. A., Ishihara, T., Crosswhite, L. H., and Hauschka, T. S.: Comparison of chromosome constitution in chronic myelocytic leukemia and other myeloproliferative disorders. *Blood, The Journal of Hematology,* 20:393-423, October 1962.

Sandberg, A. A., Kikuchi, Y., and Crosswhite, L. H.: Mitotic ability of leukemic leukocytes in chronic myelocytic leukemia. *Cancer Research,* 24:1468-1473, September 1964.

122 / TRUJILLO et al.

Sandberg, A. A., Takagi, N., Sofuni, T., and Crosswhite, L. H.: Chromosomes and causation of human cancer and leukemia. V. Karyotypic aspects of acute leukemia. *Cancer,* 22:1268-1282, December 1968.

Spiers, A. S. D., and Baikie, A. G.: Cytogenetic evolution and clonal proliferation in acute transformation of chronic granulocytic leukaemia. *British Journal of Cancer,* 22:192-204, June 1968.

Tjio, J. H., Carbone, P. P., Whang, J., and Frei, E., III: The Philadelphia chromosome and chronic myelogenous leukemia. *Journal of the National Cancer Institute,* 36:567-584, April 1966.

Todaro, G. J., and Martin, G. M.: Increased susceptibility of Down's syndrome fibroblasts to transformation by SV_{40}. *Proceedings of the Society for Experimental Biology and Medicine,* 124:1232-1236, April 1967.

Tough, I. M., Court Brown, W. M., Baikie, A. G., Buckton, K. E., Harnden, D. G., Jacobs, P. A., and Williams, J. A.: Chronic myeloid leukaemia: Cytogenetic studies before and after splenic irradiation. *Lancet,* 2:115-120, July 21, 1962.

Trujillo, J. M., Hart, J., Freireich, E. J, Frei, E., III, and Cork, A.: Unpublished data.

Trujillo, J. M., and Ohno, S.: Chromosomal alteration of erythropoietic cells in chronic myeloid leukemia, *Acta haematologica,* 29:311-316, January-June 1963.

Whang, J., Frei, E., III, Tjio, J. H., Carbone, P. P., and Brecher, G.: The distribution of the Philadelphia chromosome in patients with chronic myelogenous leukemia. *Blood, The Journal of Hematology,* 22:664-673, December 1963.

Whang-Peng, J., Canellos, G. P., Carbone, P. P., and Tjio, J. H.: Clinical implications of cytogenetic variants in chronic myelocytic leukemia (CML). *Blood, The Journal of Hematology,* 32:755-766, November 1968.

Winkelstein, A., Goldberg, L. S., Tishkoff, G. H., and Sparkes, R. S.: Leukocyte alkaline phosphatase and the Philadelphia chromosome. *Archives of Internal Medicine,* 119:291-296, March 1967.

Histopathology of Malignant Lymphomas and Hodgkin's Disease

JAMES J. BUTLER, M.D.

Department of Anatomical Pathology, The University of Texas M. D. Anderson Hospital and Tumor Institute at Houston, Houston, Texas

THE NUMBER OF DIFFERENT CLASSIFICATIONS proposed for malignant lymphomas and related diseases is a reflection of the difficulties encountered in morphologic characterization of these processes. The tendency of different authors to apply the same terms to different entities has compounded the problem of communicating the diagnosis and of comparing results of therapy. In this paper, the three chief sources of difficulty in making or communicating the diagnosis of these diseases will be covered briefly, and illustrations of the histopathologic types will be presented.

A discussion of the difficulties in establishing or transmitting the histopathologic diagnosis of malignant lymphoma and Hodgkin's disease is believed to be justified since a benign process that is interpreted as malignant or a malignant process that is not accurately diagnosed cannot be classified correctly. A diagnostic term that is easily misinterpreted by an informed clinician is a poor one.

Problems in establishing diagnoses may be attributable to technical factors or may represent errors in interpretation (Butler, 1969a). One or more of the following technical factors may be responsible: (1) poor selection of the biopsy site, (2) poor selection of a lymph node or nodes at the chosen site, (3) improper removal of the lymph node or nodes by the surgeon, (4) poor fixation of the specimen, (5) improper cutting of the section, and (6) improper staining of the section.

It is the pathologist's duty to see that the clinicians, who control the first three of these factors, are aware of their significance so that the difficulties to which they may lead may be reduced to a minimum. Since the members of the clinical staff at The University of Texas M. D. Anderson Hospital and Tumor Institute at Houston have become impressed with the importance of all these factors, the number of cases in which the clinical diagnosis and the initial pathological diagnosis have differed has strikingly decreased. The selection of a biopsy site is a problem only if more than one anatomic area is involved. If this problem arises, it is better to remove a lower cervical or axillary lymph node and to avoid the submandibular, parotid, and inguinal lymph nodes; the latter nodes often exhibit atypical changes secondary to the low-grade inflammatory processes that they commonly drain.

If one is to be reasonably certain that a disease process, whether inflammatory or neoplastic, is represented, the largest node present should be removed. In my experience, surgeons tend to remove the most accessible lymph nodes rather than the largest, if not instructed otherwise. Slaughter, Economou, and Southwick (1958) have shown that, in patients with Hodgkin's disease, normal lymph nodes or those exhibiting only a slight degree of atypia may be found adjacent to nodes having diagnostic features and the only gross indication that a node is representative is its size. We also have found this to be true in reactive processes as well as in all types of lymphoma.

It is important that the entire node be removed in one piece with the capsule intact, since the pathologist should evaluate the relationship of the normal anatomic structures to each other and to any disease process that may be present. Disturbing areas in benign hyperplastic lymph nodes are evaluated much more easily in the intact lymph node than in one or more segments of a fragmented node; in the latter case, they might be interpreted incorrectly as malignant. Also, if the question arises as to whether the malignant process is histiocytic reticulum cell sarcoma or metastatic poorly differentiated carcinoma, an intact lymph node may provide the answer; if a lymph node is incompletely filled with carcinoma, the sinusoids usually will be prominently involved.

The last three technical factors are the responsibility of the pathologist. A detailed discussion of this subject given elsewhere (Butler, 1969a) can be summarized by the statement that one needs technically excellent sections of lymph nodes to appreciate the cytologic features that are an essential part of any study of the reticuloendothelial system.

The difficulties in interpretation arise from failure to apply the basic principles of the histologic study of lymph nodes listed below. All of these principles have been discussed previously in detail (Butler, 1969a).

1. Technically excellent sections are essential.

2. The frozen-section technique and needle biopsy should be used to evaluate lymph nodes only if the presence of lymphoma is unlikely. Sufficiently thin sections cannot be cut by the frozen-section technique, even with the use of the cryostat. Also, because of the changes produced by freezing, it is impossible subsequently to obtain a satisfactory section by the paraffin-embedding technique. As a rule, the needle biopsy specimen is too

small to be representative, it cannot be related to normal anatomic land-marks, and it usually is distorted because of the very nature of the technique.

3. A normal lymph node is a reacting one; the pattern of reaction depends on the stimulus and its reacting counterpart. Since too few studies have been made of lymph nodes in known diseased states, the range of reaction in lymph nodes is not clearly understood. Also, the reacting capability of lymph nodes generally is not considered. Certainly, the usual pattern of reaction in a lymph node in a person in the first two decades of life differs from that in a person over 60 years of age. Similarly, if the hematopoietic system cannot respond normally because of either disease or nutritional deficiency or damage by drugs, radiation, or some other cytotoxic agent, the reaction to a given stimulus will differ from that expected. Thus, atypical cytologic changes in a lymph node may represent the response of an inadequate or damaged hematopoietic system rather than a primary neoplastic process.

4. Reactive processes may obscure the nodal architecture.

5. Every pattern of lymphoma may be simulated by a reactive process.

6. The criteria for malignant disease in other tissues cannot be applied in the study of lymph nodes. Although the presence of mitoses, invasion, or abnormal individual cells generally indicates a malignant process in soft tissues or epithelium, all these changes may be present in benign conditions of the lymph nodes (Fig. 1).

Fig. 1.—Mitotic figure and reactive histiocytes with large nucleoli in lymph node exhibiting postvaccination lymphadenitis. Hematoxylin-eosin; × 400.

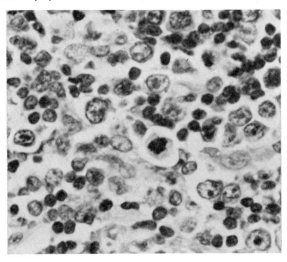

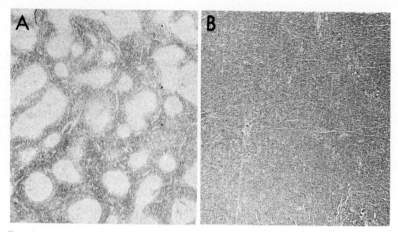

Fig. 2.—*A*, nodular lymphoma. Nodules of lymphomatous cells are separated by uninvolved lymphoid tissue. Hematoxylin-eosin; × 9. *B*, diffuse lymphoma. The proliferation of one cell type throughout the lymph node produces a homogeneous pattern. Hematoxylin-eosin; × 30.

7. The size of a lymph node is no criterion for malignant disease.

8. A malignant lymphoma is essentially a proliferation of a single cell type and is a cytologic entity. The growth pattern of the cells may be nodular or diffuse (Fig. 2). The cells may vary somewhat in size and shape although all are of the same type.

9. Lymph nodes in Hodgkin's disease present a polymorphic cellular infiltrate in which Reed-Sternberg cells must be present to establish the diagnosis. The diagnostic Reed-Sternberg cell has a lobulated nucleus or is multinucleated; at least one lobe or one nucleus contains a nucleolus that is at least one quarter of the size of the nucleus or lobe in question (Fig. 3, *A* and *B*). In reactive processes, one may find mononuclear cells with relatively large nucleoli (Fig. 1). Fortunately, reactive processes do not produce polyploidy as well as large nucleoli.

10. The diagnosis of lymphoma or Hodgkin's disease must be based on

Fig. 3.—*A* and *B*, lobulated and multinucleated Reed-Sternberg cells. Hematoxylin-eosin; × 400. *C*, an atypical histiocyte with a large nucleolus. *D*, reactive histiocytes having small nuclei containing small nucleoli. Hematoxylin-eosin; × 400.

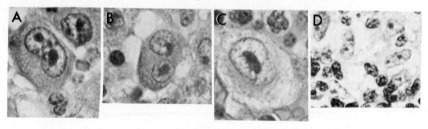

morphologic, rather than clinical findings, upon positive criteria, rather than upon the process of exclusion.

11. The study of lymph nodes must be approached systematically, with consideration of the differential diagnostic features discussed elsewhere (Butler, 1969a).

Although the foregoing diagnostic problems are fundamental, their solution has been more successful than have efforts to promote the adoption of a uniform terminology. Basic to this continuing problem is the fact that most physicians persist in using the first classification they learn unless they are presented with compelling reasons for making a change. The terminology employed at our hospital during the past eight years follows the one introduced by Gall and Mallory in 1942, with modifications to conform to the observations by Rappaport, Winter, and Hicks (1956) on nodular lymphoma. The terminology used by many of the staff, residents, and physicians, however, continues to be a mixture of this classification and older ones that they have used previously.

Table 1 compares the classification of lymphomas used at our hospital with the most common terms formerly employed. The author's view concerning the current confusion of terminology is derived from the evidence presented by this table and from experience in reviewing a large number of cases of lymphoma at Anderson Hospital and the Armed Forces Institute of Pathology.

As indicated in Table 1, "lymphosarcoma" is the most questionable term still being applied to the lymphomatous diseases. The term may be used as a synonym for malignant lymphoma (Rosenberg, Diamond, Jaslowitz, and Craver, 1961), may designate the entire group of diffuse lymphocytic lymphomas (Custer and Bernhard, 1948; Callender, 1934) which may or may not be subclassified as lymphocytic or lymphoblastic in type, or may designate a specific cell type (Rappaport, 1966). Jackson and Parker (1947) also used the term to indicate a highly malignant solitary tumor composed of mature or immature lymphocytes. More important than the terms used is the manner in which they are applied. In the author's experience, "lymphoblastic lymphoma" and, less often, "lymphosarcoma" are used to refer to tumors composed of any large cells with scant cytoplasm, including poorly differentiated lymphocytic lymphoma, undifferentiated reticulum cell sarcoma, blastic granulocytic leukemia, and undifferentiated (stem cell) leukemia. It is not surprising that some clinicians despair of correlating cellular morphology with clinical behavior. To eliminate this problem, both of these terms should be abandoned. The term "lymphoblastic lymphoma" has been replaced largely by the term "poorly differentiated lymphocytic lymphoma," which is equally descriptive and does not include the suffix "blastic"; the latter term seems to invite its use to indicate any large cell with little cytoplasm. Unfortunately, the term "lymphosarcoma," the con-

TABLE 1.—The Anderson Hospital Classification for Lymphomas and the Most
Common Terms Previously Used

Common Terms Previously Used		Anderson Hospital Classification
Lymphosarcoma (Rosenberg, Diamond, and Craver, 1961)	Lymphoblastoma (Berman, 1953)	Malignant lymphoma
	Brill-Symmers disease (Canderviotis, 1952)	A. Nodular
	Giant follicle lymphoma (Jackson and Parker, 1947)	1. Lymphocytic
		a. Well-differentiated
		b. Poorly differentiated
	Follicular lymphoma (Berman, 1953; Gall and Mallory, 1942)	2. Mixed
		3. Histiocytic (RCS)
		4. Undifferentiated (RCS)
	Follicular lymphoblastoma (Custer and Bernhard, 1948)	a. Type A (Burkitt's)
	Lymphosarcoma (Custer and Bernhard, 1948)	B. Diffuse
Lymphocytoma (Jackson and Parker, 1947)	Lymphocytic (Berman, 1953; Gall and Mallory, 1942)	1. Lymphocytic
		a. Well-differentiated
Lymphoblastoma (Jackson and Parker, 1947)	Lymphoblastic (Berman, 1953; Gall and Mallory, 1942)	b. Poorly differentiated
Clasmatocytic (Gall and Mallory, 1942)	RCS (Custer and Bernhard, 1948; Jackson and Parker, 1947)	2. Histiocytic (RCS)
Stem cell (Gall and Mallory, 1942)		3. Undifferentiated (RCS)
		a. Type A (Burkitt's)
		b. Type B

Abbreviation: RCS, reticulum cell sarcoma.

fusing nature of which was first discussed by Jackson and Parker in 1947, survives. If this term is used, the cell type to which it refers should be defined. Gall (1955), Lukes (1968), and Rappaport (1966) similarly have deplored the use of the term "reticulum cell sarcoma." In this author's opinion, the term is too entrenched in medical literature to be changed; a change is not necessary if one designates the type, as is done in the present classification. The real problem is the use of "reticulum cell sarcoma" as a wastebasket term for poorly differentiated malignant neoplasms, particularly those involving lymph nodes. No change in terminology will prevent lesions such as blastic granulocytic leukemia, metastatic alveolar rhabdomyosarcoma, or metastatic oat cell bronchogenic carcinoma from being misinterpreted as reticulum cell sarcoma. In our classification, "reticulum cell sarcoma" is indicated in parentheses so that those who prefer to use the terms "histiocytic lymphoma" and "undifferentiated lymphoma" may do so. The terms "histiocytic reticulum cell sarcoma" and "undifferentiated reticulum cell sarcoma" continue to be employed because they are more acceptable to our clinical staff. I hope to trade my use of "reticulum cell sarcoma" for their discarding of the term "lymphosarcoma."

Malignant Lymphomas

In our classification, lymphomas are described as nodular or diffuse, depending on the low-power growth pattern of the malignant cells. In nodular lymphoma, the cells grow in a nodular pattern (Fig. 2*A*), which is best appreciated under the scanning power of the microscope. The microscopic picture of diffuse lymphoma is that of a homogeneous growth of lymphoma cells (Fig. 2*B*). This classification differs from that used by Rappaport (1966) only in that the nodular and diffuse lymphomas are listed separately to emphasize the nodular group. In the author's experience, too many cases of nodular lymphoma still are not recognized as such by pathologists. Since this nodular group is so important because of its natural history and response to therapy, as discussed by Shullenberger (1970, see pages 143 to 148, this volume), this emphasis is believed to be justified. For simplicity, the term "diffuse" is not used in the diagnosis at this hospital; a lymphoma is considered diffuse if it is not designated as nodular.

Whereas the nodular and diffuse groups are similar with respect to their subtypes (Table 1), except for the absence of the mixed type in the diffuse group, this similarity is actually theoretical. In the author's experience, almost all nodular lymphomas are of either the poorly differentiated lymphocytic, mixed, or histiocytic reticulum cell sarcoma types. In addition, only in patients with poorly differentiated lymphocytic lymphomas do a significant number of diffuse lymphomas appear to originate as nodular lymphomas. These observations are believed to indicate that all lymphomas do not begin as the nodular type. They also suggest that each of the subtypes of nodular lymphomas may represent a distinctive neoplasm arising from follicular cells at the different stages of maturation recently described by electron microscopic studies (Mori, Ishii, and Onoe, 1969).

Sequential biopsy and autopsy specimens from patients with nodular lymphoma show that the tumors either retain the nodular pattern throughout the patient's life or progress to diffuse lymphoma of the same cell type (Rappaport, Winter, and Hicks, 1956). Initially, the nodules of lymphoma cells are separated by normal lymphoid tissue. If the disease progresses to the diffuse form, an increasing number of lymphoma cells develop in the internodular lymphoid tissue until the nodular origin of the disease may be difficult to determine. Recognition of the nodular pattern, even where the process is largely diffuse, seems important; some patients with tumors of this type appear to have a better prognosis than do those with a diffuse lymphoma of the same cell type, although this has not been proved by controlled studies.

From the foregoing definition of malignant lymphoma, it is clear why the author does not include mixed lymphomas in the classification of diffuse

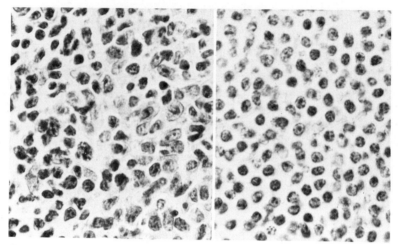

Fig. 4 (left).—Nodular lymphoma, mixed type. Small cells resembling lymphocytes are mixed with large cells resembling histiocytes. Hematoxylin-eosin; × 400.

Fig. 5 (right).—Well-differentiated lymphocytic lymphoma. The lymphocytes are remarkably uniform in size and shape. Hematoxylin-eosin; × 400.

lymphomas. In a significant number of cases of nodular lymphoma, the nodules are composed of large and small cells (Fig. 4). Either because of distortion of the cells incident to compression resulting from their growth in the nodular fashion, or because of the difference in histogenesis of nodular lymphomas previously referred to (or both), it is not possible to be certain whether the small cells are lymphocytes or small histiocytes and whether the large cells are histiocytes or large lymphocytes. The finding by Rappaport, Winter, and Hicks (1956) that approximately 90 per cent of mixed nodular lymphomas develop into diffuse histiocytic reticulum cell sarcomas suggests that the small cells are actually small malignant histiocytes. Until the cells can be identified with certainty, however, use of the term "mixed nodular lymphoma" must be continued.

Aside from this exception and the previously mentioned fact that well-differentiated lymphocytic lymphoma and undifferentiated reticulum cell sarcoma rarely, if ever, are nodular, the cell types of the nodular and diffuse tumors are similar and will be described together.

The cytologic classification used for the lymphomas gives the erroneous impression that each group is a relatively homogeneous one in which the cytologic findings vary only slightly. This, of course, is not true; each type of lymphoma in the classification covers a relatively wide range of cytologic variations although the biologic behavior of each group is similar. This is well illustrated by well-differentiated lymphocytic lymphoma, the classical histologic finding of which is a monotonous field of lymphocytes all the same size and shape with a narrow rim of cytoplasm (Fig. 5), much like a cross-section of a can of uniform English peas. However, the size of the cell, the size and the shape of the nucleus, and the amount of cytoplasm may vary widely although the small lymphocyte remains the predominant cell type (Fig. 6). On the contrary, a poorly differentiated lymphocytic lymphoma exhibits a pronounced variation in the size and shape of the cells and their nuclei; small nucleoli commonly are observed (Fig. 7). Also, mitotic figures are characteristic of poorly differentiated lymphocytic lymphoma, whereas in the well-differentiated type they are rare.

The cells of a histiocytic reticulum cell sarcoma vary widely from one patient to another and within the same patient with respect to the size of the nucleus as well as the amount of cytoplasm present. Typically, the cells are large and have a large nucleus and a relatively large acidophilic nucleolus. Usually, the cytoplasm is abundant and not well delineated. (Fig. 8).

The term "undifferentiated reticulum cell sarcoma" actually includes two different entities, as described by Lukes (1968). They are closely related since type A, the Burkitt's type, is believed to be a neoplasm of the primitive or undifferentiated reticular cell and type B is believed to represent a neoplasm of the undifferentiated hematopoietic cell (Rappaport, 1966). Common to histiocytic, type A undifferentiated, and some type B undiffer-

Fig. 6 (left).—Well-differentiated lymphocytic lymphoma. The lymphocytes exhibit a moderate variation in size and shape; the small lymphocyte is the predominant cell. Hematoxylin-eosin; × 100.

Fig. 7 (right).—Poorly differentiated lymphocytic lymphoma. The lymphocytes vary widely in size and shape, and a mitotic figure is present. Hematoxylin-eosin; × 400.

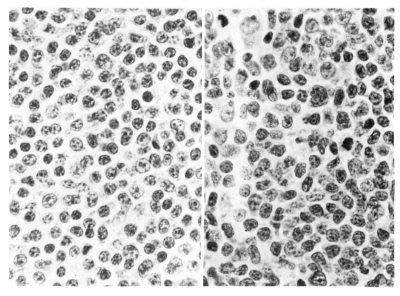

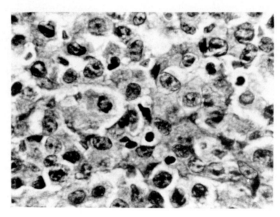

FIG. 8.—Histiocytic reticulum cell sarcoma. The malignant histiocytes have large nuclei and abundant cytoplasm. Hematoxylin-eosin; × 400.

entiated reticulum cell sarcomas, as well as some cases of blastic granulocytic leukemia, is the "starry-sky" appearance (Fig. 9A), which is attributable to benign phagocytic histiocytes scattered throughout the tumor (Bennett et al., 1969). Initially, it was believed that the starry-sky pattern was diagnostic of Burkitt's tumor; additional study, however, has shown that this is not the case (Bennett et al., 1969).

The cytologic characteristics of type A undifferentiated reticulum cell sarcoma have been described recently in detail (Bennett et al., 1969). Briefly, the cells are relatively uniform in size and are no larger than the nucleus of the benign phagocytic histiocytes (Fig. 9, A and B). The nucleus has a coarsely reticulated chromatin and two to five small nucleoli. The cytoplasm is well defined and stains like that of plasma cells, i.e., it is basophilic and stains in varying shades of red with methyl green pyronine. The cytoplasm contains small vacuoles which stain for neutral fat.

Type B undifferentiated reticulum cell sarcoma is recognized best in the lymph nodes where its infiltrating character can be suspected because of the residual normal lymph node structures isolated by sheets of tumor cells. However, this finding is not diagnostic of this type of lymphoma; the same features may be seen in histiocytic reticulum cell sarcoma and in some instances of blastic granulocytic leukemia. When viewed with high magnification, the tumor cells generally appear to have little or no cytoplasm, and the nucleus varies in size and is frequently folded or has a cleft. The nucleus contains finely dispersed chromatin and the nucleoli are small and seldom prominent (Fig. 10). In the author's experience, this tumor develops most often in children and usually leads to leukemia if the patient survives a sufficient length of time. In a recent study of lymphomas in

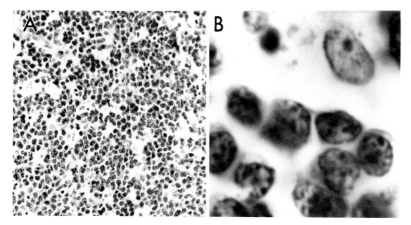

FIG. 9.—Undifferentiated reticulum cell sarcoma, type A. *A*, the starry-sky appearance is produced by phagocytic histiocytes scattered rather uniformly throughout the tumor. Hematoxylin-eosin; × 200. *B*, the tumor cells are smaller than the nucleus of the reactive histiocyte (top, right); the sharply demarcated cytoplasm contains small vacuoles. Hematoxylin-eosin; × 1,000.

children (Butler, unpublished data), the lymph node biopsy specimens from all those with lymphoma were studied. It was found that leukemia developed within two years after the biopsy in all except three of the patients with this type of lymphoma. Two of three patients who died before leukemia developed were examined at autopsy; in both, the bone marrow was diffusely involved. Many of those not found to be leukemic at or shortly after the biopsy initially had normal bone marrow. In the majority of these children, the leukemia was undifferentiated or of the stem cell type. Undoubtedly, some of these cases would be classified by others as acute lym-

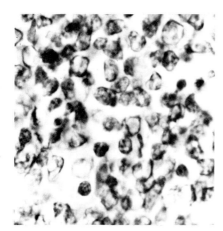

FIG. 10.—Undifferentiated reticulum cell sarcoma, type B. The nuclei vary greatly in size and shape, nuclear folding being common; little or no cytoplasm is evident. Hematoxylin-eosin; × 400.

TABLE 2.—Relationships of Lymphomas and Leukemias

Lymphoma Diffuse or Nodular	Leukemic Counterpart
Lymphocytic, WD	Chronic lymphocytic
Lymphocytic, PD	Leukosarcoma cell
Histiocytic (RCS)	Monocytic (Schilling's) histiocytic
Undifferentiated (RCS)	Stem cell
Type A	Undifferentiated
Type B	Acute lymphocytic

Abbreviations: PD, poorly differentiated; RCS, reticulum cell sarcoma; WD, well-differentiated.

phocytic leukemia of childhood.

The types of lymphomas and their leukemic counterparts are listed in Table 2. Cells in the peripheral blood of a patient with a lymphoma are believed to be another manifestation of the basic disease, just as a metastatic bronchogenic carcinoma to another site is considered to be a manifestation of bronchogenic carcinoma. In neither instance is the true nature of the disease changed.

Hodgkin's Disease

As previously indicated, the diagnosis of Hodgkin's disease can be made only if Reed-Sternberg cells (Fig. 3, *A* and *B*) are present. Mononuclear cells with large nucleoli (Fig. 3*C*) also are commonly found in Hodgkin's disease; they are not diagnostic of the disease, however, since similar cells (Fig. 1) may be produced by viral infections. In contrast to these atypical histiocytic cells, normal histiocytes also are present in some forms of Hodgkin's disease; they have abundant acidophilic cytoplasm and a relatively small nucleus containing a small nucleolus (Fig. 3,*D*). At times, these reactive histiocytes may be grouped so as to resemble a granuloma.

Our histologic classification of Hodgkin's disease (Table 3) follows that of Lukes and Butler (1966), as modified at the 1965 symposium on Hodgkin's disease held at Rye, New York (Lukes *et al.*, 1966). The relationship between these two classifications and that of Jackson and Parker (1947)

TABLE 3.—Classification of Hodgkin's Disease

A. Lymphocytic predominance
B. Nodular sclerosis
C. Mixed cellularity
D. Lymphocytic depletion

is given in Figure 11. Basically, the classification of Lukes and Butler reflects the inverse relationship existing between the number of lympho-cytes and the number of Reed-Sternberg cells in Hodgkin's disease. Since this classification depends on the number of lymphocytes present, a lymph node should be subclassified with strict reservations (if at all) when the patient previously has received chemotherapy or radiotherapy to the biopsy region, both causing lysis of lymphocytes.

The lymphocytic predominance type of Hodgkin's disease may exhibit a nodular or diffuse pattern. In the nodular pattern (Fig. 12A), which was described by Rappaport, Winter, and Hicks (1956) as the nodular form of Hodgkin's disease, the nodules usually vary widely in size; in reticulin stains, they are outlined by reticulin, as are the nodules of nodular lym-phoma. The nodules are composed of a diverse mixture of lymphocytes, benign histiocytes, and atypical histiocytes (Fig. 12B). The diffuse form of this disease may be composed either exclusively of lymphocytes (Fig. 13) or of a mixture of lymphocytes and benign histiocytes together with atypical histiocytes, as in the nodular form. Reed-Sternberg cells are found with difficulty in both the nodular and diffuse lymphocytic predominance type. Plasma cells may be numerous in this and other types of Hodgkin's disease. If the histologic sections are not technically excellent, some examples of the diffuse lymphocytic predominance type of Hodgkin's disease may be misinterpreted as well-differentiated lymphocytic lymphoma. In a recent study of Hodgkin's disease in 58 children (Butler, 1969b), three cases ini-tially had been misinterpreted in this way.

FIG. 11.—Comparison of different classifications of Hodgkin's disease.

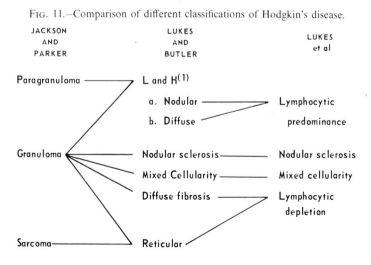

(1) Lymphocytic and / or histiocytic

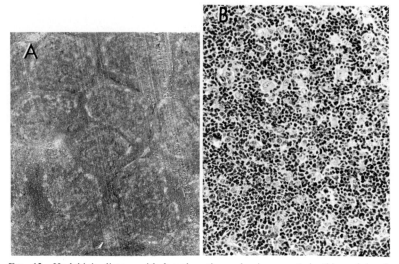

FIG. 12.—Hodgkin's disease with lymphocytic predominance. *A,* in this nodular form, the nodules are large and are well visualized only under the scanning power of the microscope. Hematoxylin-eosin; × 9. *B,* the nodules are composed of both lymphocytes and histiocytes; Reed-Sternberg cells are rare. Hematoxylin-eosin; × 100.

FIG. 13.—Hodgkin's disease with lymphocytic predominance. In this diffuse example, lymphocytes predominate. Hematoxylin-eosin; × 150.

FIG. 14.—Hodgkin's disease with mixed cellularity. The number of lymphocytes is decreased, and the number of Reed-Sternberg cells is increased; eosinophils, histiocytes, and plasma cells also are present. Hematoxylin-eosin; × 200.

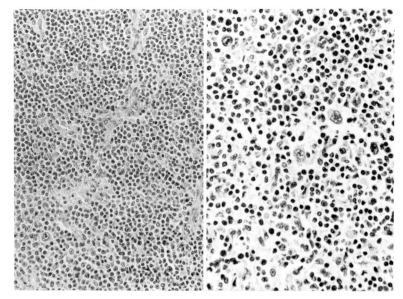

The *mixed cellularity* type of Hodgkin's disease is characterized by a decrease in the number of lymphocytes, areas of necrosis, a significant infiltration of eosinophils, and an increase in the number of Reed-Sternberg cells (Fig. 14). This is the type that most closely corresponds to the textbook description by Jackson and Parker of Hodgkin's granuloma (1947); as the name implies, it is composed of all the types of cells found in lymph nodes of patients with Hodgkin's disease. Although eosinophils appear in most cases of this form of disease, their presence is not essential. At times, the areas of necrosis in this and other forms of Hodgkin's disease may be surrounded by histiocytes and the Langhans' type of giant cells.

The *lymphocytic depletion* type of Hodgkin's disease has two histologic patterns; in both, lymphocytes are decreased in number. In the form designated "diffuse fibrosis" in the classification by Lukes and Butler (1966), a progressive decrease in lymphocytes and, to a lesser extent, all other cells is exhibited. In the end stage, an acellular or almost acellular lymph node containing only a rare Reed-Sternberg cell against a background of proteinaceous material deposited on the connective tissue framework of the lymph node can be seen (Fig. 15). This type may develop spontaneously or may be

FIG. 15 (left).—Hodgkin's disease with lymphocytic depletion. In this example, only a few cells remain in what appears to be proteinaceous material deposited on the connective tissue framework of the lymph node. Hematoxylin-eosin; × 100.
FIG. 16 (right).—Hodgkin's disease with lymphocytic depletion. In this variant, Reed-Sternberg cells are notably increased. Hematoxylin-eosin; × 100.

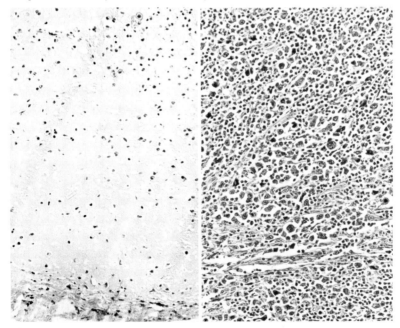

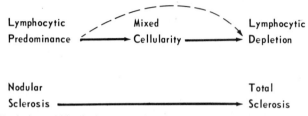

F1G. 17.—Evolution of histologic process in patients with Hodgkin's disease. In some patients, the nodular sclerosis type has a tendency to progress to total sclerosis; however, its evolution has not otherwise been clearly determined.

produced by previous local radiotherapy or systemic chemotherapy. It represents the histologic type most often found at autopsy in previously treated patients. The second form of Hodgkin's disease included under the lymphocytic depletion type was described by Lukes and Butler (1966) as the "reticular type," in which an increase in atypical histiocytes and Reed-Sternberg cells is pronounced (Fig. 16).

The foregoing three types of Hodgkin's disease are related in that they represent histologic stages, based upon the inverse relationship between lymphocytes and Reed-Sternberg cells, through which the disease, theoretically, may progress (Fig. 17). The nodular sclerosis type of Hodgkin's disease is a distinctive type, described by Lukes and Butler (1966), which does not enter into this orderly progression. Thus far, studies (Keller, Kaplan, Lukes, and Rappaport, 1968; Lukes and Butler, unpublished data) have failed to relate any histologic features with the difference in clinical stages of disease and prognosis in patients with nodular sclerosing Hodgkin's disease.

Diagnosis of the *nodular sclerosis* type is based on the presence of collagen septa in various stages of development which tend to subdivide the lymphoid tissue into nodules (Fig. 18*A*) containing atypical cells lying in spaces or lacunae (Fig. 18*B*). The fibrous septa vary in thickness from thin ones that project into the lymphoid tissue from the capsule without producing distinct nodules (Fig. 19) to the classic thick bands of collagen that surround well-defined islands of lymphoid tissue (Fig. 18*A*). Atypical reticulum cells are numerous in the nodular sclerosis form of the disease; usually lobulations of their nuclei are prominent. Paradoxically, Reed-Sternberg cells are often difficult to identify. At times, the atypical cells in lacunae are so numerous that few, if any, intervening lymphocytes are present (Fig. 20); in such cases, the disease may be misinterpreted as metastatic seminoma or possibly metastatic carcinoma, particularly if fibrosis is prominent, unless the reviewer is familiar with this variant. Eosinophils are often present in the nodular sclerosis form of the disease, as are areas of necrosis.

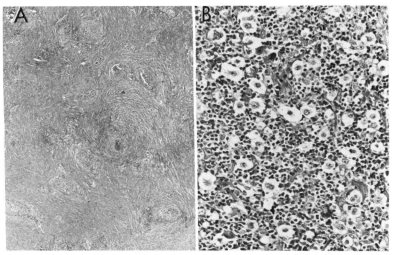

FIG. 18 (above).—Hodgkin's disease with nodular sclerosis. *A*, wide bands of collagen surround small nodules of lymphoid tissue in this example of advanced sclerosis. Hematoxylin-eosin; × 9. *B*, the atypical histiocytes of nodular sclerosis frequently exhibit pronounced lobulations of their nuclei and lie in apparent lacunae. Hematoxylin-eosin; × 100.

FIG. 19 (below left).—Hodgkin's disease with nodular sclerosis. This is an early example; only a rudimentary collagen septum is present. Hematoxylin-eosin; × 3.

FIG. 20 (below right).—Hodgkin's disease with nodular sclerosis. The center of a lymphoid nodule is composed almost exclusively of atypical histiocytes in lacunae. Hematoxylin-eosin; × 100.

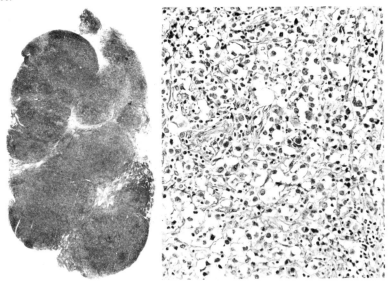

Unfortunately, the histologic findings from only classical or closely allied examples of the nodular sclerosis form of Hodgkin's disease have been illustrated in papers on the subject (Hanson, 1964; Franssila, Kalima, and Voutilainen, 1967; Keller, Kaplan, Lukes, and Rappaport, 1968), thus implying that the spectrum is much narrower than it is in reality. Figures 18A and 19 represent the ends of the spectrum of this type of disease, *i.e.*, from very early (Fig. 19) to late (Fig. 18A).

The separation of cases of Hodgkin's disease into the various types is subjective; no hard and fast dividing line enables one to place every case in one of the described categories without question. In a small number of cases, it is difficult to decide whether a tumor belongs in the mixed cellularity or the lymphocytic depletion group, or, less commonly, in the lymphocytic predominance or mixed cellularity group, or in the nodular sclerosis or mixed cellularity group. An attempt is made to keep the prognostically significant groups (*i.e.*, the lymphocytic predominance, nodular sclerosis, and lymphocytic depletion groups) as pure as possible, as illustrated by Lukes' (personal communication) triangle (Fig. 21). Admittedly, the mixed cellularity group is less clearly defined in that it includes cases which range from those closely resembling the lymphocytic predominance group to those closely related to the lymphocytic depletion group, as well as cases of the nodular sclerosis type in which the changes in the lymph nodes are not characteristic.

The transitions observed in lymphomas and Hodgkin's disease are of

FIG. 21.—Lukes' triangle, showing a schematic representation of the relationship between the three prognostically significant and histologically more distinct groups, and the histologically less well-defined mixed cellularity type of Hodgkin's disease.

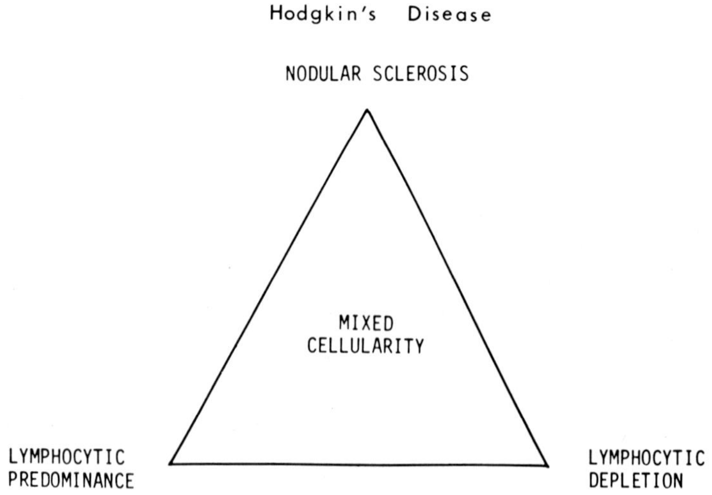

Hodgkin's Disease

NODULAR SCLEROSIS

MIXED CELLULARITY

LYMPHOCYTIC PREDOMINANCE

LYMPHOCYTIC DEPLETION

TABLE 4.—CLASSIFICATION OF HODGKIN'S DISEASE AND
MALIGNANT LYMPHOMA BASED ON CLINICAL BEHAVIOR

I. Stable or slowly progressive

Hodgkin's disease with lymphocytic predominance
Lymphocytic lymphoma, well-differentiated
Hodgkin's disease with nodular sclerosis
Nodular lymphoma (all types)

II. Moderately progressive

Hodgkin's disease with nodular sclerosis
Hodgkin's disease with mixed cellularity
Lymphocytic lymphoma, poorly differentiated

III. Rapidly progressive

Hodgkin's disease with lymphocytic depletion
Reticulum cell sarcoma (all types)

three types: (1) Nodular lymphoma may progress to a diffuse lymphoma of the same cell type. (2) Hodgkin's disease of one type may progress to a more aggressive type, as manifested histologically by a decrease in the number of lymphocytes and an increase in the number of Reed-Sternberg cells (*e.g.* progression of the lymphocytic predominance type to the mixed cellularity type). (3) Leukemia may develop according to the cellular types indicated in Table 2.

One of the aims of the classification presented in this paper is to permit the physician to relate the cytologic subgroups to behavior and, hopefully, to response to therapy. A clinical classification of these entities based on the rate of progression of the disease is presented in Table 4. Obviously, this table refers to the behavior of the various entities as groups since the clinical behavior of the disease in individual patients may differ from that of the group as a whole.

REFERENCES

Bennett, J. M., Berard, C., Butler, J. J., Dorfman, R., Gerard-Marchant, R., Hamlin, I., Hartsock, R. J., Lennert, K., Liberman, P. R., Linsell, C. A., Lukes, R. J., O'Conor, G. T., Osunkoya, B. O., Rappaport, H. H., Rebuck, J., Thomas, L. B., Torloni, H., and Wright, D. H.: Histopathological definition of Burkitt's tumour. *Bulletin of the World Health Organization,* 40:601-607, April 1969.

Berman, L.: Malignant lymphomas: Their classification and relation to leukemia. *Blood, The Journal of Hematology,* 8:195-210, March 1953.

Butler, J. J.: Non-neoplastic lesions of lymph nodes of man to be differentiated from lymphomas. In Stanton, M. F., Ed: *Comparative Morphology of Hematopoietic Neoplasms,* National Cancer Institute Monograph 32, Washington, D. C., U. S. Government Printing Office, 1969a, pp. 233-255.

_____: Hodgkin's disease in children. In *Neoplasia in Childhood,* A Collection of Papers Presented at the 12th Annual Clinical Conference on Cancer, 1967, at The University of Texas M. D. Anderson Hospital and Tumor Institute at Houston. Chicago, Illinois, Year Book Medical Publishers, Inc., 1969b, pp. 267-279.

_____: Unpublished data.

Callender, G. R.: Tumors and tumor-like conditions of the lymphocyte, the myelocyte, the erythrocyte and the reticulum cell. *American Journal of Pathology,* 10:443-465, July, 1934.

Candreviotis, N.: Histologische Untersuchungen über das Wesen des grossfollikularen Lymphoblastoms: Sarcoma lymphoides folliculare, Brill-Symmersche Krankheit. *Deutsche medizinische Wochenschrift,* 77:1115-1117, September 1952.

Custer, R. P., and Bernhard, W. G.: The interrelationship of Hodgkin's disease and other lymphatic tumors. *American Journal of Medical Sciences,* 216:625-642, December 1948.

Franssila, K. O., Kalima, T. V., and Voutilainen, A.: Histologic classification of Hodgkin's disease. *Cancer,* 20:1594-1601, October 1967.

Gall, E. A.: Enigmas in lymphoma: Reticulum cell sarcoma and mycosis fungoides. *Minnesota Medicine,* 38:674-681, October 1955.

Gall, E. A., and Mallory, T. B.: Malignant lymphoma: A clinico-pathologic survey of 618 cases. *American Journal of Pathology,* 18:381-429, May 1942.

Hanson, T. A. S.: Histological classification and survival in Hodgkin's disease. A study of 251 cases with special reference to nodular sclerosing Hodgkin's disease. *Cancer,* 17:1595-1603, December 1964.

Jackson, H., Jr., and Parker, F., Jr.: *Hodgkin's Disease and Allied Disorders.* New York, New York, Oxford University Press, 1947, 177 pp.

Keller, A. R., Kaplan, H. S., Lukes, R. J., and Rappaport, H.: Correlation of histopathology with other prognostic indicators in Hodgkin's disease. *Cancer,* 22:487-499, September 1968.

Lukes, R. J.: The pathologic picture of the malignant lymphomas. In Zarafonetis, C. J. D., Ed.: *Proceedings of the International Conference on Leukemia-Lymphoma,* The University of Michigan, Ann Arbor, Michigan, 1967. Philadelphia, Pennsylvania, Lea & Febiger, 1968, pp. 333-354.

_____: Personal communication.

Lukes, R. J., and Butler, J. J.: The pathology and nomenclature of Hodgkin's disease. *Cancer Research,* 26:1063-1081, June 1966.

_____: Unpublished data.

Lukes, R. J., Craver, L. F., Hall, T. C., Rappaport, H., and Ruben, P.: Report of the nomenclature committee. *Cancer Research,* 26:1311, June 1966.

Mori, M., Ishii, Y., and Onoe, T.: Studies on the germinal center. I. Ultrastructural study of germinal centers in human lymph nodes with correspondence to the zonal differentiation. *Journal of the Reticuloendothelial Society,* 6:140-157, April 1969.

Rappaport, H.: *Tumors of the Hematopoietic System.* Washington, D. C., Armed Forces Institute of Pathology, 1966, 442 pp.

Rappaport, H., Winter, W. J., and Hicks, E. B.: Follicular lymphoma: A re-evaluation of its position in the scheme of malignant lymphoma, based on a survey of 253 cases. *Cancer,* 9:792-821, April 1956.

Rosenberg, S. A., Diamond, H. D., Jaslowitz, B., and Craver, L. F.: Lymphosarcoma: A review of 1269 cases. *Medicine,* 40:31-84, February 1961.

Shullenberger, C. C.: Natural history patterns in leukemia and lymphoma as related to clinicopathologic classification. In *Leukemia-Lymphoma,* A Collection of Papers Presented at the 14th Annual Clinical Conference on Cancer, 1969, at The University of Texas M. D. Anderson Hospital and Tumor Institute at Houston. Chicago, Illinois, Year Book Medical Publishers, Inc., 1970, pp. 143-148.

Slaughter, D. P., Economou, S. G., and Southwick, H. W.: Surgical management of Hodgkin's disease. *Annals of Surgery,* 148:705-710, October 1958.

Natural History Patterns in Leukemia and Lymphoma as Related to Clinicopathologic Classification

C. C. SHULLENBERGER, M.D.

Section of Hematology, Department of Medicine, The University of Texas M. D. Anderson Hospital and Tumor Institute at Houston, Houston, Texas

THE LEUKEMIAS AND LYMPHOMAS are clinical and histopathological spectrums. Clinicians who evaluate large numbers of patients with these diseases have come to recognize certain hallmarks and patterns which bear directly upon diagnosis, prognosis, and selection of therapy. It is my purpose here to review these major patterns, using relatively broad terms in the space allotted; many of the gaps necessarily left will be filled in during other presentations in this conference.

Acute Leukemia

The clinical spectrum of acute leukemia separates in a remarkable way, based upon the ages of the patients. In childhood, there is a great preponderance of that cell type referred to as stem cell, or lymphoblastic. At puberty, this preponderance disappears and granulocytic and monocytic types, or morphologic combinations of the two, make up the major proportion of cases. Between the ages of 14 and 30, the acute lymphocytic variety appears to compose only about 10 per cent of the total incidence; past the age of 30 this falls to 2 per cent or less. There is now some evidence that the monocytic variety is on the increase among more elderly adults (Meyers, 1968).

This separation, based on patient age and cell type, also sets aside the responsive from the unresponsive in terms of therapeutic results. In the stem cell, or lymphoblastic type, in childhood the initial remission rate currently approaches 100 per cent, and the median survival approximates two and one-half years. In types other than stem cell, conversely, the median survival appears to be less than one-half that. It is of interest, however, that Zuelzer (1968) has noted among long survivors in his series (in excess of five years) that the myelomonocytic types were proportionally equal to the stem cell types.

Remissions in acute leukemia in the adult are much more difficult to achieve and are of shorter duration, paralleling the preponderance of the myelomonocytic cell types. The median survival, in various reports, now appears to be in the neighborhood of six to eight months.

In any event, from all studies in both children and adults, a salient feature emerges; relatively long survival depends almost wholly upon the rapid production of an initial complete remission and its maintenance for as long as possible. Stated another way, once relapse occurs, successive remissions are more difficult to produce and are shorter.

A second feature of great importance is exhibited in those cases in which a chromosomal aberration is identified, marking the leukemic cell line as a clonal phenomenon. Though cells thus marked may disappear with remission status, the identical aberration reappears with relapse even in instances where remissions had extended over a period of years (Zuelzer, 1968).

A third point of major significance has been the demonstration of the existence of nonproliferating segments within the leukemic cell population, leading to the speculation that these may be relatively secure against drug effects, lying dormant, as it were, in undetectable foci only to emerge and begin proliferation at a future time following a prolonged clinical and hematologic remission.

Chronic Granulocytic Leukemia

Chronic granulocytic leukemia has its highest incidence in the age group of 25 to 45 years with a peak incidence at about 40 years. It is characterized by an early, easily treatable phase in which response to adequate therapy is virtually 100 per cent; then follows a late phase of variable nature and duration which is relatively unresponsive to therapy and terminates usually within a few months. Median survival of patients with this disease currently appears to be in the range of three and one-half to four years (Fernandez, Trujillo, and Shullenberger, unpublished data; Haut, Abbott, Wintrobe, and Cartwright, 1961).

Two salient features must be borne in mind concerning the progression of this disease, i.e., its more or less "natural course."

1. Considering it in the light of a clonal abnormality, of which the Philadelphia chromosome is the marker, it serves as a prime example of the

impregnable nature of such clones. Cells marked in this manner are not eradicable by means of therapy; they remain, easily identifiable, when a patient may meet all other requirements of remission status, and they remain in the terminal phases of the disease, when the whole clinical and histopathological pattern changes. We may be in the dark as to whether this chromosome abnormality causes the leukemia *per se,* but we are not presently in doubt as to whether we can make it disappear as a result of therapy.

2. Analysis of the features of the terminal phase of chronic granulocytic leukemia indicates that the so-called blastic crisis is by no means the only terminal pattern. A recent review of 68 patients observed in The University of Texas M. D. Anderson Hospital and Tumor Institute at Houston showed bone marrow failure to be the preponderant histologic feature of the terminal phase in 17.6 per cent; though clusters of immature cells, primarily myeloblasts, were easily demonstrated, the outstanding features of these marrows were hypocellularity and diffuse fibrosis (Fernandez, Trujillo, and Shullenberger, unpublished data).

Thus, some of the most serious challenges to the investigator and the therapist with regard to chronic granulocytic leukemia lie in the terminal patterns of this disease. How shall we more intelligently investigate and manage the clinical patterns of blastic transformation and bone marrow failure with fibrosis?

Chronic Lymphocytic Leukemia

The age incidence of chronic lymphocytic leukemia is concentrated between 45 and 70 years, with its peak in the 60 to 70 segment.

It appears certain that chronic lymphocytic leukemia can exist for years in some patients with only minimal tendency to progression and virtually no discernible damage to the host, whereas in others a more aggressive and relentless course ensues after diagnosis. Indeed, it has been suggested that there are two types of the disease, one of which is relatively benign and the other of which has much greater neoplastic potential. Even between these two extremes there are various gradations of histologic and clinical behavior. These features, suggesting a spectrum of disease, rather than a single pattern, probably account for the difficulty in actually defining the disease and in determining survival patterns. If there is a typical pattern of chronic lymphocytic leukemia and we define it as being a disease of later years, with a preponderance of mature lymphocytes in the peripheral blood, a histologic picture designated "malignant lymphoma, well-differentiated lymphocytic type" in the lymph nodes and minimal or absent visceromegaly, then we may well be defining the disease which exhibits a median survival for a period of time in the neighborhood of 9 to 10 years (Boggs, Sofferman, Wintrobe, and Cartwright, 1966).

The borderline between chronic lymphocytic leukemia and other forms of malignant lymphoma with leukemic blood patterns is often dim, and a partial explanation for the use of such terms as "lymphosarcoma cell leukemia" is probably found in this obscure area. The lymphocytosis *per se* often impresses the clinician as being of no particular moment; the character of tissue and organ infiltrates or of nodular, proliferating foci of lymphocytic elements may be of much greater importance in evaluation and prognosis.

The progression of chronic lymphocytic leukemia toward termination has two more outstanding features: (1) autoimmune hemolytic anemia, occurring probably in 10 to 15 per cent of cases and (2) progressive hypogammaglobulinemia, occurring in more than 60 per cent of cases in some published series (Ultmann, Fish, Osserman, and Gellhorn, 1959; Ultmann, 1964). This latter feature is associated with the high incidence of recurrent infections characteristic of the end stage of the disease.

Malignant Lymphoma and Hodgkin's Disease

At one end of the spectrum of malignant lymphomatous disease stands, rather to itself, the entity of follicular lymphoma, alias giant follicle lymphoma, alias Brill-Symmers disease. It stands somewhat apart primarily because of its benign course as compared to other lymphomas. The salient features of this disease are summarized as follows: (1) Nodular histologic pattern, (2) marked response to initial therapy, (3) long remissions from initial treatment, either by radiotherapy or chemotherapy, often extending over periods of years, and (4) terminal progression to diffuse lymphomatous disease, often with the histologic pattern changing to that of one of the more aggressive malignant lymphomas.

In evaluating the patient with malignant lymphoma (or with Hodgkin's disease), one tries to bring together in the most meaningful way the histologic features and the clinical pattern, or distribution, of the disease. This points the way to prognosis and to selection of the therapeutic program. In the lymphomas (aside from Hodgkin's disease), it still appears, although we as clinicians do not dwell upon it as heavily as formerly, that leukemic and/or "leukemoid" patterns give some clue to the possible generalization of the disease process. Therefore, it is well to attempt to line up the histologic pattern with leukemic potentiality. A brief summary of this correlation follows:

1. With the histologic pattern of malignant lymphoma, well-differentiated lymphocytic type, the leukemic potentiality is marked and the peripheral blood picture is most commonly that of chronic lymphocytic leukemia.

2. With the histologic pattern of malignant lymphoma, poorly

differentiated lymphocytic type, the leukemic potentiality is only moderate; very commonly, the peripheral blood pattern is that of lymphosarcoma cell leukemia.

3. With the histologic pattern of reticulum cell sarcoma, the leukemic potential appears to be minimal; when seen, the peripheral blood pictures may include the monocytic and leukemic reticuloendotheliosis varieties.

In the case of localized or regional lymphomatous disease, another point of prime importance is the likely direction or route of spread if the disease leaves the local area and disseminates. Much of current thought regarding therapy is based on this consideration as applied to the pattern of recurrence after initial treatment. The reason for this is well summarized in an analysis of the recurrence patterns in series of patients with Hodgkin's disease, lymphosarcoma, and reticulum cell sarcoma published by Peters, Hasselback, and Brown (1968), from which the data in Table 1 below are taken.

Finally, in the case of Hodgkin's disease, the preponderance of current thought is in terms of histologic patterns as they relate to certain well-defined clinical features which include extent and distribution of disease and the status of immunologic functions. These correlations, again, form the bases for prognosis and planning of therapy. In general terms, some of these major relationships may be summarized as follows:

1. The histologic pattern of Hodgkin's disease with lymphoid predominance is characteristically associated with (a) localized disease, (b) preservation of immunologic functions, and (c) long survival.

2. The histologic pattern of Hodgkin's disease with lymphoid depletion is characteristically associated with (a) disseminated disease, (b) loss of immunologic functions, and (c) short survival.

3. The histologic patterns of nodular sclerosis and mixed cellularity display clinical features occupying a middle ground between the extremes outlined above.

In conclusion, one may observe, at the risk of over-simplification, that these diseases are telling us their whole story in the evolution of their clinical patterns. Our understanding is improving, but slowly, by reason of

TABLE 1.—PATTERN OF RECURRENCE AFTER INITIAL
THERAPY OF LOCALIZED DISEASE

SITE	HD	LSC	RCS
Adjacent	71%	73%	80%
Distant	29%	27%	20%

Abbreviations: HD. Hodgkin's disease; LSC, lymphosarcoma; RCS, reticulum cell sarcoma.

constant and recurrent analyses of those patterns and by the concentration of our thought and investigations upon the challenges yet posed by traditional puzzles and past defeats.

REFERENCES

Boggs, D. R., Sofferman, S. A., Wintrobe, M. M., and Cartwright, G. E.: Factors influencing the duration of survival of patients with chronic lymphocytic leukemia. *American Journal of Medicine*, 40:243-254, February 1966.

Fernandez, M. N., Trujillo, J. M., and Shullenberger, C. C.: Unpublished data.

Haut, A., Abbott, W. S., Wintrobe, M. M., and Cartwright, G. E.: Busulfan in the treatment of chronic myelocytic leukemia. The effect of long term intermittent therapy. *Blood, The Journal of Hematology*, 17:1-19, January 1961.

Meyers, M. C.: Treatment of acute leukemia in adolescents and adults. In Zarafonetis, C. J. D., Ed.: *Proceedings of the International Conference on Leukemia-Lymphoma*, The University of Michigan, Ann Arbor, Michigan, 1967. Philadelphia, Pennsylvania, Lea and Febiger, 1968, pp. 463-468.

Peters, M. V., Hasselback, R., and Brown, T. C.: The natural history of the lymphomas related to the clinical classification. In Zarafonetis, C. J. D., Ed.: *Proceedings of the International Conference on Leukemia-Lymphoma*, The University of Michigan, Ann Arbor, Michigan, 1967. Philadelphia, Pennsylvania, Lea and Febiger, 1968, pp. 357-370.

Ultmann, J. E.: Generalized vaccine in a patient with chronic lymphocytic leukemia and hypogammaglobulinemia. *Annals of Internal Medicine*, 61:728-732, October 1964.

Ultmann, J. E., Fish, W., Osserman, E., and Gellhorn, A.: The clinical implications of hypogammaglobulinemia in patients with chronic lymphocytic leukemia and lymphocytic lymphosarcoma. *Annals of Internal Medicine*, 51:501-516, September 1959.

Zuelzer, W. W.: Therapy of acute leukemia in childhood. In Zarafonetis, C. J. D., Ed.: *Proceedings of the International Conference on Leukemia-Lymphoma*, The University of Michigan, Ann Arbor, Michigan, 1967. Philadelphia, Pennsylvania, Lea and Febiger, 1968, pp. 451-461.

Host Defense Mechanisms
in Lymphoma and Leukemia*

EVAN M. HERSH, M.D.,
JOHN E. CURTIS, M.D.,
JULES E. HARRIS, M.D.,†
CHARLES McBRIDE, M.D.,
RAYMOND ALEXANIAN, M.D., AND
ROGER ROSSEN, M.D.

*Departments of Developmental Therapeutics, Medicine, and Surgery,
The University of Texas M. D. Anderson Hospital and Tumor Institute at Houston,
and Department of Microbiology, Baylor College of Medicine, Houston, Texas*

THE RELATIONSHIP of altered host defense mechanisms to the etiology and pathogenesis of malignant disease in man is still uncertain in spite of intense investigation (Chase, 1966). The possibility that immunological deficiency permits the development of malignancy stems from four observations. (1) Prior immunosuppression either accelerates or increases the incidence of spontaneous, transplanted, and carcinogen- and virus-induced tumors in rodents (Allison and Taylor, 1967; Reiner and Southam, 1967). (2) Tumor-specific antigens and tumor-specific immune responses (usually ineffective) occur in man (Hellström, Hellström, Pierce, and Bill, 1968). (3) There is an increased incidence of malignant disease in patients undergoing chronic immunosuppressive therapy (Penn, Hammond, Brettschneider, and Starzl, 1969). (4) Many patients with different types of cancer have immu-

*Supported by United States Public Health Service Contract No. PH 43-68-949 from the Collaborative Research Program, National Institute of Allergy and Infectious Diseases, National Institutes of Health; Grants No. CA-05831 and No. FR-05511 from the Department of Health, Education and Welfare; General Clinical Research Center Grant No. RR-00350 and Training Center Grant No. HE-05435 from the United States Public Health Service; and by the Veterans Administration.

†Present address: Department of Medicine, The University of Ottawa School of Medicine, Ottawa, Ontario, Canada.

nological deficiency, at least during periods of active disease (Hersh and Freireich, 1968).

Previous studies of host defense mechanisms in cancer patients have indicated that distinct patterns of immunological deficiency are associated with specific categories of malignant disease in human beings (Hersh and Freireich, 1968). Thus, patients with chronic lymphocytic leukemia (CLL) and multiple myeloma are described as having normal cellular immunity, but impaired ability to make antibody (Shaw *et al.*, 1960; Fahey, Scoggins, Utz, and Szwed, 1963). Patients with Hodgkin's disease and reticulum cell sarcoma mainly have been described as having impaired cellular immunity (Aisenberg, 1962; Hersh and Oppenheim, 1965). Patients with metastatic solid tumors also have impaired cellular immunity (Gross, 1965). Immunological abnormalities are not usually found in patients with acute leukemia (Hersh and Freireich, 1968). Recently, however, a number of these concepts have been challenged (Brown *et al.*, 1967; Block, Haynes, Thompson, and Neiman, 1969; Chase, 1966; Lytton, Hughes, and Fulthrope, 1964; Salmon and Fudenberg, 1969; Hersh *et al.*, in press).

To more precisely define the immunological deficiency in patients with cancer and to define simultaneously the relationship in these patients between cellular and humoral immunity, their primary immune responses to a strong protein antigen were studied. The results were correlated with other parameters of immunity. Also, in selected patients with CLL, the immunological competence of the thoracic duct and peripheral blood lymphocytes was compared as a further evaluation of immunological deficiency.

Materials and Methods

The clinical material included 13 patients with Hodgkin's disease, 13 patients with CLL, and 22 patients with multiple myeloma or localized plasmacytoma. The last 22 patients will be reported on in greater detail elsewhere (Harris, Alexanian, Migliore, and Hersh, in preparation). The results of the studies on the 26 lymphoma and leukemia patients were compared to similar studies done on patients with localized or disseminated solid tumors and normal subjects which have been reported on in detail elsewhere (Curtis *et al.*, in press). The patients used for comparison included 14 normal volunteer subjects, nine patients with no evident disease after surgical excision of primary malignant melanoma (designated group 1), and 11 patients with metastatic solid tumors (designated group 2).

•The patients with Hodgkin's disease, CLL, multiple myeloma, and localized plasmacytoma all had active disease and were not on chemotherapy during the study period. Ten of the entire group of 48 patients had received chemotherapy in the prestudy period, but at least one month prior to immunization.

Specific immunity was measured in several ways. The induction of new delayed hypersensitivity was studied by measuring the delayed hypersensitivity response to 100 μg of keyhole limpet hemocyanin (KLH) injected intradermally three weeks after primary subcutaneous immunization with 5 mg. KLH. Results from the skin tests were read at 24 and/or 48 hours and recorded as the average induration measured in two directions at right angles. The KLH was prepared by the method of Campbell and colleagues (Campbell, Garvey, Cremer, and Sussdorf, 1964).

In addition to these measurements of cellular immunity in vivo, lymphocyte function was studied in vitro by measuring the blastogenic responses of the patients' lymphocytes to mitogenic agents. These agents included phytohemagglutinin-M* (PHA), streptolysin-O* (SLO), streptokinase-streptodornase†, vaccinia‡, and various doses of KLH. The in vitro lymphocyte responses were measured by ^{3}H-thymidine incorporation (Curtis et al., in press; Hersh and Harris, 1968).

The primary antibody response to KLH was measured by passive hemagglutination using either the tanned (Stravitsky, 1954) or chromic chloride-treated (Gold and Fudenberg, 1967) red blood cell method. This procedure has been described in detail previously (Curtis et al., in press). IgM and IgG antibody responses were determined by testing their sensitivity to 2-mercaptoethanol (2-ME) and by ultracentrifugation. Antibody titers were expressed as $\log_2$ of the highest positive serial twofold dilution.

The plan of study was to measure established delayed hypersensitivity and lymphocyte responses in vitro during the first visit, to immunize the patients with KLH at this time, and to follow the subsequent lymphocyte and antibody responses during the next seven weeks.

Three patients with CLL also were studied by means of thoracic duct cannulation and short-term drainage. The objective of cannulation procedures in these patients was to deplete them of abnormal cells mechanically. Simultaneous blood and lymph lymphocyte counts and cultures were done serially during the drainage procedure. The results of these studies were compared to similar studies done on two hematologically normal subjects.

Results

PRIMARY ANTIBODY RESPONSES

The responses of the three main groups of patients were abnormal and distinct from each other and from those of the three control groups. The results are shown in the figures.

---

*Difco Laboratories, Detroit, Michigan.
†Varidase, Lederle Laboratories, Pearl River, New York.
‡Dryvax, Wyeth, Philadelphia, Pennsylvania.

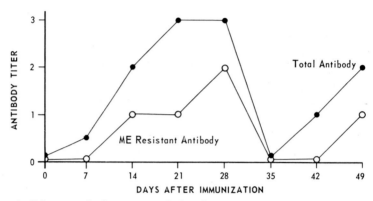

FIG. 1.—Primary antibody response of 13 patients with untreated Hodgkin's disease to keyhole limpet hemocyanin (KLH). Antibody titer in this and all subsequent figures is expressed as $\log_2$ of the reciprocal of the last positive tube of a serial two-fold dilution. Antibody was measured by passive hemagglutination. Total and 2-ME-resistant antibody responses are depicted.

In patients with Hodgkin's disease (Fig. 1), antibody production was delayed one week in half of the patients, but by two weeks after immunization, all but one of the patients were making antibody. The median peak titer was only 3 (1:8) at 28 days. Antibody resistant to 2-ME was observed in more than half of the patients by two weeks, but four of the 13 never made this class of antibody. Every patient made some antibody eventually, but after 28 days, antibody titers dropped to low levels. They tended to rise again after the skin test, which was usually done on that day.

In patients with CLL (Fig. 2), antibody production was also delayed; at seven days after immunization, eight of the 13 patients had no detectable antibody against KLH. In contrast to the patients with Hodgkin's disease, one third of the CLL patients still had no antibody at 21 days. After that time, antibody production gradually increased. Examination of the patients' sera for 2-ME-resistant antibody revealed that the appearance of this antibody also was delayed. Only after 35 days did it appear in half of the subjects, and it never reached the normal level. In contrast to the patients with Hodgkin's disease, the total antibody titers tended to rise gradually and progressively and achieved a normal level by day 42.

The pattern of antibody response in the patients with multiple myeloma (Fig. 3) was quite different from that in patients with CLL and Hodgkin's disease. Again, there was a one-week delay in the onset of antibody production. Also, peak median antibody titer was diminished, as compared to that for controls (4 or 1:16). This peak occurred early, however, and was noted

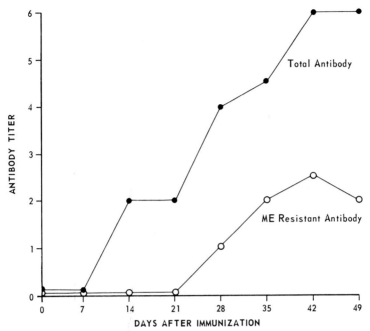

FIG. 2.—Primary antibody response to KLH of 13 patients with CLL.

FIG. 3.—Primary antibody response of 22 patients with multiple myeloma and localized plasmacytoma.

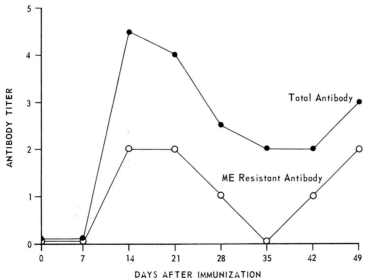

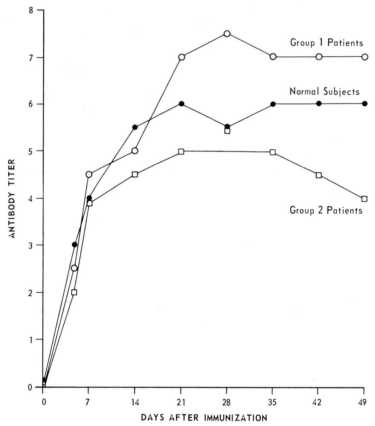

FIG. 4.—Primary antibody response of control groups to KLH. These groups include 14 completely normal volunteers (normal subjects), nine patients with no evident disease after excision of primary melanoma (group 1) and 11 patients with metastatic solid tumors (group 2). The total antibody response is represented.

between days 14 and 21. After day 21, the titers tended to decline. Another interesting finding in the multiple myeloma patients was an accelerated switchover from 2-ME-sensitive to 2-ME-resistant antibody production. Thus, by 14 days, more than half of the subjects had an ME-resistant antibody titer of at least 2. This compared to the level seen at 28 days in the normal patients and those with Hodgkin's disease, and 35 days in the patients with CLL. However, the ME-resistant antibody titer was not maintained and fell to a median value of 0 at 35 days. As in the patients with Hodgkin's disease, the titers rose again after the skin test.

The abnormal results in the patients with lymphoproliferative disorders were contrasted with the results in patients of groups 1 and 2 and in normal control subjects (Figs. 4, 5, and 6). In all these individuals, antibody was

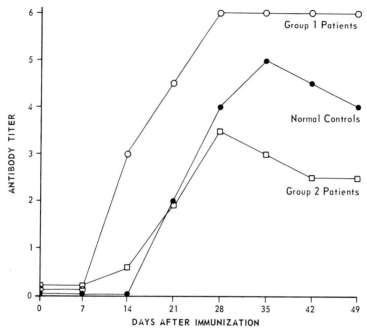

FIG. 5.—2-ME-resistant antibody responses to KLH of three control groups.

detectable by seven days after immunization, antibody titers had reached a maximum level between days 21 and 28, and they plateaued thereafter. There was no significant fall in the antibody titers by 49 days.

Figure 7 shows the development of circulating memory cells for the KLH antigen in the normal and comparison patient groups. The presence of these cells was detected in vitro by measuring the blastogenic response of the patients' lymphocytes to the antigen. In group 2 patients (those with metastatic solid tumor), the memory cells appeared promptly but rose slowly to the normal maximum (at 28 days). The patterns of appearance of these cells in the blood of the patients with the lymphoproliferative disorders were grossly abnormal (Fig. 8). In the multiple myeloma patients the peak antigen response was noted in cells collected between 14 and 21 days after immunization. After 21 days, there was a profound fall in the number of antigen-responsive lymphocytes. In contrast to these patients, the appearance of antigen-reactive lymphocytes was very slow in patients with both CLL and Hodgkin's disease, but the cells continued to increase in number throughout the 49-day study period. Thus, on day 49, the normal group showed approximately 13,000 counts per minute per 10^6 lymphocytes, the multiple myeloma patients showed 600 counts per minute, the

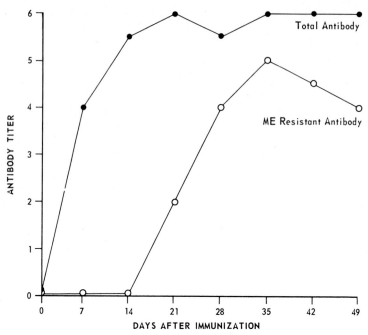

FIG. 6.—Primary antibody response of normal subjects to KLH.

FIG. 7.—Development of circulating memory cells after KLH immunization of control groups as detected by the in vitro blastogenic response to the antigen. Response is measured as counts per minute per 10⁶ lymphocytes with ³H-thymidine incorporation during the last two hours of a five-day culture period.

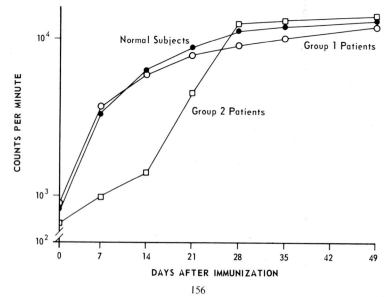

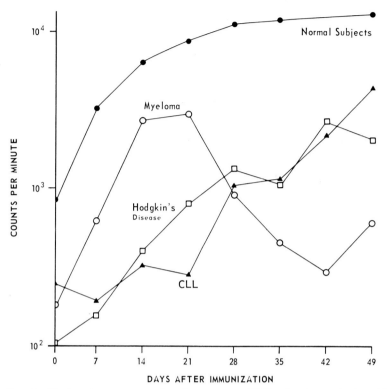

Fig. 8.—Blastogenic responses of study groups to KLH after immunization. Normal control curve is included for comparison.

patients with Hodgkin's disease showed 2,000 counts per minute, and the patients with CLL showed 4,200 counts per minute. The contrast between these groups also was very apparent at 28 days, when the normal subjects showed 11,000 counts per minute, the multiple myeloma patients showed 900 counts per minute, and the patients with Hodgkin's disease and CLL showed 1,350 and 1,060 counts per minute, respectively. The abnormality in the multiple myeloma patients was seen in those with fully developed disease only. In patients with localized plasmacytoma, the antigen-responsive lymphocyte counts were normal (Fig. 9).

These results are put into better perspective by examining the blastogenic response of these patients' lymphocytes to the nonspecific mitogen PHA and the specific mitogenic antigen SLO (Table 1). The PHA responses of the patients with Hodgkin's disease and multiple myeloma were close to those of the normal patients and those with solid tumors. Less than one third of the patients with Hodgkin's disease and multiple myeloma had responses outside the normal range. Even among the patients with CLL, only half showed responses to PHA outside the normal range. In contrast to these results, the specific antigen responses of all three groups with lymphoproliferative disorders were notably deficient, and less than one third of the patients in each group had responses in the normal range. These differences between the antigen responses of the study and control groups were all statistically significant.

Results from skin tests with KLH also are of interest in regard to the already outlined studies (Table 2). All of 14 normal subjects and nine patients with surgically removed solid tumors developed delayed hypersensitivity to KLH after immunization. Also, the majority of the patients with advanced solid tumors had positive skin reactions. Of the study

FIG. 9.—Blastogenic responses of normal subjects and patients with multiple myeloma compared to responses of patients with localized plasmacytoma.

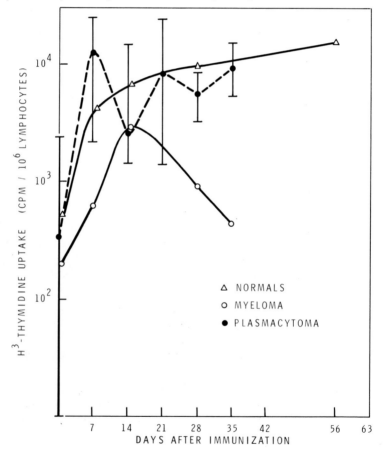

TABLE 1.—Blastogenic Responses of PHA- and SLO-Stimulated
In Vitro Lymphocyte Cultures of Control and Study Groups

Disease Category	PHA* Response		SLO* Response	
	Median	Range	Median	Range
Normal	35.0	18.0-89.0	15.5	19.0-54.0
Solid tumor	40.8	2.6-166.0	11.2	0.0-51.0
Hodgkin's disease	25.0	1.7-96.0	0.33	0.0-10.0
Multiple myeloma	46.0	14.0-115.0	0.60	0.0-38.0
Chronic lymphocytic leukemia	17.5	2.1-43.5	0.50	0.0-4.3

*Response is shown in counts per minute per 10^6 lymphocytes $\times$ 10^3.
Abbreviations: PHA, phytohemagglutinin; SLO, streptolysin-O.

TABLE 2.—Delayed Hypersensitivity Responses
of Control and Study Groups to Challenge with KLH

Diagnosis	No. Tested	No. Positive	% Positive	Reaction Diameter	
				Median	Range
Normal	14	14	100	10.3	5-30
Group 1	9	9	100	15.7	5-25
Group 2	11	9	85	8.0	0-15.5
Hodgkin's disease	13	6	46	4.8	0-20
Multiple myeloma	22	18	82	6.5	0-15.5
Chronic lymphocytic leukemia	13	12	92	8.6	0-13.0

Abbreviation: KLH, keyhole limpet hemocyanin.

patients, those with multiple myeloma and localized plasmacytoma developed almost normal delayed hypersensitivity to KLH. About 90 per cent of the CLL patients had detectable skin sensitivity to KLH after immunization. Failure to develop delayed hypersensitivity was most pronounced in patients with Hodgkin's disease; approximately only half showed this parameter of immunity.

A unique approach to the analysis of the immunological deficiency of patients with CLL has been a comparative study of their thoracic duct and peripheral blood lymphocytes. This approach was prompted by the apparent disparity between the relatively normal in vivo lymphocyte function (near-normal delayed hypersensitivity) and abnormal in vitro lymphocyte function in these patients.

In a hematologically normal patient with a solid tumor, the absolute lymphocyte counts in blood and thoracic duct lymph were found to be similar (Fig. 10); this is true even when a previously hematologically normal patient is made lymphopenic by means of thoracic duct drainage (Fig. 11). In contrast, patients with CLL have much lower lymphocyte counts in their

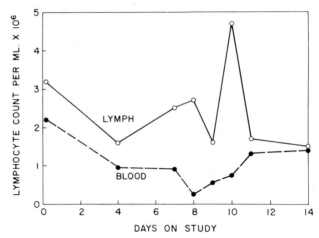

Fig. 10.—Simultaneous absolute lymphocyte counts in peripheral blood and thoracic duct lymph of a hematologically normal patient with a solid tumor during 14 days of thoracic duct cannulation.

Fig. 11.—Simultaneous absolute lymphocyte counts in blood and lymph of a patient undergoing thoracic duct drainage as preparation for an organ graft.

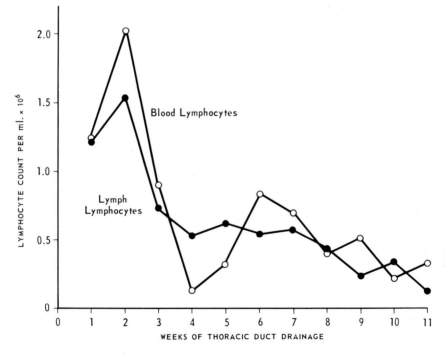

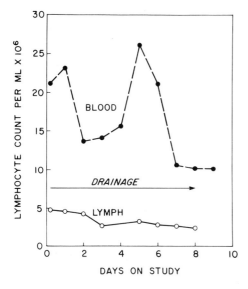

FIG. 12.—Simultaneous absolute lymphocyte counts in peripheral blood and thoracic duct lymph of a patient with CLL.

thoracic duct lymph than in their blood (Figs. 12, 13, and 14); this suggests that the abnormal cells may not get into the lymph from the blood.

Results of studies on the simultaneous collection of blood and lymph lymphocyte cultures confirmed and extended this suggestion. In the normal subjects, the PHA responses of the blood and lymph lymphocytes were

FIG. 13.—Simultaneous absolute lymphocyte counts in peripheral blood and thoracic duct lymph of a patient with CLL during thoracic duct drainage.

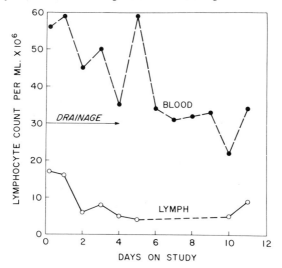

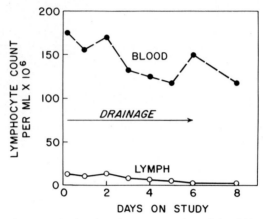

Fig. 14.—Simultaneous absolute lymphocyte counts in peripheral blood and thoracic duct lymph of a patient with CLL.

identical, whereas the antigen responses were either the same or diminished in the lymph, as compared to the blood (Fig. 15). In contrast to the normal situation, both the PHA and antigen responses of the lymphocytes of patients with CLL were much more vigorous in the lymph (Fig. 16). This observation, together with the data presented above (Figs. 12, 13, and 14), suggests that the abnormal cells in patients with CLL cannot get from the blood through the nodes into the lymph. Therefore, the lymphocyte counts are lower and the blastogenic responses greater in the lymph than in the blood.

Discussion

These studies were designed to elucidate further the mechanisms involved in the immunological deficiency associated with the lymphoid or lymphoreticular malignant diseases. Two unique approaches, not used previously in such studies, were undertaken. The first was the study of the primary immune response by using an antigen which elicits antibody production, delayed hypersensitivity, and circulating memory cells detectable by in vitro blastogenesis (Curtis *et al.*, in press). The second was to compare the function of simultaneously collected peripheral blood and thoracic duct lymphocytes (Hersh *et al.*, in press).

Patients with three types of lymphoproliferative disease (Hodgkin's disease, CLL, and multiple myeloma) were compared to normal subjects, patients with metastatic solid tumors, and patients who had had primary tumors removed surgically. This comparison was believed to be necessary since nonspecific factors associated with neoplasia, such as cachexia, infection, prior chemotherapy, and lymph node involvement, might have

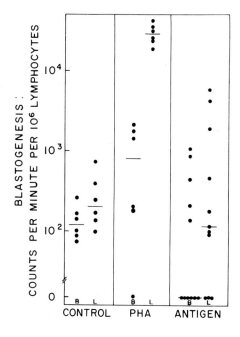

Fig. 15.—Blastogenic responses to mitogenic stimulation in vitro of simultaneously collected and cultured blood and lymph lymphocytes from a hematologically normal subject. *PHA*, phytohemagglutinin; *SLO*, streptolysin-O; *VAR*, varidase (streptokinase-streptodornase); *POX*, small pox vaccine.

Fig. 16.—Blastogenic response of simultaneously collected and cultured blood and lymph lymphocytes from a patient with CLL.

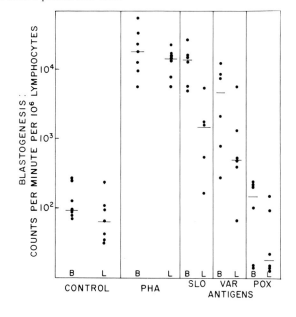

influenced the results. The comparison indicated that there are unique patterns of immunological deficiency in patients with the lymphoreticular disorders. Patients with multiple myeloma produced antibodies and circulating memory cells promptly, but both immunological reactants disappeared from the circulation relatively rapidly. The disappearance of antibody was not an unexpected finding in view of the fact that increased catabolism of immunoglobulins has been observed in patients with this disease (Soloman, Waldmann, and Fahey, 1963). However, the rapid decline in detectable circulating memory cells (as measured by blastogenesis in vitro was unexpected and suggested that these cells might have impaired immunological memory. Most of these patients had a positive reaction to skin tests with KLH at four weeks. It might be anticipated that, if retested after some period of time, these patients would have a negative reaction to the skin test.

The patterns of appearance of circulating memory cells in the patients with Hodgkin's disease and CLL were both abnormal, but were similar to each other. Although there was a notable delay, there was a slow, steady rise in the blastogenic response to KLH. Neither group, however, achieved a normal level during the study period. Although their blastogenic responses were similar, the antibody production of the patients with Hodgkin's disease was deficient. The peak occurred at the normal time; however, it was not maintained and declined to low levels rapidly. In contrast, the patients with CLL, although slow to produce antibody, had total antibody titers which eventually reached a normal level; they never produced normal levels of 2-ME-resistant antibody.

The question of whether immunological deficiency precedes or follows the development of the malignant disease is answered partially by these studies. In the patients with solid tumors who had no evident disease after surgical treatment, the immune response was actually slightly greater than normal. In those with metastatic solid tumors, it was slightly lower than normal. This clearly suggests that the deficiency develops as the disease progresses. This same progression of immunological deficiency has been observed by others in studies on serial solid tumor patients (Krant, Manskopf, Brandrup, and Madoff, 1968), and on patients with Hodgkin's disease (Brown et al., 1967; Hersh and Irwin, in press). In the latter group, immunological deficiency is most prominent in patients with stages III and IV disease, particularly in patients who are in group B (Hersh and Oppenheim, 1965). Also, in patients who have received radiotherapy and whose disease has gone into remission, the in vitro lymphocyte responses and in vivo delayed hypersensitivity are nearly normal (Hersh and Irwin, in press). In patients with CLL, host defense failure, as manifested by hypogammaglobulinemia and increased rate of infection, is apparent late in the disease, particularly in patients who are refractory to chemotherapy. Indeed, in patients with CLL, cellular immunity probably is nearly normal. This is believed to be so because these patients develop normal, new delayed hypersensitivity to KLH and other antigens (Block, Haynes, Thompson, and Neiman, 1969) and their lymphocytes successfully transfer immunity to nonimmune subjects (Curtis, Hersh, and Freireich, in preparation). This possibility is confirmed by the current observation of two populations of lymphocytes in patients with CLL: (1) a normally responsive population which circulates from blood through lymph nodes to thoracic duct lymph and back to blood and (2) a population which is immunologically unresponsive and has difficulty in circulating out of the blood vascular system. These populations can be identified by the fact that the thoracic duct lymphocytes in CLL patients are significantly more responsive to in vitro mitogens than are the peripheral blood lymphocytes. The response of the latter to mitogens is masked by the large numbers of unresponsive leukemic lymphocytes.

Current studies suggest that there are at least two major components of the mammalian immune system: (1) a system of cells under the influence of gut-associated central lymphoid tissue and (2) a system of cells under the influence of the thymus. In addition, the antibody-producing cell population is apparently derived from the bone marrow (Mosier and Coppleson, 1968). It has been suggested that immunological deficiency associated with some of the malignant states described is caused by failure or abnormality in one or the other of the systems (Miller, 1967). This might fit the hypothesis that immunological deficiency precedes neoplasia. However, the overall results of various studies suggest that deficient antibody production, deficient functioning of circulating lymphocytes, and defects in the delayed hypersensitivity response are late events and manifestations of advanced disease. The survival rate of patients with these defects often is poor compared to that of those who are immunologically normal (Krant, Manskopf, Brandrup, and Madoff, 1968).

Thus, the mechanism which causes these immunological defects remains unknown. With a complex configuration such as the lymphoid system, changes in the production of precursor cells, effector cells, or immune reactants may play a role in the development of the immunological deficiency. Defects in antigen uptake, processing, and storage also may be important. Investigation of these phenomena in cancer patients will be an important and exciting task for the future.

Acknowledgments

The authors wish to acknowledge the excellent technical assistance of Miss April Durrett, Miss Sarah Dyre, Mrs. Donna Storms, and Mr. Charles Geschwind.

REFERENCES

Aisenberg, A. C.: Studies on delayed hypersensitivity in Hodgkin's disease. *Journal of Clinical Investigation,* 41:1964-1970, November 1962.

Allison, A. C., and Taylor, R. B.: Observations on thymectomy and carcinogenesis. *Cancer Research,* 27:703-707, April 1967.

Block, J. B., Haynes, H. A., Thompson, W. L., and Neiman, P. E.: Delayed hypersensitivity in chronic lymphocytic leukemia. *Journal of the National Cancer Institute,* 42:973-980, June 1969.

Brown, R. S., Haynes, H. A., Foley, H. T., Godwin, H. A., Berard, C. W., and Carbone, P. P.: Hodgkin's disease: Immunologic, clinical, and histologic features of 50 untreated patients. *Annals of Internal Medicine,* 67:291-302, August 1967.

Campbell, D. H., Garvey, J. S., Cremer, N. E., and Sussdorf, D. H.: *Methods in Immunology.* New York, New York, W. A. Benjamin, Inc., 1964, 263 pp.

Chase, M. W.: Delayed-type hypersensitivity and the immunology of Hodgkin's disease, with a parallel examination of sarcoidosis. *Cancer Research,* 26:1097-1120, June 1966.

Curtis, J. E., Hersh, E. M., and Freireich, E. J: Characteristics of the transfer of immunity in man with peripheral blood leukocytes. (In preparation.)

Curtis, J. E., Hersh, E. M., Harris, J. E., McBride, C., and Freireich, E. J: The human primary immune response to keyhole limpet hemocyanin: Interrelationships of delayed hypersensitivity, antibody response and in vitro blastogenesis. *Clinical and Experimental Immunology.* (In press.)

Fahey, J. L., Scoggins, R., Utz, J. P., and Szwed, C. F.: Infection, antibody response and gamma globulin components in multiple myeloma and macroglobulinemia. *American Journal of Medicine,* 35:698-708, November 1963.

Gold, E. R., and Fudenberg, H. H.: Chromic chloride: A coupling reagent for passive hemagglutination reactions. *Journal of Immunology,* 99:859-865, November 1967.

Gross, L.: Immunological defect in aged population and its relationship to cancer. *Cancer,* 18:201-204, February 1965.

Harris, J. E., Alexanian, R., Migliore, P., and Hersh, E. M.: Abnormal immune response in multiple myeloma to keyhole limpet hemocyanin. (In preparation.)

Hellström, I. E., Hellström, K. E., Pierce, G. E., and Bill, A. H.: Demonstration of cell-bound and humoral immunity against neuroblastoma cells. *Proceedings of the National Academy of Sciences of the U.S.A.,* 60:1231-1238, August 1968.

Hersh, E. M., and Freireich, E. J: Host defense mechanisms and their modification by cancer chemotherapy. In *Methods in Cancer Research.* New York, New York, and London, England, Academic Press, 1968, Vol. IV, pp. 355-451.

Hersh, E. M., Guinn, G. A., Wallace, S., Rose, S., Rossen, R., and Freireich, E. J: Two populations of lymphocytes in chronic lymphocytic leukemia (CLL). *Proceedings of the IVth Annual Leukocyte Culture Conference,* June, 1969. New York, New York, Appleton-Century-Crofts, Inc. (In press.)

Hersh, E. M., and Harris, J. E.: Macrophage-lymphocyte interaction in the antigen-induced blastogenic response of human peripheral blood leukocytes. *Journal of Immunology,* 100:1184-1194, June 1968.

Hersh, E. M., and Irwin, W. S.: Blastogenic responses of lymphocytes from patients with untreated and treated lymphomas. *Lymphology.* (In press.)

Hersh, E. M., and Oppenheim, J. J.: Impaired in vitro lymphocyte transformation in Hodgkin's disease. *New England Journal of Medicine,* 273:1006-1012, November 4, 1965.

Krant, M. J., Manskopf, G., Brandrup, C. S., and Madoff, M. A.: Immunologic alterations in bronchogenic cancer. *Cancer,* 21:623-631, April 1968.

Lytton, B., Hughes, L. E., and Fulthrope, A. J.: Circulating antibody response in malignant disease. *Lancet,* 1:69, January 11, 1964.

Miller, D. G.: Immunological deficiency and malignant lymphoma. *Cancer,* 20:579-588, April 1967.

Mosier, D. E., and Coppleson, L. W.: A three-cell interaction required for the induction of the primary immune response in vitro. *Proceedings of the National Academy of Sciences of the U.S.A.,* 61:542-547, October 1968.

Penn, I., Hammond, W., Brettschneider, L., and Starzl, T. E.: Malignant lymphomas in transplantation patients. *Transplantation Proceedings*, 1:106-112, March 1969.

Reiner, J., and Southam, C. M.: Increased growth of tumor isotransplants after immunosuppression of the recipient mice by methotrexate or 5-fluoro-2'-deoxyuridine. *Journal of the National Cancer Institute*, 38:753-759, May 1967.

Salmon, S. E., and Fudenberg, H. H.: Abnormal nucleic acid metabolism of lymphocytes in plasma cell myeloma and macroglobulinemia. *Blood, The Journal of Hematology*, 33:300-312, February 1969.

Shaw, R. K., Szwed, C., Boggs, D. R., Fahey, J. L., Frei, E., III, Morrison, E., and Utz, J. P.: Infection and immunity in chronic lymphocytic leukemia. *Archives of Internal Medicine*, 106:467-478, October 1960.

Solomon, A., Waldmann, T. A., and Fahey, J. L.: Metabolism of normal 6.6S γ-globulin in normal subjects and in patients with macroglobulinemia and multiple myeloma. *Journal of Laboratory and Clinical Medicine*, 62:1-17, July 1963.

Stavitsky, A. B.: Micromethods for the study of proteins and antibodies. I. Procedure and general application of hemagglutination and hemagglutination-inhibition reactions with tannic acid and protein-treated red blood cells. *Journal of Immunology*, 72:360-367, May 1954.

Paralymphomatous Disease: The Syndrome of Macroglobulinemia*

STEPHAN E. RITZMANN, M.D.,
JERRY C. DANIELS, M.A., AND
WILLIAM C. LEVIN, M.D.

Division of Hematology-Immunology, Shriners Burns Institute, and Division of Hematology, Department of Medicine, The University of Texas Medical Branch at Galveston, Galveston, Texas

THE NATURE OF MACROGLOBULINEMIA can be appreciated best in the context of the historical background of the related disorder, myeloma. In 1846, multiple myeloma was first reported in a tradesman complaining of lassitude and weakness of 13 months' duration (Dalrymple, 1846; MacIntyre, 1850); he suffered from "mollities ossium" (soft bones) and urine containing large quantities of "animal matter," the peculiar characteristics of which were described by Dr. Henry Bence Jones as belonging to an unusual protein or "modified albumin" (Bence Jones, 1848). This is the first report of an "abnormal" immunoglobulin in a patient with presumptive myeloma (Clamp, 1967).

In 1889, Kahler described four cardinal findings in patients with multiple myeloma: bone pain, fragility and deformity of bones, Bence Jones proteins, and cachexia. In 1900, Wright discovered the now well-established association of plasma cell proliferation within the bone marrow of patients with multiple myeloma. Subsequently, the production of "abnormal" globulins by proliferating plasma cells was documented (Vasquez, 1958; Dutcher and Fahey, 1960; Curtain and O'Dea, 1959; Zucker-Franklin, Franklin, and Cooper, 1962).

In 1944, Waldenström recognized another entity within the group of malignant plasma cell disorders. This disease is characterized by discrete

*Supported by Program Grants No. DHEW 1P01 AI 09278-01, No. DHEW 5P01 HE 10893-03, and No. DHEW 5M01 FR 0073-07, and Grants NAS 9-8258 and NAS 9-8122.

lymphadenopathy and splenomegaly, absence of bone pain or osteolytic lesions, proliferation of plasma cells in the bone marrow, and large amounts of macroglobulins in the serum; hence, the disorder has been called Waldenström's macroglobulinemia.

NORMAL IMMUNOGLOBULINS

Proteins exhibiting antibody characteristics may be classified either on the basis of predominant electrophoretic mobility (gamma[γ]-globulins) or on the basis of function and structure (immunoglobulins [Ig]). Five classes of normal human immunoglobulins have been described: γG-globulins (IgG), γA-globulins (IgA), γM-globulins (IgM), γD-globulins (IgD), and γE-globulins (IgE). Together these immunoglobulins constitute 20 to 25 per cent of the total serum proteins (Heremans, 1960; Grabar and Burtin, 1964; Franklin and Lowenstein, 1964; *Nomenclature for Human Immunoglobulins,* 1964; Ritzmann and Levin, 1969). Figure 1 shows serum electrophoresis with immunoglobulin distribution and relative concentrations. The basic structure of immunoglobulins includes four polypeptide chains linked by disulfide and hydrogen bonds (Fig. 2). Two of the chains, with a molecular weight of 20,000 to 25,000 each, are light chains; these are linked to two heavy chains with molecular weights of 50,000 to 70,000. The light chains common to all immunoglobulins may be of either type K (kappa [κ] light chains) or type L (lambda [λ] light chains). Heavy chains are unique for

FIG. 1.–Normal serum electrophoresis indicating the migration ranges and relative concentrations of IgG, IgA, IgM, and IgD. (Reproduced with kind permission of Fahey, 1965.)

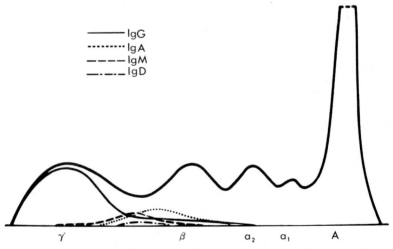

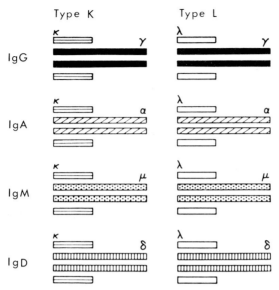

Type K   Type L

κ   γ   λ   γ
IgG

κ   α   λ   α
IgA

κ   μ   λ   μ
IgM

κ   δ   λ   δ
IgD

Fig. 2.–Diagrammatic presentation of the basic structure of IgG, IgA, IgM, and IgD. (Reproduced with kind permission of Osserman and Fahey, 1968.)

each class of immunoglobulins. Heavy chains of IgG, IgA, IgM, IgD, and IgE are termed γ(gamma), α(alpha), μ(mu), δ(delta), and ε(epsilon) chains, respectively. The high molecular weight (approximately 900,000, 19S) IgM molecules consist of five subunits, each of which consists of two light chains and two μ heavy chains (Miller and Metzger, 1965, 1966). A low molecular IgM, sedimenting at 7S to 8S in the ultracentrifuge, has recently been recognized (Rothfield, Frangione, and Franklin, 1965; Stobo and Tomasi, 1967; Solomon and Kunkel, 1967).

In normal adults, the immunoglobulin classes are present at different serum concentrations (mg./100 ml. ± 2 SD range): IgG, 1,200 mg./100 ml. (700 to 1,700); IgA, 210 mg./100 ml. (70 to 350); IgM, 140 mg./100 ml. (70 to 210); IgD, 3 mg./100 ml., and IgE, <0.3 mg./100 ml. (for references, see Ritzmann and Leyin, 1969). The various immunoglobulin classes possess different antibody properties. IgG contains most antibacterial, antiviral, and antitoxic antibodies. IgA constitutes the main antibody class in secretory fluids. IgM possesses most of the natural antibodies, including ABO-blood group isoantibodies; cold agglutinins; rheumatoid factors; Wassermann, heterophile, and saline Rh antibodies; antibodies to gram-negative microorganisms; and others. The antibody function of IgD is unknown. IgE contains antibodies which elicit the Prausnitz-Küstner reaction (for references, see Ritzmann and Levin, 1969).

"ABNORMAL" IMMUNOGLOBULINS

The term "paraprotein" was introduced by Apitz (1940) to denote foreign proteins in the blood, urine, or tissues produced by myeloma cells. Gutman (1948) coined the term "M protein" for the discrete proteins demonstrable by electrophoresis in sera of patients suffering from myeloma (Fig. 3). Riva (1957) applied this term to the narrow bands seen by serum electrophoresis which also were associated with macroglobulinemia.

"Monoclonal gammopathy" was suggested by Waldenström (1961, 1962) as a more comprehensive term for such abnormal immunoglobulins and their associated clinical conditions. Criteria for monoclonal gammopathies have been suggested (Osserman and Takatsuki, 1965): (1) neoplastic proliferation of plasma cells without an apparent antigenic stimulus, (2) elaboration of eletrophoretically homogeneous serum γ-globulin and/or compara-

FIG. 3.—Diagram of the immunoelectrophoretic (center panel) and ultracentrifugal (bottom panel) characteristics of M proteins on electrophoresis (top panel). The detection of an M protein on electrophoresis necessitates further characterization by immunoelectrophoresis and, occasionally, by analytic ultracentrifugation. Immunoelectrophoretically, M proteins resulting from IgM are indicated by greatly enlarged and deformed IgM precipitin lines. On ultracentrifugation, IgM monoclonal gammopathy is characterized by increased 19S components and the occurrence of heavier components (22 to 24S, 32S, and >32S).

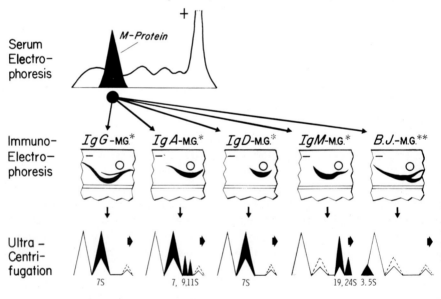

* Monoclonal Gammopathy
** Bence Jones Monoclonal Gammopathy

tively homogeneous γ-globulin subunits, and often (3) a deficiency of normal immunoglobulins. Such monoclonal immunoglobulins can be either IgG, IgA, IgD, IgE, IgM, free light chains (*i.e.,* Bence Jones proteins), or free heavy chains (*i.e., γ, α,* and *μ* chains) (for references, see Ritzmann and Levin, 1969).

The clonal concept—that myeloma may be considered the result of unlimited autonomous proliferation of one specific colony, or clone, of plasma cells—is based upon Burnet's hypothesis (Burnet, 1959). Waldenström (1961, 1962) extended this hypothesis and included all types of electrophoretically narrow-banded hyper-γ-globulinemic conditions in the monoclonal group. In contrast, electrophoretically broad-based, diffuse hyper-γ-globulinemia is regarded as polyclonal in origin.

Diagnostic Criteria of Macroglobulinemia

Although Waldenström's macroglobulinemia may be suspected on clinical grounds, its diagnosis is dependent upon the demonstration of monoclonal IgM in the serum, which is strongly supported by evidence of proliferating lymphoid plasma cells seen either by bone marrow aspiration or biopsy examination of lymphoid organs.

Because of the protein nature of immunoglobulins, it is not surprising that the laboratory diagnosis of immunoglobulin abnormalities utilizes techniques of classical protein chemistry such as electrophoresis (paper, cellulose acetate, *etc.*) and analytical ultracentrifugation. Recognition and characterization of immunoglobulinopathies have been enhanced greatly during the past decade by the application of the newer technique of immunoelectrophoresis, which combines the detection of physicochemical properties with that of antigenic characteristics. Other special tests for particular physicochemical characterization of specific proteins or biological activity of serum components are useful in individual cases.

SERUM PROTEIN ANALYSIS

ELECTROPHORESIS: M PROTEINS.—On serum electrophoresis (Fig. 3, top panel), M proteins may occur as definite spikes anywhere within the entire migration range of immunoglobulins, *i.e.* between the γ- and α_2-globulin positions. Less commonly, the abnormality may appear not as a distinct peak or spike, but as a subtle asymmetry of one of the normal electrophoretic components; thus, careful analysis of the electrophoretic pattern is required for the identification of M proteins. Statistically, most M proteins are found in the γ-globulin area, fewer in the β-globulin range, and still fewer in the α_2-globulin position. Since the immunoglobulins overlap in these regions, electrophoresis does not permit the identification of the immunoglobulin classes of the M proteins.

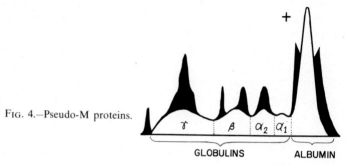

FIG. 4.—Pseudo-M proteins.

DIFFERENTIAL DIAGNOSIS: PSEUDO-M PROTEINS.—Conditions other than monoclonal gammopathies are characterized by serum protein patterns, on electrophoresis, which mimic M proteins. These proteins have been termed "pseudo-M proteins" (Ritzmann and Levin, 1967) (Fig. 4). The types of pseudo-M proteinemia include the following: (1) Bisalbuminemia, or double albuminemia (Scheurlen, 1955; Knedel, 1957; Wuhrmann, 1957; Waldmann, 1964), shows a split albumin peak which simulates a fast-moving M protein either preceding or following the albumin. (2) Hyperlipidemia (Riva, 1957; Ritzmann and Levin, 1967), because of increased serum concentrations of lipoproteins, produces spikes in the α_2-globulin position which are dissipated by mixing the serum with an equal volume of ether and allowing the mixture to stand at 4°C for five minutes. (3) Hyper-α_2-M-globulinemia (Kunkel, 1960; Eriksen, 1958) with an elevated 19S component on ultracentrifugation, usually in association with hypoalbuminemia as in the nephrotic syndrome (Riva, 1957; Wuhrmann and Märki, 1963; Sunderman, 1964), may produce an α_2-globulin spike. (4) Hemolysis of the serum sample may cause a tall spike in the β-globulin region. (5) Fibrinogen migrates as a noticeable peak in the slower β-globulin region. (6) Notable bacterial contamination or desiccation of serum samples may produce breakdown products with electrophoretic mobility in the slower β-globulin region (Ritzmann and Levin, 1967). (7) Hypertransferrinemia, associated with chronic iron-deficiency anemia, can cause a spike in the slow β-globulin region (Zawadzki and Edwards, 1969; Daniels, Levin, and Ritzmann, in press). (8) γ-Globulin complexes may migrate as peaks in the β-γ-globulin range (Ritzmann and Levin, 1967). (9) Hypermuramidasemia (hyperlysozymemia), resulting from renal insufficiency or other causes, may produce a spike in the post-γ-globulin region (Osserman and Lawlor, 1966). Although electrophoresis is useful for screening sera for the presence of M proteins, confirmation by immunoelectrophoresis with specific antisera is necessary for the identification of M proteins associated with myeloma, macroglobulinemia, or other conditions.

IMMUNOELECTROPHORESIS: DIAGNOSTIC PATTERNS OF MACROGLOBU-
LINEMIA.—Immunoelectrophoresis is the method of choice for the precise
immunochemical characterization of M proteins (Heremans, 1960; Grabar
and Burtin, 1964; Osserman and Lawlor, 1961; Roulet et al., 1961; Fahey,
1962; Bachmann and Laurell, 1963; Ritzmann and Levin, 1967, 1969). By
using appropriate antisera, the diagnosis of monoclonal gammopathies
can be established in almost all instances (Fig. 3, center panel). Monoclonal
gammopathies described to date include those resulting from over production of IgG, IgA, IgM, IgD, and IgE, and of free light chains (i.e. Bence
Jones proteins, light chain disease) and free heavy chains (i.e., γ, α, and μ
chains, heavy chain diseases). Characteristically, IgM monoclonal gammopathy is reflected by a heavy and distorted IgM precipitin line (Fig. 3, center
panel). Light chain typing indicates that the abnormal IgM is either of the K
or L type (McKelvey and Fahey, 1965; Imhof, Ballieux, Mul, and Poen,
1966).

ULTRACENTRIFUGATION: DIAGNOSTIC PATTERNS OF MACROGLOBU-
LINEMIA.—Analytical ultracentrifugation of serum occasionally may be
required for confirmation of the diagnosis of macroglobulinemia. IgM
monoclonal gammopathy is characterized by large, tall 19S components
(termed M_1) and heavier 22 to 24S components (termed M_2) (Fig. 3, bottom
panel). Occasionally, additional heavier fractions may occur, i.e. M_3 (approximately 32S) and M_4 (greater than 32S) (Heremans, 1963; Laurell,
1961; Imhof, Ballieux, and Mijnlieff, 1960; Korngold, 1961; Jahnke and
Scholtan, 1960). Rarely, a component slightly lighter than the 19S M_1 component (i.e. M'_1 component) is encountered which sediments with about
17.6S (Filitti-Wurmser, Gentou, and Hartmann, 1964; Jahnke and Scholtan,
1960).

ADDITIONAL TECHNIQUES.—In addition to total serum protein quantitation, serum protein electrophoresis, immunoelectrophoresis, quantitative
immunodiffusion techniques, and ultracentrifugation, other techniques
have been employed to detect and characterize macroglobulinemia M proteins, particularly to differentiate them from myeloma M proteins. In general, these methods have been disappointing as screening tests for macroglobulinemia because of their lack of specificity and/or sensitivity. Such
techniques include the following:

1. The Sia test (also called water test, euglobulin test, Ray test [Ray,
1921]) was introduced by Sia (Sia and Wu, 1924) and Brahmachari and
Seu (1923) for the detection of kala-azar. Waldenström (1952) recommended this test for the detection of primary macroglobulinemia (Ritzmann
and Levin, 1969). A positive test consists of precipitation or flocculation
on addition of one drop of serum to a tube of demineralized water. Positive Sia tests have been reported, however, in patients with multiple my-

eloma and polyclonal gammopathies and in patients whose sera have high rheumatoid factor activity. Also, the test may be negative in known cases of Waldenström's macroglobulinemia (Ritzmann and Levin, 1969).

2. The formolgel test is based upon the condition for gel formation by macroglobulinemic sera treated with formaldehyde (Wuhrmann and Märki, 1963; Riva, 1957; Kanner, 1964; Gaté and Papacostas, 1920; Bing, 1940). This test is not specific for macroglobulins and may be positive in patients with either monoclonal or polyclonal gammopathies.

3. In the Rivanol test, Rivanol(TM) (ephacridine lactate) supposedly precipitates macroglobulinemia M proteins, but not normal β-globulins, γ-globulins, or myeloma proteins (Kaldor, Saifer, Terry, and Vecsler, 1962; Saifer and Gerstenfeld, 1962). Saifer (1964) and Kahn (1967) suggested in vitro Rivanol treatment of sera, in conjunction with paper electrophoresis, to differentiate macroglobulinemia from myeloma. Subsequent studies (Ritzmann, Cobb, and Levin, 1967) have demonstrated Rivanol precipitation of myeloma proteins and the failure of Rivanol to precipitate certain macroglobulinemia proteins.

4. In the penicillamine test, the in vitro treatment of sera with d,1-penicillamine reportedly shifted paper electrophoretic mobility of macroglobulinemia, but not that of myeloma M proteins (Leder, 1967); however, some sera from patients with IgA myeloma exhibit similar shifts, and some sera from those with Waldenström's macroglobulinemia do not (Ritzmann, Cobb, and Levin, 1967).

5. The acid gel test consisting of the addition of dilute hydrochloric acid to serum in a 1:2 (acid-to-serum) ratio has been reported to produce rapid gel formation in sera containing M proteins (Schoen, Glover, and Labiner, 1965; Schoen, 1967), but subsequent studies (Huhnstock and Grossman, 1967; Daniels, Cobb, Levin, and Ritzmann, in press) have demonstrated that this test is nonspecific.

6. Notable rouleaux formation and accelerated erythrocyte sedimentation rates may be diagnostic clues of the presence of monoclonal gammopathy, although they are not pathognomonic (Levin and Ritzmann, 1966; Jeannet and Hässig, 1964).

In conclusion, immunoelectrophoresis with appropriate antisera, and ultracentrifugation, when indicated, constitute the methods of choice for precisely identifying M proteins.

Our experience is based upon 442 instances of monoclonal gammopathy at The University of Texas Medical Branch at Galveston studied between 1962 and 1969 (Table 1). A total of 71 cases of IgM monoclonal gammopathy have been studied, including four instances of IgM monoclonal gammopathy associated with Bence Jones proteins and one case with IgG-IgM biclonal gammopathy. These represent approximately 16 per cent of all

TABLE 1.—Cases of Monoclonal Gammopathy at
The University of Texas Medical Branch
from 1962 to 1969

	Ig Categories	No.	Total No.	%
1	IgG-M.G.	238		
	IgG + B.J.-M.G.	25	263	59.5
2	IgA-M.G.	51		
	IgA + B.J.-M.G.	22	73	16.6
3	IgD-M.G.	1	1	0.2
4	IgM-M.G.	66		
	IgM + B.J.-M.G.	4	70	15.8
5	B.J.-M.G. (light chain disease)	34	34	7.7
6	IgG + IgM-B.G.	1	1	0.2
	Total		442	100.0

Abbreviations: B.G., bioclonal gammopathy; B.J., Bence Jones protein; M.G., monoclonal gammopathy.

cases of monoclonal gammopathy seen at this institution (Ritzmann and Levin, 1969). The same relative incidence is apparent from the tabulation of the published series comprising 3,336 cases of monoclonal gammopathy (Ritzmann and Levin, 1969). The results of ultracentrifugal analysis of 57 cases of IgM monoclonal gammopathy are shown in Table 2. In all 57 instances, the M_1 and M_2 components were present. The M_1 component was predominant without exception, followed in incidence and concentration by the M_3, M'_1, and M_4 components. These data confirm earlier observations (Heremans, 1963; Laurell, 1961; Imhof, Ballieux, and Mijnlieff, 1960; Kappeler, Krebs, and Riva, 1958) that: (1) M components appear with a certain periodicity, *i.e.* at 19S, 22S to 24S, 32S, and higher, and (2) the concentrations of the M components decrease, in general, from M_1 to M_4. The finding of a lighter M'_1 component (about 17.6S) in approximately 9 per cent of cases, is interesting, but the significance of this fraction is unknown.

TABLE 2.—Results of 57 Sera Analyzed by Ultracentrifugation

Macroglobulin Components	M'_1	M_1	M_2	M_3	M_4
$S^°_{20,w}$—values	17.6	19	22-24	approx. 32	>32
No. of components present	5	57	57	29	2
Per cent of components present	9	100	100	51	3.5

Hematological Criteria and Bone
Marrow Characteristics

Patients with macroglobulinemia often develop some degree of anemia. The anemia usually is the result of suppression of erythropoiesis and is of the normocytic and normochromic type (Martin, 1969; Levin and Ritzmann, 1966; Kappeler, Krebs, and Riva, 1958); however, hemolytic anemia (Fankhauser, Arnold, Schaub, and Lapp, 1956) or blood loss with microcytic-hypochromic anemia may be encountered (Fahey, Barth, and Solomon, 1965; Levin and Ritzmann, 1966; Ritzmann, Thurm, Truax, and Levin, 1960; Martin, 1969). In some instances of anemia of unknown origin, the routine application of serum electrophoresis has led to the diagnosis of monoclonal gammopathy.

Examination of the bone marrow of a patient with macroglobulinemia reveals proliferation of lymphocytoid plasma cells (Fig. 5), which are often indistinguishable morphologically from atypical lymphocytes or normal small lymphocytes and can lead to diagnoses such as lymphoproliferative disorders, lymphosarcoma, chronic lymphocytic leukemia, *etc.* Occasionally, sheets of plasmacytoid cells indistinguishable from multiple myeloma cells (Brecher, Tanaka, Malmgren, and Fahey, 1964) may be seen. Proliferation of cells intermediate in morphology between lymphocytes and plasma

Fig. 5.—Bone marrow pattern of patient with macroglobulinemia. × 70.

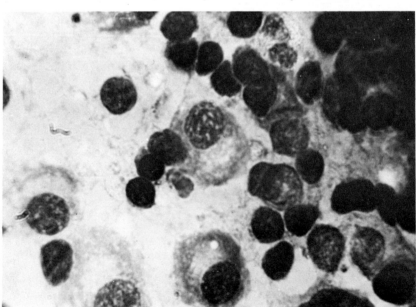

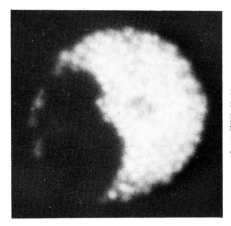

FIG. 6.—IgM-containing immunocyte from bone marrow of patient with macroglobulinemia; immunofluorescence pattern. Obtained by direct immunofluorescence techniques using fluorescein-isothiocyanate-conjugated anti-μ-chain antiserum.

cells may be present (Zucker-Franklin and Mullaney, 1964; Solomon, Fahey, and Malmgren, 1963). In the same patient, such variations may be encountered at different sampling times or at different sampling locations. No definite correlations can be drawn between the cell type and the immunoglobulins produced (Levin and Ritzmann, 1965). The predominant type of plasma cells in the bone marrow of patients with macroglobulinemia are lymphoid plasma cells (Fig. 5). These cells have been shown to contain IgM globulins (Fig. 6).

HISTOPATHOLOGICAL CRITERIA—SPLEEN AND LYMPH NODE PATTERNS

In contrast to myeloma, the lymphatic organs often became infiltrated by IgM-producing plasma cells in patients with Waldenström's macroglobulinemia. The histopathological features may be inconclusive. As shown in lymph node biopsy specimen in Figure 7, "round-cell" infiltration can be significant in the lymphatic organs, and often, in the liver (Cohen, Solomon, Paronetto, and Popper, 1963). Such cells are easily classified as lymphocytoid in nature, leading to a pathological diagnosis of lymphosarcoma. By electron microscopy, these cells reveal endoplasmic reticulum and Golgi structures characteristic of plasma cells (Cohen, Solomon, Paronetto, and Popper, 1963).

Clinically, patients with macroglobulinemia often appear to have a lymphoma, although immunoglobulin-producing plasma cells and, consequently, disorders of the humoral defense mechanisms (Fahey and Lawrence, 1963; McKelvey and Fahey, 1965; Fahey, Scoggins, Utz, and Szwed, 1963; Ballieux et al., 1968) are associated with the disease. For these reasons, the term "paralymphomatous disease" has been suggested (Shullenberger, personal communication).

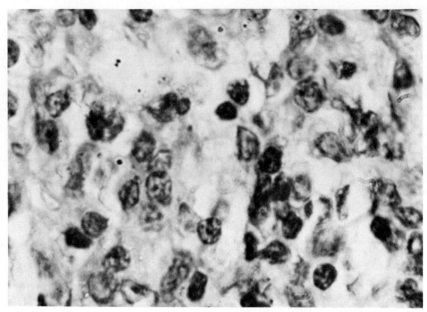

FIG. 7.—Histopathological pattern of lymph node biopsy specimen from patient with macroglobulinemia.

CHROMOSOMAL ABERRATIONS

In 1961, Bottura and colleagues (Bottura, Ferrari, and Veiga, 1961) described a unique chromosomal abnormality consisting of a submetacentric (subterminal) supernumerary chromosome in the AB size range or larger in a patient with Waldenström's macroglobulinemia. During the same year, German and associates (German, Biro, and Bearn, 1961) reported the occurrence of a metacentric supernumerary chromosome larger than any other in the cell in another patient with Waldenström's macroglobulinemia. These two chromosomal abnormalities, the submetacentric of at least AB size range and the large metacentric, have provided the prototypes for numerous additional cases of Waldenström's macroglobulinemia associated with karyotypic aberrations (Benirschke, Brownhill, and Ebaugh, 1962; Pfeiffer, Kosenow, and Bäumer, 1962; Elves and Israëls, 1963; Ferguson and Mackay, 1963; Heni and Siebner, 1963; Nowell and Hungerford, 1964; Seligmann, Danon, and Mihaesco, 1965; Siebner et al., 1965; Moretti et al., 1965; Houston, Ritzmann, and Levin, 1967a, b). In the reported cases, the submetacentric variety of abnormality has been predominant over the metacentric variety. The cytogenetics of this disorder were recently reviewed by Broustet (1966). Figure 8 presents a comparison of these distinct types of aberrations. Inasmuch as similar defects have been identified in patients with both IgG and IgA monoclonal gammopathy (MG) (Houston, Ritzmann, and Levin, 1967a, b), these abnormal chromosomes more recently have been termed "MG chromosomes." Although the morphological appearance of MG chromosomes is indistinguishable in patients with IgG, IgA, and IgM monoclonal gammopathies, it is of interest that, in a comparative study of the chromosomal aberrations common to these three classes of monoclonal gammopathies (Houston, Levin, and Ritzmann, 1967), MG chromosomes occurred as supernumeraries in most patients with macroglobulinemia and IgA myeloma, with one exception in each category. This was in contrast to IgG myeloma patients, who demonstrated, again with a single exception, MG chromosomes as constituents of pseudodiploid cells. MG chromosomes do not appear to be pathognomonic of monoclonal gammopathies, since indistinguishable chromosomes have been observed in a patient with acute myeloblastic leukemia and in two patients with acute

FIG. 8.—Aberrant chromosomal pattern in patient with macroglobulinemia. (Reproduced with kind permission of Mrs. E. M. Houston, research associate, Cytogenetic Laboratory, Division of Hematology, Department of Medicine, The University of Texas Medical Branch at Galveston, Galveston, Texas.)

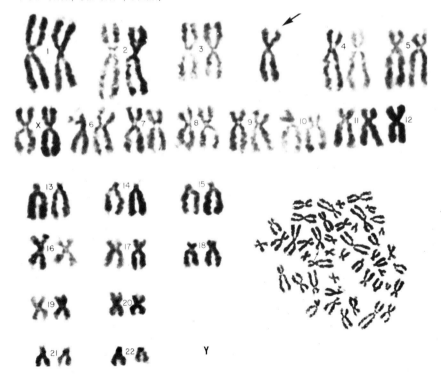

lymphoblastic leukemia (Sandberg, Ishihara, Kikuchi, and Crosswhite, 1964).

In addition to the MG chromosomes, a high incidence of abnormalities in pair 12 chromosomes of group C has been documented in karyotypic studies of patients with Waldenström's macroglobulinemia (Fig. 8) (Houston, Ritzmann, and Levin, 1967a, b). These heterogeneous abnormalities, including deleted or supernumerary chromosomes as well as structural derangements, again were not confined to macroglobulinemia patients but also were distributed among patients with IgG and IgA monoclonal gammopathy. Statistical analysis, by which this vulnerability of pair 12 chromosomes was identified, also suggested that pairs 5 and 20, and possibly pair 22, represented additional sensitive foci.

Predictably, in karyotypes of Waldenström's macroglobulinemia, patients with numerous nonspecific abnormalities are observed, including poor matching attributable to differences in the degree of coiling, deletions or translocations of chromatin material, polyploidy, chromatid or isochromatid gaps or breaks, and occasional endoreduplication (Houston, Ritzmann, and Levin, 1967b; Houston, Levin, and Ritzmann, 1964).

The variety of aberrations in a single patient and the variation in morphology of MG chromosomes from patient to patient is such that simple causal relationship between any chromosomal abnormality and the etiology of monoclonal gammopathy appears unlikely. Rather, it is postulated that some unidentified defect(s) common to all three types of monoclonal gammopathy contributes to the formation of MG chromosomes. One suggestion (Houston, Ritzmann, and Levin, 1967) has been that the abnormal chromosome patterns seen in patients with Waldenström's macroglobulinemia and the IgG and IgA varieties of myeloma may be secondary to the cellular environment, which conceivably could be altered sufficiently by the persistent presence of abnormal immunoglobulins to reflect deleterious effects on sensitive chromosomal foci through interference with cellular metabolism. The precise relationships between the underlying etiological and pathogenetic mechanisms of Waldenström's macroglobulinemia and the chromosomal abnormalities associated with this disorder are yet to be delineated.

Clinical Manifestations and Management of Macroglobulinemia

GENERAL MANIFESTATIONS OF MACROGLOBULINEMIA

Macroglobulinemia often develops insidiously and is accompanied by discrete lymphadenopathy, splenomegaly, bone marrow infiltration by lymphoid plasma cells, and by telangiectases, bleeding diathesis, increased susceptibility to infections, *etc.*

Idiopathic, Asymptomatic IgM Monoclonal Gammopathy

DEFINITION.—The presence of an M protein has long been considered to be a consequence of either multiple myeloma or Waldenström's macroglobulinemia. In recent years, however, an increasing number of patients with monoclonal gammopathies unassociated with myeloma or macroglobulinemia at the time of recognition of M proteins have been identified. A certain percentage of such individuals eventually may develop one or more clinical manifestations of multiple myeloma (Wallerstein, 1951; Waldenström, 1968; Hobb, 1969; Nørgaard, 1957; Osserman, 1958; Osserman and Lawlor, 1955; Stevens, 1965; Kyle and Bayrd, 1966; Seligmann and Basch, 1968) or macroglobulinemia (Osserman, 1961). Such cases appropriately may be termed "premyeloma" (Waldenström, 1942), "preclinical myeloma" (Nørgaard, 1964), or "preclinical macroglobulinemia."

In addition, there are patients with M proteins who almost certainly do not have multiple myeloma or macroglobulinemia (Osserman and Takatsuki, 1963). Even with long-standing follow-up studies (Michaux and Heremans, 1969; Axelsson and Hällén, 1968; Rádl and Masopust, 1964; Laurell, Laurell, and Waldenström, 1957) and at autopsy examination (Waldenström, 1964; Dubi, 1965; Riva, 1964), no evidence of myeloma or macroglobulinemia has been demonstrated.

SYNONYMS.—In 1952, Waldenström (1952) coined the term "essential hyperglobulinemia" to describe patients who had had M proteins for several years without clinical evidence of myeloma. Subsequently, other terms were suggested, as shown in Table 3.

Waldenström (1964) emphasized certain points which distinguish patients with the idiopathic, asymptomatic forms from those with the classical, symptomatic forms of monoclonal gammopathies. In patients with idiopathic asymptomatic disease, (1) the M protein concentrations were 3.0 g./100 ml. or less, (2) the M protein levels remained stable for several years, (3) the anemia was minimal, (4) the albumin concentrations were essentially normal, and (5) the plasma cell content of the bone marrow was usually 3 to 5 per cent, although sometimes higher.

These criteria apply chiefly to IgG and IgA monoclonal gammopathies, but in general, they also are applicable to patients with IgM monoclonal gammopathies. It must be realized, however, that the clinical classification into asymptomatic or symptomatic macroglobulinemia often is impossible.

The relative incidence of idiopathic, asymptomatic monoclonal gammopathies is variously estimated at from less than 10 per cent to more than 60 per cent (Ritzmann and Levin, 1967), with a modal frequency of about 25 to 30 per cent.

TABLE 3.—SYNONYMS OF MONOCLONAL GAMMOPATHIES

SYNONYMS	AUTHORS*	YEAR
I. "Classical" symptomatic monoclonal gammopathies		
1. "Obligate" paraproteinemia	Spengler *et al.*	1961
2. "Grosse" paraproteinemia	Märki and Siegenthaler	1964
3. Primary malignant monoclonal immunoglobulin disorders	Michaux and Heremans	1969
II. "Idiopathic" asymptomatic monoclonal gammopathies		
1. Essential hyperglobulinemia	Waldenström	1952
2. Essential, monoclonal benign hypergammaglobulinemia	Waldenström	1961
3. Benign paraproteinemia	Olhagen and Liljestrand	1955
4. Nonmyelomatous paraproteinemia	Smith	1957
5. γ1-Syndrome	Knedel	1958
6. Dysgammaglobulinemic syndrome	Hammack, Bolding, and Frommeyer	1959
7. Atypical dysproteinemia	Creyssel, Fine, and Morel	1959
8. Cryptogenetic paraproteinemia	Schobel and Wewalka	1961
9. Essential hyperdysglobulinemia	Olmer, Mongin, Muratore, and Denizet	1961
10. "Facultative" paraproteinemia	Spengler *et al.*	1961
11. Monoclonal gammopathy of unknown etiology	Osserman and Takatsuki	1963
12. Rudimentary paraproteinemia	Märki and Wuhrmann	1963
13. Secondary paraproteinemia	Videbaek and Drivsholm	1964
14. Idiopathic paraproteinemia	Rádl and Masopust	1964
15. Idiopathic and "Begleit" paraproteinemia	Riva	1964
16. "Symptom-poor" paraproteinemia	Huhnstock, Meiser, and Weicker	1964
17. Pseudo-myelomatous dysproteinemia	Laroche *et al.*	1964
18. Essential or isolated paraproteinemia	Brittinger and König	1965
19. Essential and atypical dysglobulinemia	Derycke, Fine, and Boffa; Fine, Derycke, Bilski-Pasquier, and Marchal	1965 1964
20. Atypical paraproteinemia	Klemm, Hunstein, and Harwerth	1965
21. Discrete gammaglobulin (M) components	Hällén	1966
22. Asymptomatic monoclonal hypergammaglobulinemia	Allensmith and Chandor	1966
23. Lanthanic dysimmunoglobulinemia	Zawadzki and Edwards	1967

24. Secondary and primary benign
monoclonal immunoglobulin
disorders

Michaux and
Heremans

1969

*Complete references to authors cited are as follows:

Allensmith, M., and Chandor, S.: Asymptomatic monoclonal IgA hypergammaglobulinemia. *American Journal of Medicine*, 41:486-490, September 1966.

Brittinger, G., and König, E.: Zur Klinik der Paraproteinämien. *Schweizerische medizinische Wochenschrift*, 95:1584-1588, November 13, 1965.

Creyssel, R., Fine, J.-M., and Morel, P.: Étude biochimique de quelques formes atypiques de dysproteinémies. *Revue d'hematologie*, 14:238-249, July-September 1959.

Derycke, C., Fine, J.-M., and Boffa, G. A.: Dysglobulinémies "essentielles" chez les sujets agés. *Nouvelle Revue Francaise d'Hematologie*, 5:729-738, September-October 1965.

Fine, J.-M., Derycke, C., Bilski-Pasquier, G., and Marchal, G.: Dysglobulinémies atypiques et dysglobulinémies essentielles. *Abstracts, Xth Congress of the International Society of Haematology*, Stockholm, Sweden, 1964, p. D:12.

Hällén, J.: Discrete gammaglobulin (M-) components in serum: Clinical study of 150 subjects without myelomatosis. *Acta medica scandinavica*, 179 (Suppl. 462):1-127, 1966.

Hammack, W. J., Bolding, F. E., and Frommeyer, W. B., Jr.: The dysgammaglobulinemic syndrome. *Annals of Internal Medicine*, 50:288-299, February 1959.

Huhnstock, K., Meiser, J., and Weicker, H.: Biochemische und cytoligische Kontrolluntersuchungen bei symptomenarmen Paraproteinämien. *Verhandlungen der deutschen Gesellschaft für Innere Medizin*, 70:227-231, 1964.

Klemm, D., Hunstein, W., and Harwerth, H. G.: Zur Klassifizierung atypischer paraproteinämischer Hämoblastosen. *Blut*, 11:208-233, July 1965.

Knedel, M.: Vortrag vor der Medizinischen Fakultät München, 1958. As cited by Schettler, G., and Neikes, K.: Die Bedeutung der Serumeiweisskörper in der Klinischen. *Diagnostik Medizinische Klinik*, 55:960-968, 1960.

Laroche, C., Nenna, A., Seligmann, M., Richet, G., Caquet, R., and Bognon, J.: Dysprotéinémie psuedomyélomateuse au cours de pyonéphroses. *La presse médicale*, 72:2833-2837, November 14, 1964.

Märki, H. H., and Siegenthaler, R.: Über eine unter dem Bilde einer Paraleukoblastenleukämie verlaufende Form der Makroglobulinämie. *Schweizerische medizinische Wochenschrift*, 94:1557-1561, October 31, 1964.

Märki, H. H., and Wuhrmann, F.: Rudimentäre Paraproteinämie. Eine Frühform des multiplen Myeloms?

Schweizerische medizinische Wochenschrift, 93:1381-1387, September 28, 1963.

Michaux, J. L., and Heremans, J. F.: Thirty cases of monoclonal immunoglobulin disorders other than myeloma or macroglobulinemia. A classification of diseases associated with the production of monoclonal-type immunoglobulins. *American Journal of Medicine*, 46:562-579, April 1969.

Olhagen, B., and Liljestrand, A.: Persistently elevated erythrocyte sedimentation rate with good prognosis. *Acta medica scandinavica*, 151:441-449, 1955.

Olmer, J., Mongin, M., Muratore, R., and Denizet, D.: *Myélomes, Macroglobulinémies et Dysglobulinémies Voisines*. Paris, France, Masson et Cie, 1961, 339 pp.

Osserman, E. F., and Takatsuki, K.: Plasma cell myeloma: Gamma globulin synthesis and structure. A review of biochemical and clinical data, with the description of a newly-recognized and related syndrome. Hγ2-chain (Franklin's) disease. *Medicine*, 42:357-384, November 1963.

Rádl, J., and Masopust, J.: Idiopathische Paraproteinämie, *Schweizerische medizinische Wochenschrift*, 94:961-967, July, 1964.

Riva, G.: Idiopathische und Beglietparaproteinämien. *Helvetica medica acta*, 31:285-297, November 1964.

Schobel, B., and Wewalka, F.: Paraproteinämie ohne klinisch nachweisbarem Plasmocytom oder Morbus Waldenström. *Deutsches Archiv für Klinische Medizin*, 207:85-108, 1961.

Smith, E. W.: Nonmyelomatous paraproteinemia. (Abstract) *Clinical Research*, 5:158, 1957.

Spengler, G. A., Roulet, D. L. A., Ricci, C., Schnider, U., Schoop, W., Kappeler, R., and Riva, G.: Paraproteinämie bei chronischer Lymphadenose. *Schweizerische medizinische Wochenschrift*, 91:984-996, August 26; 1025-1029, September 2, 1961.

Videbaek, A., and Drivsholm, A.: Sekundaer paraproteinaemi. *Nordisk Medicin*, 71:124, 1964.

Waldenström, J.: Abnormal proteins in myeloma. *Advances in Internal Medicine*, 5:398-440, 1952.

————: Studies on conditions associated with disturbed gamma globulin formation (gammopathies). *The Harvey Lectures*, Series 56:211-231, 1960-1961.

Zawadzki, Z. A., and Edwards, G. A.: Dysimmunoglobulinemia in the absence of clinical features of multiple myeloma and macroglobulinemia. *American Journal of Medicine*, 42:67-88, January 1967.

CLASSICAL, SYMPTOMATIC IgM MONOCLONAL GAMMOPATHY

DEFINITION.—Patients with the clinical syndrome of macroglobulinemia display the usual classical clinical manifestations of primary macroglobulinemia and high serum concentration of M proteins.

SPECTRUM OF CLINICAL MANIFESTATIONS.—The clinical course in the majority of these patients is relentlessly progressive. The clinical manifestations of macroglobulinemia depend upon (1) the stage of the disease and (2) the special properties of the abnormal IgM.

A frequent complication in patients with classical monoclonal gammopathy is the hyperviscosity syndrome (Fahey, Barth, and Solomon, 1965; Ritzmann, Thurm, Truax, and Levin, 1960; Somer, 1966; Hemodynamic disturbances in macroglobulinemia and myeloma, 1969; Williams, 1968; Kopp, MacKinney, and Wasson, 1969), which is directly attributable to increased serum viscosity, with attendant changes in hemodynamics. Its manifestations, which are aggravated by exposure to cold, include: anorexia, lassitude, dizziness, mucous membrane bleeding, telangiectasia, blurred vision with sausage-shaped retinal veins, Meniere's syndrome, and often, bizarre nervous system involvement.

Hyperviscosity syndrome.—In approximately 25 to 30 per cent of macroglobulinemia patients, the abnormal macroglobulins gel upon cooling (cryogelglobulinemia), as shown in Figure 9. Such cryoglobulins often lead to the serum hyperviscosity syndrome, as do elevated levels of serum viscosity not leading to actual gelling.

CASE 1.—B.Y. (UH#129731-M), a 60-year-old Caucasian male, was in good health until 1960, when he noted weakness, malaise, fatigue, anorexia, dizziness, occasional numbness of toes and tingling of the hands, anterior chest pain exacerbated by exertion, mild dyspnea, and intolerance to cold. Later, he experienced severe epistaxes and urinary tract infections. In 1961, an abnormal serum globulin was identified, and the marrow was infiltrated by lymphoreticular cells. The diagnosis of macroglobulinemia was established by the appropriate studies. The patient was treated with penicillamine, but this agent was discontinued after 10 days because of untoward drug effects. Alkeran was administered for two months, and Leukeran for five months; however, no improvement ensued. In July 1962, severe hepatitis and urticaria developed. All drugs were discontinued until October 1962, when urethan was given for two months without relief. In November 1962, severe hematuria developed in the patient. In December 1962, he was referred to this

FIG. 9.—Macrocryogelglobulinemia, in which the abnormal macroglobulins gel upon cooling.

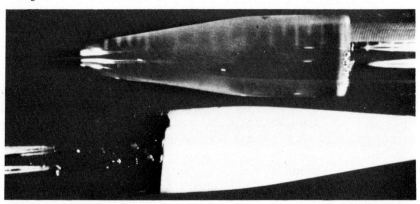

clinic. At that time clinical symptoms were melena, retinal hemorrhages with sausage-like engorgement of the retinal veins, occasional diplopia, decreased visual acuity, facial telangiectases, right-sided deafness, splenomegaly, periorbital and dependent edema, a 30-lb. weight loss, and numbness and tingling of toes and hands. After transfusions and treatment with mercaptopyridoxine for one month, the patient improved considerably with notable regression of weakness, dyspnea, and hemorrhagic manifestations. The serum viscosity (relative to saline viscosity) at $13\,°C$ (η rel $^{13\,°C}$) decreased from 44 to that of 25. Several days later, agranulocytosis developed, and the marrow revealed complete absence of myeloid elements and plasma cells. During the next month, erythromycin, streptomycin, tetracycline, Colymycin, neomycin, kanamycin, Mycostatin, multiple transfusions, and γ-globulin injections were required for the management of infectious complications. White blood cell counts remained low, but the patient improved and was discharged in February 1963, only to be readmitted in May 1963, with severe epistaxis when chilled, weakness, and dyspnea. The patient remained fairly well until September 1963, at which time sudden weakness, malaise, dizziness, and syncope developed. He had moderate lymphadenopathy, but no splenomegaly. After plasmapheresis with 14 units in one month, he was discharged. Two months later, cold weather precipitated the onset of dizziness, exertional dyspnea, weakness, malaise, melena, epistaxis, and visual blurring. Transfusions and plasmapheresis numerous times induced a good clinical remission. Since January 1964, plasmapheresis has been done more than 600 times (Fig. 10). He was monitored by observation of his clinical status and by periodic serum viscosity determinations. He has been maintained almost free of symptoms by regular plasmapheresis on a paramedical basis and long-term chlorambucil (2 mg./day) administration. In 1965, he was able to tolerate herniorrhaphy without incident. He was seen last in November 1969, when he exhibited no clinical complications of Waldenström's macroglobulinemia or hyperviscosity syndrome.

Following the classical description of Wintrobe and Buell (1933), states of hyperviscosity have been observed in patients with a variety of disorders associated with abnormalities of immunoglobulins (Wuhrmann, 1956; Bing and Neel, 1936; Smith, Kochwa, and Wasserman, 1965; Fahey, Barth, and Solomon, 1965; Ritzmann, Coleman, and Levin, 1960; Felten, Regli, and Frick, 1963; Schwab, Okun, and Fahey, 1960; Solomon and Fahey, 1963; Skoog, Adams, and Coburn, 1962; Somer, 1966; Waldenström, 1944, 1952). These include monoclonal gammopathies, especially Waldenström's macroglobulinemia, and certain polyclonal gammopathies, such as rheumatoid arthritis and ill-defined, bizarre collagen diseases.

Mercaptanes have been proposed (Ritzmann, Coleman, and Levin, 1960; Bloch, Prasad, Anastasi, and Brigg, 1960) for the management of manifestations of hyperviscosity associated with Waldenström's macroglobulinemia, but toxicity (Levin and Ritzmann, 1963) and unpredictability of beneficial effects have been observed subsequently. Schwab and associates (Schwab and Fahey, 1960; Schwab, Okun, and Fahey, 1960) demonstrated that the technique of plasmapheresis (Abel, Rowntree, and Turner, 1914) was effective in alleviating clinical manifestations attribut-

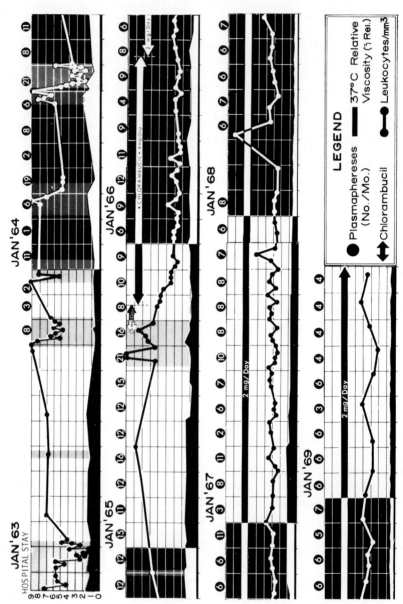

FIG. 10—Synopsis of effects of long-term plasmapheresis upon relative serum viscosity at 37°C and leukocytes.

able to hyperviscosity. Subsequent confirmations (Smith, Kochwa, and Wasserman, 1965; Fahey, Barth, and Solomon, 1965; Solomon and Fahey, 1963; Fahey, 1963; Skoog, Adams, and Coburn, 1962; Kopp, Beirne, and Burns, 1967; Cohen, Bohannon, and Wallerstein, 1966; Hoffmann and Ritzmann, 1965) suggest that this form of management is feasible. Concomitant chemotherapy with clorambucil, melphalan, cyclophosphamide, *etc.*, may suppress the formation of abnormal immunoglobulins and either obviate the need for or reduce the frequency of plasmapheresis.

The therapeutic response in the case study presented is impressive. Almost immediately after initiation of plasmapheresis, listlessness, tiredness, and dizziness disappeared, and the patient experienced a sense of well-being. The bleeding tendency decreased and transfusion requirements were diminished significantly. During the last several years, no blood transfusions have been required. Facial telangiectases receded, engorgement and segmentation of retinal veins disappeared, and visual acuity improved. Two to three months after plasmapheresis was initiated, the spleen no longer could be palpated. Fahey and associates (Fahey, Barth, and Solomon, 1965) studied the frequency and types of symptoms attributable to hyperviscosity in 25 patients with macroglobulinemia. Plasmapheresis was used successfully to reduce the concentration of serum macroglobulins and excessive viscosity, to control symptomatology resulting from hyperviscosity, and to induce subjective and objective improvement. Patient B.Y. also responded favorably to regular plasmaphereses over a prolonged period of time. Disappearance of palpable splenomegaly during the plasmapheresis period without chemotherapy cannot be explained readily.

During the last four years of the plasmapheresis program, the number of bacterial infections experienced by the patient decreased considerably. Inguinal herniorrhaphy was performed without unnecessary loss of blood after hyperviscosity had been reduced. Side effects attributable to plasmapheresis were not observed. The removal of two to four units of plasma once or twice a week was well tolerated. Removal of large amounts of serum proteins with the removal of approximately 180 liters of plasma after undergoing plasmapheresis more than 600 times did not produce adverse clinical manifestations during the 80-month period of plasmapheresis. The loss of approximately 4 kg. of albumin and 15 kg. of abnormal IgM was well tolerated. Paradoxically, the serum albumin concentration after long-term intensive plasmapheresis was slightly higher than at the beginning of treatment.

Thrombocytopenia may be a contraindication to plasmapheresis therapy (Solomon and Fahey, 1963). In our initial evaluation of plasmapheresis, a transient decrease of platelets and leukocytes was seen occasionally. Preservation and reinfusion of the buffy coat layer prevented the appearance of these transient episodes of thrombocytopenia and leukopenia. Furthermore, plasmaphereses performed in several patients with notable thrombocytopenia have not produced untoward effects.

Determination of the frequency of plasmapheresis required by a given patient depends in part upon the "symptomatic" threshold (Fahey, Barth, and Solomon, 1965) or "critical level" of serum viscosity peculiar to that patient. In general, this critical level is below η rel of 10 at 37°C (*i.e.* 10 η rel[37°C]), but often reduction to 5 η rel[37°C] or less is required to maintain the patient in an asymptomatic state. The critical level in the patient described was between 7 and 8 η rel[37°C].

The η rel[37°C] appears to be a reliable guide in planning the schedule of plasmapheresis. Determination of the relative serum viscosity, using an Ostwald's viscosimeter (Ritzmann, Coleman, and Levin, 1960; Fahey, Barth, and Solomon, 1965; Barth, 1964) (Fig. 11), is a simple and reliable technique which can be performed on an outpatient basis.

Technique of viscosimetry. The flow time of freshly obtained serum may be determined by using a viscosimeter of 2- or 5-ml. capacity, and may be calibrated with a corresponding volume of 0.9% saline at 37°C in a waterbath. The viscosity of a given serum usually is expressed in terms relative to the viscosity of normal saline:

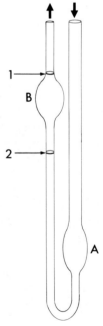

FIG. 11.—Diagram of Ostwald's viscosimeter. The tube is immersed in a 37°C water bath and serum is delivered into reservoir *A*. After equilibration at 37°C, suction is applied until the upper meniscus of the serum is above mark 1. The serum is then allowed to flow freely back into reservoir *A*. The time required for the upper meniscus of the serum to pass between marks 1 and 2 is measured with a stopwatch.

$$\frac{\text{flow time for serum (in seconds)}}{\text{flow time for saline (in seconds)}} = \eta \ rel^{37°C}$$

Normal serum possesses η rel$^{37°C}$ of 1.6 to 1.9. Certain myeloma and macroglobulinemia sera exhibit a relatively high η rel$^{37°C}$, particularly at lower temperatures.

When the critical level of relative viscosity is exceeded in a given patient, the first manifestations are usually increased fatigue and tiredness, recurrence of bleeding, visual and otic disturbances, *etc.* Since the "target" organs (Fahey, Barth, and Solomon, 1965) affected by hyperviscosity are not the same in all patients, it is obvious that such symptoms and signs are specific for the individual patient; hence, these must be evaluated individually.

Concomitant chemotherapy may be useful in that it may decrease the production rate of abnormal immunoglobulins. This may be sufficient to lower serum viscosity, thus decreasing the frequency of, or even obviating the necessity for plasmapheresis. Chlorambucil on a low-dosage, long-term basis has been reported to be beneficial in the treatment of patients with Waldenström's macroglobulinemia (Clatanoff and Meyer, 1963; McCallister, Bayrd, Harrison, and McGuckian, 1967). After the addition of chlorambucil to the therapeutic regimen in this patient, the plasmapheresis requirements were decreased during the last 50 months. Initially, removal of three to four units of plasma was required weekly, but subsequent to supplementary chlorambucil administration, two plasmapheresis procedures per week were sufficient to maintain η rel below the critical level. In December 1967, the plasmapheresis requirements were reduced further to one and two procedures during alternate weeks.

Thermoprotein properties of IgM-M proteins.—The abnormal IgM in patients with macroglobulinemia may exhibit temperature-dependent behavior. Thermoproteins are those immunoglobulins (Wert, 1964) with unusual physical characteristics at temperatures below or above 37°C; these include (1) cryoglobulins, (2) pyroglobulins, and (3) Bence Jones proteins. The presence of such proteins in the serum frequently indicates an underlying monoclonal gammopathy. The IgM of macroglobulinemia often possesses such characteristics.

1. Cryoglobulins (Lerner and Watson, 1947; Hansen and Faber, 1947) are immunoglobulins which gel or precipitate, usually reversibly, at low temperatures (Fig. 9). At least five categories of cryoglobulins have been identified (Meltzer and Franklin, 1966; LoSpalluto, Dorward, Miller, and Ziff, 1962; Auscher and Guinand, 1964; Kritzman, Fudenberg, and Liss, 1966; Ritzmann and Levin, 1969; Peetoom and van Loghem-Langereis, 1965; Lewis, Ommen, and Page, 1966; Wager, Mustakallio, and Räsänen, 1968). They include: (1) 7S IgG, usually in association with multiple my-

eloma, (2) 19S IgM, usually associated with Waldenström's macroglobulinemia or lymphosarcoma, (3) rare instances of IgA, (4) Bence Jones proteins, and (5) mixed types of cryoglobulins including IgA-IgG, IgM-lipoproteins, and 19S IgM-7S IgG.

Cryoglobulinemia was encountered 15 times among 48 of our cases of macroglobulinemia examined, *i.e.,* an incidence of approximately 30 per cent. Clinical manifestations of the hyperviscosity syndrome were found in three of the 48 patients as well as in two others without cryoglobulinemia, *i.e.* in approximately 10 per cent of all cases with macroglobulinemia. In temperate climates, this incidence may be higher.

2. Pyroglobulins are immunoglobulins which irreversibly precipitate or gel at 56°C (Martin and Mathieson, 1953; Martin, Mathieson, and Eigler, 1959; Solomon and Steinfield, 1965; Ritzmann, Thurm, and Levin, 1963). Like the cryoglobulins, pyroglobulins may appear as M proteins on serum electrophoresis. The clinical significance of pyroglobulinemia is unknown. Pyroglobulinemia usually is detected when inactivating serum complement at 56°C for serological testing for syphilis (anticomplementary activity).

Of the 48 patients with macroglobulinemia examined, pyroglobulinemia was found in four; both cryoglobulinemia and pyroglobulinemia were found in one of these four.

3. *Bence Jones* proteins (Bence Jones, 1848; Osserman, Takatsuki, and Talal, 1964; Kyle and Bayrd, 1961; Bernier and Putnam, 1964), in contrast to pyroglobulins, are reversibly precipitable between 40 and 60°C. In patients with plasmacytic dyscrasias, testing the urine for Bence Jones proteins is an integral part of protein analysis. The detection of Bence Jones proteins may be a diagnostic clue to an underlying amyloidosis, since the association of this condition with Bence Jones proteins has been noted frequently.

Bence Jones proteins, or free light chains, were encountered in four of our 71 patients with IgM monoclonal gammopathy. In these, there was no definite evidence of associated renal impairment or amyloidosis. In fact, in one idiopathic, asymptomatic macroglobulinemia patient, Bence Jones proteinuria was detected.

In other patients with macroglobulinemia, the chief clinical manifestations may be the result of antibody activity of the abnormal IgM. In 47 macroglobulinemia sera, seven instances of high cold agglutinin titers (up to 2,000,000) and seven instances of high titers of rheumatoid factor activity (up to 163,000) were found (Table 4). None of the latter seven patients exhibited clinical manifestations of rheumatoid arthritis. This is an interesting observation, since the IgM rheumatoid factors constitute autoantibodies to IgG (Franklin, Holman, Müller-Eberhard, and Kunkel, 1957). They tend to form IgG-IgM complexes, which often lead to hyperviscosity and cryoglobulinemia. The abnormal macroglobulins harboring the

TABLE 4.—SEROLOGICAL ACTIVITY OF SERA FROM
14 OF 47 PATIENTS WITH MACROGLOBULINEMIA

PATIENTS	COLD AGGLUTININS (RECIPROCAL TITERS, 4°C)	PATIENTS	RHEUMATOID FACTORS (RECIPROCAL LATEX TITERS)
W.D.	2,000,000	H.S.	163,840
M.H.	2,000,000	A.T.*	40,960
H.D.	262,144	E.P.*	40,960
A.J.	131,072	R.A.*	20,480
C.C.	65,536	H.B.*	10,240
M.S.*	32,768	F.W.*	10,240
E.M.	16,384	M.S.†	5,120

*Positive for cryoglobulins. †Positive for pyroglobulins.

high cold agglutinin or rheumatoid factor antibody activities may be considered to be the products of unique IgM-cell clones which specialize in the formation of these antibodies. Consequently, such patients may be considered to represent cases of unique clonal forms of macroglobulinemia, namely the "rheumatoid factor clonal form" and the "cold agglutinin clonal form" of macroglobulinemia (Levin and Ritzmann, 1966).

Cold agglutinin disease.—An example of the cold agglutinin clonal form of macroglobulinemia, or *cold agglutinin disease,* is as follows:

CASE 2.—W.D. (UH#21433-M) was a 65-year-old Caucasian male who experienced cyanosis, numbness, pain, and coldness of the fingers upon exposure to cold, symptoms which were relieved by warming. In 1956, he experienced episodic passage of dark urine. In February 1956, the patient was admitted to John Sealy Hospital. The hemoglobin concentration was 8 g./100 ml. and the cold agglutinin titer was 1:2,000,000. The marrow revealed erythroid hyperplasia and a slight increase in lymphoid elements. Diverticulosis of the colon was demonstrated radiographically. During the next several years, the patient required multiple blood transfusions and symptomatic treatment of hemolytic crises precipitated by chilling. In 1957, corticosteroids were administered. The serum protein electrophoresis pattern revealed a γ-globulin spike of 33 per cent of a total serum protein concentration of 5.3 g./100 ml. Persistent hepatosplenomegaly and nerve deafness were observed. In May 1959, treatment with penicillamine produced a reduction of the cold agglutinin titer. In December 1959, a basal cell carcinoma of the left arm and an epidermoid carcinoma of the periauricular skin were diagnosed by examination of biopsy tissue. During this admission, bilateral herniorrhaphy was followed by chilling and a hemolytic crisis requiring multiple transfusions. In February 1961, the patient was admitted for acute cholelithiasis and received transfusions. In May 1961, he again received transfusions. In March 1962, the patient was readmitted with a history of passing red urine for about a year, intermittent chills and fever, and jaundice. Serum protein electrophoresis revealed a sharp peak in the γ-globulin fraction. This was identified as IgM by immunoelectrophoresis. The marrow revealed hyperplasia of lymphoreticular cells. The hemoglobin level was 5.7 g./100 ml., the direct Coombs test was positive, and the red cell half-life (T/2) was 13 days. There was prominent hepatosplenomegaly. Splenectomy, cholecystectomy and exploration of the common bile duct were performed. Postoperatively, the patient manifested persistent fever, jaundice, and a toxic state thought to result from bacteremia secondary to biliary exploration. A T-tube cholangiogram was within normal limits. On the sixth postoperative day, the patient's blood pressure became unstable and he exhibited muscle fasciculations. His clinical state deteriorated rapidly and he died on July 9, 1962. An autopsy was not performed.

Cold agglutinins are blood group antibodies usually of anti-I-specificity (van Loghem et al., 1962; Marsh, 1961), but rarely of the anti-H, anti-O, or anti-i variety (Marsh, 1961). I-antigen is found on erythrocytes of almost all adult human beings in low titers, whereas erythrocytes, during the first few months of life, show the i phenotype which is gradually replaced by I-antigens (van Loghem et al., 1962; Marsh, 1961). Cold agglutinins are γ-globulins on electrophoresis (Christenson and Dacie, 1957; Stats, Perlman, Bullowa, and Goodkind, 1943), sediment in the ultracentrifuge as 19S macroglobulins (Charlwood, 1957; Fudenberg and Kunkel, 1957; Ritzmann and Levin, 1962), and immunoelectrophoretically are of the IgM class (Christenson and Dacie, 1957; Gordon, 1953; Harboe and Deverill, 1964; Mehrotra, 1960). They may be depolymerized and inactivated by mercaptanes (Fudenberg and Kunkel, 1957; Leddy, Trabold, Vaughan, and Swisher, 1962; Ritzmann and Levin, 1961).

The light chain type of the monoclonal cold agglutinins in cold agglutinin disease is of the K type (Harboe et al., 1965) (i.e. monotypical), although exceptions occur (Gabl et al., 1969). This is in contrast to cold agglutinins present normally or occurring in increased titers in certain patients with mycoplasma pneumonii infections which are polyclonal in nature and consist of both K- and L-type light chains (Feizi, 1967; Harboe, 1965).

The serologic properties of cold agglutinins are characterized by a temperature-titer relationship. Maximal erythrocyte agglutination is observed at 0°C, with decreasing activity at higher temperature ranges and absence of agglutination above 30 to 32°C (Schubothe, 1966) (Fig. 12). Upon rewarming, deagglutination of erythrocytes occurs. In the presence of complement, maximum hemolysis occurs at 22°C (Schubothe, 1966). Agglutination and hemolysis are apparent at the same temperature. This "monothermic" behavior of cold agglutinins is distinct from the "bithermic" characteristics of Donath-Landsteiner cold hemolysins which require a two-temperature stepwise mechanism, i.e. antibody fixation at low temperature ranges and hemolysis at higher temperature ranges (between 30 and 40°C) (Dacie, 1962; Schubothe, 1966).

Reversible or transient increases of cold agglutinin titers with, or without acute hemolytic anemia, are observed in certain patients with *Mycoplasma*

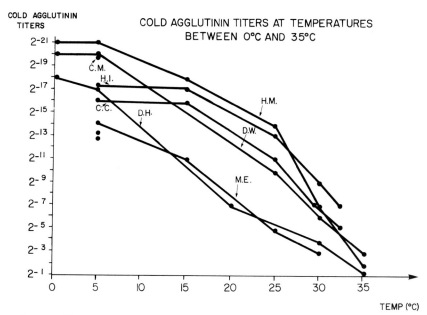

COLD AGGLUTININ
TITERS

COLD AGGLUTININ TITERS AT TEMPERATURES
BETWEEN 0°C AND 35°C

TEMP (°C)

FIG. 12.—Titer-temperature relationship of cold agglutinins in sera from patients with cold agglutinin disease.

pneumoniae infections (Dacie, 1962; Schubothe, 1966). Moderate to marked increases may be associated with certain lymphoproliferative disorders (Dacie, 1962; Schubothe, 1966). In the primary form of cold agglutinin increase, the cold agglutinin disease (Ritzmann and Levin, 1962), the cold agglutinin titers are usually high, sometimes reaching 1:2,000,000 (Table 4). In such patients, there is marked cold hypersensitivity or cryopathy (Ritzmann and Levin, 1961) reflected by pallor and/or acrocyanosis, often with numbness of ear lobes, nose, lips, *etc.* (this is reversible upon warming), seasonally fluctuating hemolytic anemia and jaundice with maxima during the winter months (Dacie, 1962; Schubothe, 1966), and hemoglobinuria. This disease must be considered in the differential diagnosis of Raynaud's phenomenon or cryopathies (Ritzmann and Levin, 1961). Usually, hepatosplenomegaly and discrete lymphadenopathy are present, a marked lymphoplasmacytic proliferation may be seen, and the bone marrow contains increased numbers of lymphoid plasma cells (Fudenberg and Kunkel, 1957; Schubothe, 1966; Ritzmann and Levin, 1962).

The age and sex distributions of cold agglutinin disease in 64 patients (Schubothe, 1966) reveal a maximum occurrence between 51 and 60 years and preponderance in males.

Cold agglutinin disease is a special form of Waldenström's macroglobulinemia (Schubothe, 1966; Ritzmann and Levin, 1962), or more specifically, a "clonal type" of macroglobulinemia (Levin and Ritzmann, 1966) *(i.e.,* a form of macroglobulinemia in which the cold agglutinin-active, lymphoid plasma cell clone is proliferating, producing a monoclonal cold agglutinin-active IgM).

The treatment of patients with cold agglutinin disease is challenging. Careful avoidance of cold temperatures and abstaining from cold drinks and foods are mandatory. Moving to warmer climates may have to be considered. Attempts at therapy using splenectomy, adrenocorticotropic hormone (ACTH), corticosteroids, cytotoxic drugs, *etc.* have failed (Dacie, 1962; Schubothe, 1966). Improvement following mercaptane administration (penicillamine, mercaptopyridoxine) has been observed (Ritzmann and Levin, 1961), although beneficial effects have not been noted by others (Dacie, 1962; Schubothe, 1966; Lind, Mansa, and Olesen, 1962). Supportive measures include blood transfusions. Long-term treatment with cyclophosphamide has been found promising (Schubothe, 1966), as in other forms of macroglobulinemia (Klemm, Schubothe, and Hunstein, 1964; Cass, Anderson, and Vaughan, 1969; Bouroncle, Datta, and Frajola, 1964), as has treatment with chlorambucil (Olesen, 1964).

Autoimmune warm-type hemolytic anemia.—Autoimmune hemolytic anemia, unrelated to cold agglutinins, may also occur in macroglobulinemia.

CASE 3.—J.C.B. (UH#37434-P) was a 61-year-old Caucasian male who was admitted to John Sealy Hospital in November 1964 with complaints of weakness, dyspnea, and massive anasarca for the previous seven months. Transient symptoms similar to these had been experienced for 10 to 15 years. Physical examination revealed diffuse matted lymphadenopathy, splenomegaly, and a gallop rhythm. Bilateral pleural effusion and cardiomegaly compatible with congestive heart failure were present. The hemoglobin was 3.4 g./100 ml. The anemia was normochromic-normocytic and a reticulosis of 11.4 per cent was seen. The direct Coombs' test and the non-γ-Coombs' test were positive. Lymph node biopsy and marrow biopsy revealed histological patterns compatible with lymphocytic lymphosarcoma. A tall homogeneous spike on serum protein electrophoresis was identified as IgM by immunoelectrophoresis and ultracentrifugation. Diagnoses of Waldenström's macroglobulinemia with severe anemia and congestive heart failure were made. Cardiac decompensation was treated with digitalis, diuretics, and transfusions, and the patient's clinical status improved. Despite transfusions, the hemoglobin level fell repeatedly. Autoimmune hemolytic anemia, responsive to prednisone, was considered to be present. The cold agglutinin titer was 1:16 and serum viscosity was at the upper limits of normal. A course of Alkeran therapy was administered. Shortly thereafter, the patient experienced manifestations of a urinary tract infection; an *Escherichia coli* bacteremia which responded to antibiotics and administration of γ-globulin was documented. In January 1966, the patient was readmitted with severe anemia (hemoglobin 4.5 g./100 ml.) and a *Pseudomonas aeruginosa* pneumonia which responded to ampicillin. The patient received transfusions and was started on Alkeran, which was discontinued shortly because of leukopenia. After recovery of the marrow, Leukeran therapy was begun. In the summer of 1966, the patient died at home without the cause of death being reported.

Hemolytic anemia of autoimmune nature is occasionally encountered in patients with macroglobulinemia (Levin and Ritzmann, 1966; Fankhauser, Arnold, Schaub, and Lapp, 1956; Wilde and Hitzelberger, 1954; Cline, Solomon, Berlin, and Fahey, 1963; McCallister, Bayrd, Harrison, and McGuckian, 1967). The judicious use of corticosteroids and the administration of chemotherapy for the macroglobulinemic process appear indicated under these circumstances. This probably is the only indication for corticosteroids in macroglobulinemia.

Multiple malignant conditions and Gram-negative septicemias.—An extraordinarily high percentage of patients with macroglobulinemia develops epithelial malignant disorders, 25 per cent in our series. Additionally, the incidence of gram-negative infections is impressive.

CASE 4.—S.K. (UH # 102588-M) was a 67-year-old Caucasian male who was first seen because of scaly encrusted lesions of the forearm and face. This was diagnosed as actinic keratosis, and basal cell carcinomas were demonstrated by biopsy of several lesions. The patient was admitted several times in 1961 and 1962 for removal of multiple basal cell carcinomas of the face, and for excision of squamous cell carcinomas of the left ear and right cheek. Residual basal cell carinomas were removed later. The hemogram was normal during this period. Late in 1962, the patient was admitted with severe anemia (hemoglobin 5.0 g./100 ml.) and pancytopenia. Recurrence of both squamous cell and basal cell carcinomas was evident. Multiple marrow aspirations and bone biopsies demonstrated proliferation of lymphoid elements. A conclusive diagnosis could not be made. The patient received many transfusions. He was admitted two months later with bleeding gums, numerous petechiae, and ecchymoses. The patient was discharged after transfusions and given prednisone and testosterone. In March 1963, the patient was admitted with complaints of dizziness and weakness, again manifesting anemia and pancytopenia. Petechiae and ecchymoses were generalized, fundoscopy revealed hemorrhages and exudates, and pitting edema, splenomegaly, and lymphadenopathy were present. The total serum proteins were 12.5 g./100 ml. A tall M protein was identified on serum electrophoresis, and immunoelectrophoresis confirmed the clinical diagnosis of macroglobulinemia. The patient required multiple transfusions and the clinical course was complicated by numerous infections. In June 1963, the patient was admitted with hypotension, fever, and symptoms of a urinary tract infection. The patient died two hours following hospitalization. Blood cultures revealed *E. coli* and *P. aeuriginosa*. Autopy findings were compatible with the diagnosis of Waldenström's macroglobulinemia, and the direct cause of death was attributed to gram-negative septicemia.

An increased incidence of epithelial cancers has been documented in patients with macroglobulinemia (Schaub, 1953; for additional references, see Ritzmann and Levin, 1967, 1969).

This incidence is remarkable since patients with myeloma do not appear to experience a high rate of such tumors (Ritzmann and Levin, 1967, 1969). It is tempting to assume that the emergence of malignant conditions in such patients is the result of the IgM deficiency, but the reverse—the development of IgM monoclonal gammopathy in response to epithelial tumors—cannot be excluded.

Patients with macroglobulinemia may display an extraordinary susceptibility to gram-negative microorganisms. IgM contains the majority of antibody activity to gram-negative germs, and the low levels of normal or residual IgM in such patients may explain this tendency. The treatment of such infectious complications requires prompt attention and the administration of the appropriate antibiotics, and in selected cases, γ-globulin substitution. Since commercially available γ-globulin preparations do not contain appreciable amounts of IgM, the use of plasma may have to be considered (Stiehm, Vaerman, and Fudenberg, 1966).

Biclonal gammopathy (IgM and IgG).—Macroglobulinemia is rarely associated with an additional M protein, *i.e.* biclonal gammopathy.

CASE 5.—C.T. (UH#54597-M) was a 66-year-old Negro male who presented with a firm mass in the right anterior chest wall and pain in the left hip and leg in 1958. Biopsies of pectoralis muscle and breast tissue revealed Hodgkin's sarcoma. There was radiologic evidence of destruction of the third rib and collapse of the fifth lumbar vertebra. Small osteolytic lesions of the skull were seen, but long bone x-ray films, intravenous pyelograms (IVP), and barium enema and upper gastrointestinal series were normal. Hemogram and urinalysis were normal and there was no evidence of Bence Jones proteinuria. Total serum protein concentration was 7.2 g./100 ml., comprised of 4.5 g./100 ml. albumin and 2.7 g./100 ml. globulins; paper electrophoresis showed no M protein spike. External irradiation of the right chest and lumbar spine induced disappearance of the mass from the chest wall and relief of bone and radicular pain. Soon thereafter the patient experienced thoracic pain, recurrence of pain in the left leg, x-ray evidence of T_3-T_4 vertebral involvement, and compression at L_3 through L_5. Additional radiotherapy was delivered to the spine. Serum paper electrophoresis again did not show definite evidence of an M protein; however, ultracentrifugation indicated an elevated 19S M_1 component and the presence of a 22S M_2 component. Immunoelectrophoresis revealed evidence of IgG myeloma protein, type L, and IgM macroglobulinemia protein, type L.* Cryoglobulin and pyroglobulin determinations were negative. Serum viscosity was normal. Subsequently, the patient developed signs of arteriosclerotic cardiovascular disease, hypertension, and eventually congestive heart failure, with aortic insufficiency, and mild Parkinsonism. In September 1969, the patient, then 77 years old, was reported to be in satisfactory condition.

The presence of two M proteins, *i.e.* biclonal gammopathy (Waldenström, 1961; Engle and Nachman, 1966; Burtin *et al.,* 1957; Sanders *et al.,* 1969), and three M proteins, *i.e.* triclonal gammopathy (Sanders *et al.,* 1969), has been reported. On serum electrophoresis, the M proteins may be inconspicuous; immunoelectrophoretic analysis is essential for their detection (Sanders *et al.,* 1969). This case demonstrates that biclonal gammopa-

---

*We are grateful to Dr. William Terry, National Cancer Institute, Immunoglobulin Reference Center, Springfield, Virginia, for confirmation of these findings.

thy may be compatible with long survival. In general, the predominant abnormal immunoglobulin appears to determine the clinical manifestations. In this case, the concentration of the IgG myeloma protein exceeded that of the IgM macroglobulinemia protein, and the clinical manifestations were those of classical myeloma. No marked progression has ensued, and the serum protein concentrations have remained relatively stable during the last decade, suggesting that the IgM component may be of the idiopathic type.

Spontaneous remission.—Macroglobulinemia is either progressive or unremittingly nonprogressive. Rarely, however, regressions do occur.

Case 6.—(Ritzmann *et al.*, in preparation).—E.P. (UH#42515-P) is a 65-year-old man who was first seen in 1965 complaining of weakness and purpuric lesions. The platelet level and bleeding and clotting times were normal, and the tourniquet test was negative. During the next few months, the patient experienced weight loss, a hemorrhagic diathesis (with epistaxis and bleeding of oral mucosa), severe anemia (hemoglobin 6.8 g./100 ml.), partial deafness, engorged "sausage-like" retinal veins, moderate axillary and inguinal lymphadenopathy, slight splenomegaly, and cryopathy. Total serum proteins were 7.0 g./100 ml. and the serum electrophoresis pattern was characterized by a conspicuous spike in the mid-γ fraction, and, on ultracentrifugation, by two broad-shouldered intermediate fractions and a large 19S M_1 and moderate 22S M_2 component. Immunoelectrophoresis exhibited a markedly increased IgM globulin precipitin line. The serum gelled at room temperature. No Bence Jones proteins could be detected in either serum or urine, and a rheumatoid factor-latex titer of 1:40,000 was present (Table 4). The bone marrow indicated a lymphoproliferative disorder. Skull films revealed nasal septal destruction, and there was radiologic evidence of involvement of the radius. Chromosomal abnormalities, characterized by aneuploidy, endoreduplication, and presence of the submetacentric monoclonal gammopathy chromosomes were seen in lymphocyte cultures. A diagnosis of Waldenström's macroglobulinemia with hyperviscosity syndrome and 19S IgM to 7S IgG complex-type cryoglobulinemia was established. Despite administration of prednisone, blood transfusions, and the performance of plasmaphereses, the serum viscosity continued to rise, and clinical evidence of the hyperviscosity syndrome (increased bleeding tendency, blurred vision, dizziness, partial deafness, stocking paralysis of both feet and hands) became predominant.

Additional plasmaphereses were followed by reduction of serum viscosity. In August 1965, the patient was discharged and continued plasmaphereses were advised. In January 1966, he experienced a severe episode of serum hepatitis, from which he gradually improved. In June 1966, the patient felt well and had regained much of his strength, except for residual weakness of both hands. At this time, there was no evidence of the hyperviscosity syndrome, the monoclonal gammopathy had disappeared (Fig. 13), and the marrow and chromosome patterns were normal. In March 1967, the serum protein pattern was normal and the rheumatoid factor-latex titer was 1:320. The serum immunoglobulin levels were: IgG, 1,659 g./100 ml.; IgA, 160 g./100 ml.; and IgM, 364 g./100 ml. In July 1969, the patient was clinically well and exhibited none of the stigmata of Waldenström's macroglobulinemia. No abnormal chromosomes were encountered. It seemed that a spontaneous remission of Waldenström's macroglobulinemia had followed the serum hepatitis.

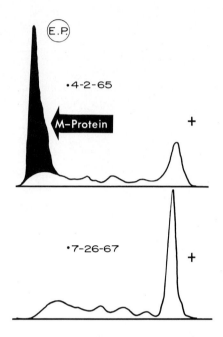

FIG. 13.—Spontaneous remission of macroglobulinemia coincident with serum hepatitis.

In this case, differential reduction studies were performed to rule out a complex disease ("pseudo"-macroglobulinemia) (Ritzmann and Levin, 1967). Serum was incubated with (1) 0.14 M NaCl (control), (2) 6 M urea, (3) pH 4.0 formate buffer, and (4) 0.1 M mercaptoethanol, as reported previously (Kunkel, Müller-Eberhard, Fudenberg, and Tomasi, 1961). The results were as follows: (1) control serum contained 1.55 g./100 ml. of 7S component, 2.96 g./100 ml. of 19S M_1 component, 1.19 g./100 ml. of 24 to 26S M_2 component, and a trace of a 32S M_3 component; (2) after incubation with 6 M urea, the M_1 component remained unchanged, the M_2 component had decreased slightly, and the M_3 component had disappeared; (3) following treatment with pH 4.0 formate buffer, the M_1, M_2, and M_3 components were unaltered; and (4) incubation with 0.1 M mercaptoethanol resulted in the disappearance of the M_3 and M_2 components with the M_1 component present as a tiny fraction; a small broad-shouldered intermediate fraction appeared concomitant with a marked increase of the 7S component (Fig. 14). These results further supported the diagnosis of a true IgM monoclonal gammopathy.

IgM molecules are readily depolymerized to smaller units of 7.4 to 7.6 $S_{20,w}^{o}$ (Albert and Johnson, 1961; Reisner and Franklin, 1961; Deutsch and Morton, 1957; Glenchur, Zinneman, and Briggs, 1958) by a number of sulfhydryl reagents which cleave the disulfide bonds in the molecule. This

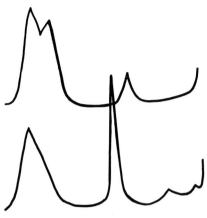

Fig. 14.—Differential reduction of macromolecular components, analyzed by serum ultracentrifugation. *Bottom panel:* control serum incubated with 0.14 M NaCl. The characteristic macroglobulinemia pattern is seen, *i.e.* large peaked 19S, moderate 24S, and small 32S components. *Top panel:* serum incubated with 0.1 M mercaptoethanol. The 19S component is markedly decreased and the 24S and 32S components have disappeared concomitantly with a corresponding increase of the 7S component. Incubation with 6 M urea and pH 4.0 formate buffer did not appreciably alter the original pattern. Such a reaction pattern of depolymerization of the macromolecular fractions supports the diagnosis of IgM monoclonal gammopathy.

process is usually accompanied by loss of antibody activity (Grubb and Swahn, 1958). IgM fractions which are dissociated by mercaptanes are usually unaffected by 6 M urea or acid buffers (Kunkel, Müller-Eberhard, Fudenberg, and Tomasi, 1961; Ritzmann and Levin, 1967). Rheumatoid factor complexes similar to those described by Kunkel, Müller-Eberhard, Fudenberg, and Tomasi (1961) of the polyclonal gammopathy type are usually cleaved by 6 M urea and acid buffers, but not by mercaptanes. These rheumatoid factor complexes may be intermediate (9 to 17S) and/or high molecular (greater than 19S). Such complexes have been observed in patients with rheumatoid arthritis, nonthrombocytopenic purpura, Sjögren's and Felty's syndromes, and bizarre collagen or autoimmune diseases (Kunkel, Müller-Eberhard, Fudenberg, and Tomasi, 1961; Tomasi, 1965; Bloch, Buchanan, Wohl, and Bunim, 1965; Ritzmann and Levin, 1967), some of which have been mistaken for chronic lymphocytic leukemia and Waldenström's macroglobulinemia (Ritzmann and Levin, 1967). "Macroglobulinemia spuria Kunkel," "spurious" or "pseudo" paraproteinemia, and pseudo-M proteins are terms which have been suggested for this condition, but which must be differentiated from true Waldenström's macroglobulinemia associated with high rheumatoid arthritis factor activity of the M protein type (*i.e.* "rheumatoid factor clonal type" of macroglobulinemia) (Ritzmann and Levin, 1967, 1969).

Characterization of isolated monoclonal IgM.—The IgM was isolated from the patient's serum* (for details, see Ritzmann *et al.*, in preparation. Anti-γ-globulin (rheumatoid factor) activity was demonstrable in the macroglobulin preparation. Strong precipitates were formed with heat-aggregated

*We are indebted to Dr. R. E. Schrohenloher, Department of Medicine, University of Alabama Medical College, Birmingham, Alabama, for the immunochemical studies.

pooled normal human γ-globulin. Anti-γ-globulin activity was also evident by the latex fixation, sensitized human cell, and sensitized sheep cell tests. Only those fractions which contained the macroglobulin components precipitated aggregated γ-globulin and agglutinated latex particles coated with human IgG. Similarly, the anti-γ-globulin activity was shown to be associated with, and confined to, the macroglobulin by preparative zone electrophoresis in starch.

The formation of a cryoglobulin fraction which contained both IgM and IgG and which was insoluble in saline suggested that the cryoprecipitate formed by the serum was of the IgM and IgG types. The high anti-γ-globulin activity of the isolated IgM proteins emphasized the fact that the IgM was the active component of the cryoprecipitate. Direct evidence that the cryoprecipitate was the reactive product of the monoclonal IgM-K with inactive IgG was provided by observation of the formation of a strong precipitate of the isolated macroglobulin and the patient's own IgG or pooled normal IgG. Additional studies on the reaction of the monoclonal IgM from this patient, with proteolytic fragments of IgG, indicated that it also reacted with structures in the Fc-fragment. These results indicate that the monoclonal IgM possessed biologic activity of the anti-γ-globulin variety.

Biologic activity of M proteins.—At present, it is unknown whether the M proteins are abnormal immunoglobulins or simply excessively increased immunoglobulins normally present in trace quantities. Increasing circumstantial evidence appears to favor the latter alternative. This is based mainly upon the finding of serological (*i.e.* specific antibody) activity in certain M proteins. Harboe (1965) has defined criteria for biologically active monoclonal IgM. These include: (1) very high titered serological activity of serum and a large homogeneous peak on zone electrophoresis, (2) demonstration, by preparative electrophoresis, of maximal serological activity in the center segments of the peak, (3) identical electrophoretic mobility of the isolated serologically active proteins and the peak, and (4) complete disappearance of the peak following absorption. Several cases of typical Waldenström's macroglobulinemia have been described in which the monocloncal macroglobulin possessed serological activity, even when judged by these strict criteria: cold agglutinin activity (Fudenberg and Kunkel, 1957), ability to fix complement in the presence of extracts of various human organs (Mackay, 1959), rheumatoid factor activity (Kritzman, Kunkel, McCarthy, and Mellors, 1961), and the ability to agglutinate stored but not fresh erythrocytes (Ozer and Chaplin, 1963; Schubothe, Klemm, and Conraths, 1965).

In patient E.P., Harboe's criteria for biologic activity of M proteins appear fulfilled. Forty-seven macroglobulinemic sera have been assayed for a variety of antibody activities, including anti-A and anti-B isohemagglu-tinins, cold agglutinins, rheumatoid factors, Wassermann, heterophile, and Rh-saline antibodies. Seven instances were found with cold agglutinin titers, and seven with rheumatoid factor activity (Table 4). None of the latter patients displayed clinical manifestations of rheumatoid arthritis. tis.

It is of interest that five of the seven sera with high rheumatoid factor activity were positive for cryoglobulins (Table 4) and one additional serum was positive for pyroglobulins. This high incidence may suggest a causal relationship. It can only be suggested that they were all of the rheumatoid factor clonal type of macroglobulinemia.The reaction between the pathological IgM and autologous IgG may be viewed as an autoim-mune process (Peetoom and van Loghem-Langereis, 1965) leading to dis-ease manifestations often more incapacitating than the underlying macroglobulinemia itself. It is of interest that the cold agglutinin clonal type of macroglobulinemia (*i.e.* cold agglutinin disease) also constitutes an au-toimmune disorder, within the boundaries of the syndrome of macroglobulinemia.

Disappearance of M proteins.—In patient E. P., a gradual disappearance of all manifestations of macroglobulinemia occurred following the recovery from a severe episode of infectious hepatitis. In general, M proteins do not regress spontaneously, although exceptions occur. Disappearance of M pro-teins has been reported without obvious cause (Nutter and Kramer, 1965; Anderson and Ferriman, 1960), following the surgical removal of a breast tumor (Bohard, 1957) and a parathyroid tumor (Clubb, Posen, and Neale, 1964), after the cure of certain infections (Michaux and Heremans, 1969; Laroche *et al.*, 1964; Hobbs, 1966; Hällén, 1966), after the correction of folic acid deficiency (Roman and Coles, 1966), and coincident with hepatitis (Osserman and Takatsuki, 1965; London, 1955; and possibly Case 9 of Cohen, Bohannon, and Wallerstein, 1966). It is tempting to implicate the hepatitic process in the induction of remission in these cases, though the mechanism responsible for such a phenomenon would be completely un-known.

MANAGEMENT OF MACROGLOBULINEMIA

The treatment for patients with macroglobulinemia requires an indi-vidualized approach. Examples of this are provided by the selected case summaries. In general, patients with idiopathic, asymptomatic forms of macroglobulinemia require no therapy, whereas those with classical, symp-tomatic macroglobulinemia need active therapy. Basically, treatment should be directed toward suppression of the proliferating IgM-producing immu-nocytes. Reduction of the number of such plasma cells is generally followed

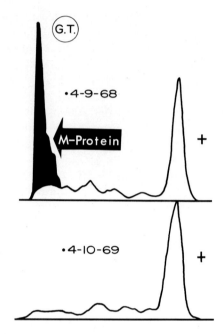

FIG. 15.—Effect of long-term chlorambucil treatment upon serum concentration of IgM M proteins.

by a corresponding decrease of the M proteins (Brecher, Tanaka, Malmgren, and Fahey, 1964).

CHEMOTHERAPY.—Chiorambucil (Bayrd, 1961; Clatanoff and Meyer, 1963; McCallister, Bayrd, Harrison, and McGuckian, 1967; Olesen, 1964; Cohen, Bohannon, and Wallerstein, 1966) and cyclophosphamide (Klemm, Schubothe, and Hunstein, 1964; Schubothe, Kitahama, Klemm, and Erpenbeck, 1965; Bouroncle, Datta, and Frajola, 1964; Cass, Anderson, and Vaughan, 1969) have been found the most effective agents for macroglobulinemia. It is necessary that these agents be administered on a low-dose, long-term basis. At least 18 months of administration should be allowed before a failure to respond is accepted. Treatment with these agents may result in a decrease or even disappearance of the M proteins. The effectiveness of chlorambucil is exemplified by Figure 15. Over a prolonged treatment period, the abnormal macroglobulin peak decreased and eventually disappeared. The patient's general condition improved remarkably.

PLASMAPHERESIS.—Plamapheresis has emerged as the treatment of choice in macroglobulinemia complicated by the serum hyperviscosity syndrome (Solomon and Fahey, 1963; Schwab and Fahey, 1960). A simple plasmapheresis technique has been developed in our institution which is applicable on a paramedical basis in the home of the patient. It can be supervised by nurses (Hoffmann and Ritzmann, 1965) (Fig. 16).

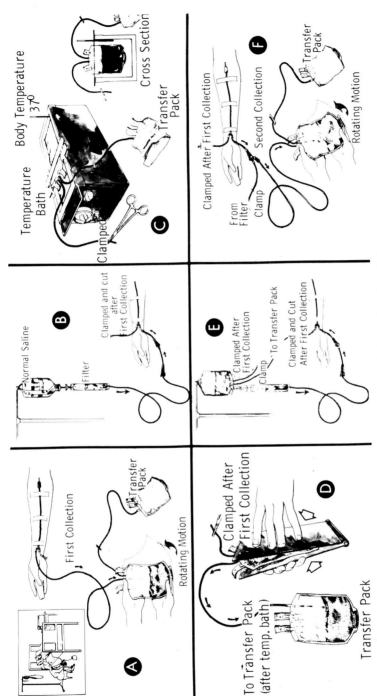

Temperature Bath

Body Temperature 37°

Cross Section

Transfer Pack

Clamped

C

Normal Saline

Filter

Clamped and cut after First Collection

B

Clamped After First Collection

Second Collection

From Filter

Clamp

Rotating Motion

Transfer Pack

F

First Collection

Transfer Pack

Rotating Motion

A

Clamped After First Collection

Clamp

To Transfer Pack

Clamped and Cut After First Collection

E

Clamped After First Collection

To Transfer Pack (after temp. bath)

Transfer Pack

D

Fig. 16.—A–F, simplified plasmapheresis technique.

Technique of plasmapheresis.—Venous blood is obtained by phlebotomy and collected by gravity into a Fenwal plasmapheresis bag. After collecting 500 ml. of blood, the bag is disconnected and placed in a 37°C waterbath for quick separation of plasma. A second and sometimes a third unit of blood may be withdrawn by inserting the needle of the plasmapheresis set into the rubber connection of the tubing used for the withdrawal of the first unit of blood. Approximately 100 ml. of 0.9 per cent sodium chloride solution is infused intravenously between the periods of blood collections. After separation, the plasma is squeezed into the transfer bag by means of a metal chart cover. The plasma volume removed per unit of blood is approximately 300 ml. After removal of the last unit of blood, the erythrocytes are rapidly reinfused. The entire plasmapheresis procedure is usually completed within one and one-half to two hours and is tolerated exceptionally well. This simplified plasmapheresis procedure has permitted its use on an outpatient basis, even in the patient's home, thus eliminating the inconvenience of frequent hospital visits and reducing the concomitant financial burden. Similarly, the η rel$^{37°C}$ was determined, either on an outpatient basis or in the patient's home, with an Ostwald's viscosimeter.

The number and frequency of plasmaphereses are based upon results of the determination of the relative serum viscosity at 37°C. To avoid the increase of serum viscosity above critical levels, maintenance plasmapheresis (the removal of one to three units of plasma weekly) may be required. The increase of serum viscosity is not proportional to the increase of M proteins, and a slight increase in M protein concentration may increase the serum viscosity disproportionately. Approach of critically high levels of relative viscosity (*i.e.*, 4 to 8 η rel$^{37°C}$) may be heralded by subjective manifestations such as listlessness, fatigue, shortness of breath, "fullness" in the head, *etc.* Patients responding to simultaneous chemotherapy treatment will require progressively fewer plasmapheresis procedures. The effectiveness of this approach is depicted in Figure 10.

CORTICOSTEROIDS.—In general, corticosteroids alone are ineffective in patients with macroglobulinemia. In special circumstances, however, they may be life-saving, as in the case of autoimmune hemolytic anemia (see Case 3).

ANTIBIOTICS.—Increased susceptibility to bacterial infections requires the judicious use of antibiotics. Gram-negative septicemias are a particularly common complication, and early clinical recognition may be essential to the survival of such patients (see Cases 1 and 4). Normal IgM contains the chief antibody activity to gram-negative microorganisms, and the low level of normal IgM in many patients probably explains the increased susceptibility. The management of such infections requires prompt administration of appropriate antibiotics, and in selected cases, γ-globulin substitution.

γ-GLOBULIN SUBSTITUTION.—Patients with IgM monoclonal gammopathies often display low levels of IgG, IgA, and normal or residual IgM. This is particularly the case in patients with the classical, symptomatic forms of macroglobulinemia. Critically low serum levels of IgG (*i.e.*, 300 to 350 mg./100 ml.) may require γ-globulin substitution. Commercially available γ-globulin contains approximately 16 per cent IgG but only trace amounts of IgA and IgM. An effective intramuscular dose consists of at least 0.3 ml./kg. (*i.e.*, 0.05 g./kg.). Presently, no IgA or IgM preparations are available for substitution therapy. In desperate situations, the intravenous use of plasma (Stiehm, Vaerman, and Fudenberg, 1966) may be indicated, despite the inevitable risk of serum hepatitis.

Incidence of Macroglobulinemia

AGE DISTRIBUTION

The age distribution of 46 patients with macroglobulinemia is shown in Figure 17. The peak incidence (37 per cent) occurs at ages 60 through 69, whereas about 24 per cent of such cases are in each of the age brackets of 50 through 59 and 70 through 79. The average age was 61.3 years (males, 59.8 years; females, 63.6 years). The peak incidence is identical with that reported by Waldenström (1968). The onset of macroglobulinemia appears to be earlier than that of myeloma (Waldenström, 1968), although the opposite view has been expressed (Martin, 1969).

FIG. 17.—Age incidence of macroglobulinemia. Cumulative number of cases diagnosed at each decade of life (total number of cases, 46).

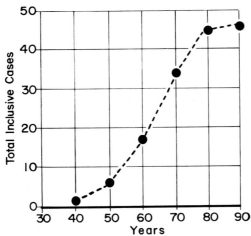

OCCURRENCE AT EARLY AGE

Case 7.*—(UH#107440-P) is a 33-year-old Caucasian female, first seen in November 1968 with a 15-year history of intermittent episodes of fever and splenomegaly. Initially, the episodes were three to six months apart with progressive decrease in frequency. Anemia and thrombocytopenia suggested hypersplenism, and this was considered to be confirmed by a ^{51}Cr erythrocyte half-life of 7.5 days and by sequestration of erythrocytes by the spleen. Total serum proteins were 12.0 g./100 ml., and serum electrophoresis demonstrated a large M protein in the γ-globulin region (7.1 g./100 ml.). An IgM monoclonal gammopathy was diagnosed by immunoelectrophoresis. Immunoglobulin quantitation by radial immunodiffusion revealed: IgG, 1,491 mg./100 ml.; IgA, 28 mg./100 ml.; and IgM, 15,872 mg./100 ml. The ultracentrifugal pattern contained a small 32S, a large peaked 22 to 24S, and a tall 19S component. A tiny 17.6S component was present. (The 7S component was increased, probably containing low molecular IgM, this accounting for the discrepancy of total serum protein and IgM values.) Pyroglobulins and cryoglobulins were negative. Relative serum viscosity was 5.0 at 37°C. Bone lesions were not identified. Marrow examination demonstrated an increase in the lymphoid series compatible with a lymphoproliferative disorder. In January 1969, a splenectomy was performed. Excisional lymph node biopsy and liver biopsy at splenectomy were consistent with the diagnosis of Waldenström's macroglobulinemia. The patient was discharged and given prednisone. During the next month, she became progressively weaker and experienced intermittent left upper quadrant pain. Wound dehiscence required readmission in April 1969. *E. coli* were cultured from the sinus tract of the dehiscence, and ampicillin treatment was begun. The patient left the hospital against medical advice.

In this patient, it was assumed that the macroglobulinemia had developed prior to the third decade of life. The occurrence of macroglobulinemia at such an early age was practically unknown until recently, when M proteins were described as occurring sporadically, even in children and infants (Hochwald and Thorbecke, 1964; Stoop, Zegers, van der Heiden, and Ballieux, 1968; Stoop, Ballieux, and Weyers, 1962; Schaller *et al.*, 1966; Dalloz, Castaing, Nezeloff, and Seligmann, 1965; Harboe *et al.*, 1966; Danon, Clauvel, and Seligmann, 1967; de Koning *et al.*, 1969; Braunsteiner *et al.*, 1968). They have been observed in infants following fetal thymic allotransplantation (Harboe *et al.*, 1966; de Koning *et al.*, 1969); in these, monoclonal IgM may develop (Braunsteiner *et al.*, 1968). In this connection, the rather frequent occurrence of M proteins in patients with thymomas (Braunsteiner *et al.*, 1968; Birch *et al.*, 1964; Lindström, Williams, and Brunning, 1968; Harley, Anido, and Gilbert, 1966; Gilbert *et al.*, 1968; Gabl *et al.*, 1969; Anderson and Vye, 1967) may be of etiologic significance. These cases re-emphasize the vital immunological functions of the thymus gland.

*The authors are grateful to F. Muñiz, M.D., Division of Hematology, Department of Medicine, The University of Texas Medical Branch at Galveston, Galveston, Texas, for permission to publish this case report.

SEX DISTRIBUTION

Of 61 patients with macroglobulinemia, 54 per cent were males and 46 per cent were females. This ratio varies somewhat from that reported by Waldenström, who encountered approximately 68 per cent males and 32 per cent females (Waldenström, 1968).

RACE INCIDENCE

The race incidence in our series was 87.5 per cent Caucasian and 12.5 per cent Negro, although the relative number of Negroes seen in our hospital exceeds this figure.

FAMILIAL INCIDENCE OF MACROGLOBULINEMIA

Familial macroglobulinemia has been observed (Seligmann, Danon, and Mihaesco, 1965; Seligmann, Danon, Mihaesco, and Fudenberg, 1967; for other references, see Ritzmann and Levin, 1969). Seligmann (1966) examined the sera of 216 close relatives of 65 patients with macroglobulinemia. In eight of 216 relatives, an IgM M protein was identified. Six of these affected individuals were apparently healthy and were more than 50 years old. Axelsson and Hällén (1965), Hällén (1963), and Axelsson, Bachmann, and Hällén (1966) surveyed nearly 7,000 sera from a normal population and found M proteins in 64 instances. Seven of the persons with M proteins of the IgG, IgA, or IgM class belonged to three families. These findings suggest a genetic predisposition to the development of monoclonal gammopathies, and, furthermore, a random expression of the class (either IgG, IgA, or IgM) of monoclonal gammopathy in such families.

RELATIVE AND ABSOLUTE INCIDENCE OF MACROGLOBULINEMIA

The relative incidence of monoclonal gammopathies has been reported to vary between 0.12 per cent and 1.1 per cent (Ritzmann and Levin, 1967) within various reported series. These figures were based upon routine serum electrophoretic analyses of patients seeking medical advice. The absolute incidence of monoclonal gammopathies cannot be determined with certainty at this time. The frequency with which monoclonal gammopathies occur has undoubtedly been underestimated in the past. In our own institution, one case of monoclonal gammopathy is diagnosed per week; this includes about nine cases of macroglobulinemia per year. Swedish authors (Axelsson, Bachmann, and Hällén, 1966) have attempted to determine the frequency of the M proteins in a random population, including most persons in one province in Sweden, above 25 years of age. Among 6,995 sera examined, 64 instances of M proteins were encountered, an incidence of

0.92 per cent. The incidence increases with age (Hällén, 1963). M proteins were detected in 9 of 294 (3 per cent) subjects who were older than 70 years and apparently in good health. Similar data have been reported by French authors (Derycke, Fine, and Boffa, 1965) who observed 15 cases of monoclonal gammopathies among 500 individuals 68 years of age or older. The relative incidence of IgM monoclonal gammopathies, among all monoclonal gammopathies, is approximately 16 per cent (Ritzmann and Levin, 1967, 1969); therefore, the absolute incidence of macroglobulinemia may be expected to be 16 per cent of the above quoted figures. However, more extensive population studies are required before these figures can be accepted as generally applicable.

Summary and Conclusions

Paradoxically, with the increasing knowledge about macroglobulinemia, it becomes more difficult to formulate a unified concept and to offer an all-inclusive definition. A decade or so ago, macroglobulinemia was diagnosed by the characteristic immunoglobulin abnormalities accompanied by the classical clinical manifestations. Asymptomatic macroglobulinemias and those with atypical clinical complications cannot be so described. Furthermore, IgM monoclonal gammopathies in association with thymomas or emerging after fetal thymic allotransplantation must also be considered. Presently, the occurrence of a monoclonal IgM is the only common denominator upon which the diagnosis of macroglobulinemia can be established.

The associated clinical manifestations embrace a wide spectrum, ranging from complete absence of symptoms to the occurrence of severe classical symptoms of lymphadenopathy, splenomegaly, anemia, and frequent infections, and accompanied by variable manifestations caused by the specific properties of the "abnormal" macroglobulins, such as hyperviscosity syndrome, cold agglutinin disease, autoimmune hemolytic anemia, *etc.* Therefore, the concept of a syndrome of macroglobulinemia appears appropriate. This disorder occurs in a relatively small but not precisely determined percentage of the population and represents about 16 per cent of monoclonal gammopathies. There is a slight preponderance in males, and there is an increase in incidence with advancing age. The apparently autonomous proliferation of immunocytes and the concomitant production of homogeneous, monoclonal macroglobulins can be decreased with chemotherapy with chlorambucil or cyclophosphamide and the various clinical complications can be treated symptomatically, *e.g.,* plasmapheresis for patients with the hyperviscosity syndrome.

Certain interesting associations include the increased occurrence of multiple malignant conditions and mesenchymal disorders (for references, see Ritzmann and Levin, 1969) which are not seen in multiple myeloma. The latter disorder is closely related to macroglobulinemia on the basis of apparently autonomous clonal proliferation productive of abnormal proteins, but it differs from the syndrome of macroglobulinemia clinically (*e.g.*, osteolysis with bone pain) as well as serologically (*i.e.*, monoclonal IgG, IgA, IgD, IgE, and/or light chains, instead of IgM). The challenge remains to identify the etiologic factors which are responsible for this type of apparently meaningless cellular proliferation and protein overproduction. These disorders may reflect pathophysiological derangements associated with biological aging of immunological control mechanisms. They also invite speculation concerning the relationships between the various anatomical and functional components of the immune system. The antibody-producing cells which proliferate in macroglobulinemia possess a considerable potential for autoantibody production, which could exert protective as well as deleterious effects.

We find ourselves still pondering the enigmatic nature of monoclonal gammopathies more than 120 years after Henry Bence Jones opened a Pandora's box which may well hold keys to basic immunologic controls of life itself.

Acknowledgments

We gratefully acknowledge the secretarial assistance of Mrs. Helen Mueller, the technical assistance of Mrs. Monica Lawrence, and the services of Mr. Ed Stephenson and Mr. Lewis Mulutin of the Medical Illustration Division.

REFERENCES

Abel, J. J., Rowntree, L. G., and Turner, B.E.: Plasma removal with return of corpuscles (plasmaphaeresis). *Journal of Pharmacology and Experimental Therapeutics,* 5:625-641, 1914.

Albert, A., and Johnson, P.: Macroglobulins. I. Studies on the isolation and physical properties of pathological macroglobulins. *Biochemical Journal,* 81:658-669, October-December 1961.

Anderson, A. B., and Ferriman, D.: Macroglobulinaemia. *British Medical Journal,* 1:277, January 23, 1960.

Anderson, E. T., and Vye, M. V.: Dysproteinemia of the myeloma type associated with a thymoma. *Annals of Internal Medicine,* 66:141-149, January 1967.

Apitz, K.: Die Paraproteinosen. (Über die Störung des Eiweissstoffwechsels bei Plasmocytom.) *Virchows Archiv für Pathologische Anatomie und Physiologie und für Klinische Medizin,* 306:631-699, 1940.

Auscher, C., and Guinand, S.: Étude d'une beta $_{2A}$-globuline cryo-précipitable. *Clinica chimica acta,* 9:40-48, January 1964.

Axelsson, U., Bachmann, R., and Hällén, J.: Frequency of pathological proteins (M-components) in 6,995 sera from adult population. *Acta medica scandinavica,* 179:235-247, February 1966.

Axelsson, U., and Hällén, J.: Familial occurrence of pathological serum-proteins of different γ-globulin groups. *Lancet,* 2:369-370, August 21, 1965.

_____: Review of fifty-four subjects with monoclonal gammopathy. *British Journal of Haematology*, 15:417-420, October 1968.

Bachmann, R., and Laurell, C.-B.: Electrophoretic and immunologic classification of M-components in serum. *The Scandinavian Journal of Clinical and Laboratory Investigation*, Suppl. 69-73:11-24, 1963.

Ballieux, R. E., Imhof, J. W., Mul, N. A. J., Zegers, B. J. M., and Stoop, J. W.: Pathology of immunoglobulins: Some aspects of monoclonal gammopathy. *Clinica chimica acta*, 22:7-13, September 1968.

Barth, W. F.: Viscosimetry of serum in relation to the serum globulins. In Sunderman, F. W., and Sunderman, F. W., Jr., Eds.: *Serum Proteins and the Dysproteinemias*. Philadelphia, Pennsylvania, and Montreal, Canada, J. B. Lippincott Co., 1964, pp. 102-109.

Bayrd, E. D.: Continuous chlorambucil therapy in primary macroglobulinemia of Waldenström: Report of four cases. *Proceedings of the Staff Meetings of the Mayo Clinic*, 36:135-147, March 15, 1961.

Bence Jones, H.: On a new protein occurring in the urine of a patient with mollities ossium. *Proceedings of the Royal Society*, 1848, p. 673.

Benirschke, K., Brownhill, L., and Ebaugh, F. G.: Chromosomal abnormalities in Waldenström's macroglobulinemia. *Lancet*, 1:594-595, March 17, 1962.

Bernier, G. M., and Putnam, F. W.: Polymerism, polymorphism, and impurities in Bence-Jones proteins. *Biochimica et biophysica acta*, 86:295-308, March 17, 1964.

Bing, J.: Further investigation on hyperglobulinemia. I. Occurrence and degree of hyperglobulinemia in the various diseases—the ratio between hyperglobulinemia, hyperproteinemia, and hypoalbuminemia—the formolgel reaction. *Acta medica scandinavica*, 103:547-583, 1940.

Bing, J., and Neel, A. V.: Two cases of hyperglobulinemia with affection of central nervous system on toxi-infectious bases. *Acta medica scandinavica*, 88:492-506, 1936.

Birch, C. A., Cook, K. B., Drew, C. E., London, D. R., Mackenzie, D. H., and Milne, M. D.: Hyperglobulinaemic purpura due to a thymic tumour. *Lancet*, 1:693-697, March 28, 1964.

Bloch, H. S., Prasad, A., Anastasi, A., and Brigg, D. R.: Serum protein changes in Waldenström's macroglobulinemia during administration of a low molecular weight thiol (penicillamine). *Journal of Laboratory and Clinical Medicine*, 56:212-217, August 1960.

Bloch, K. J., Buchanan, W. W., Wohl, M. J., and Bunim, J. J.: Sjögren's syndrome. A clinical, pathological, and serological study of sixty-two cases. *Medicine*, 44:187-231, May 1965.

Bohard, M. G.: Plasmocytosis and cryoglobulinemia in cancer. *Journal of the American Medical Association*, 164:18-21, May 4, 1957.

Bottura, C., Ferrari, I., and Veiga, A. A.: Chromosome abnormalities in Waldenström's macroglobulinaemia. *Lancet*, 1:1170, May 27, 1961.

Bouroncle, B. A., Datta, P., and Frajola, W. J.: Waldenström's macroglobulinemia: Report of three patients treated with cyclophosphamide. *Journal of the American Medical Association*, 189:729-732, September 7, 1964.

Brahmachari, U. N,., and Seu, P. B.: Globulin opacity test for kala-azar. *Indian Medical Gazette*, 58:295, 1923.

Braunsteiner, H., Gabl, F., Lederer, B., Pastner, D., Propst, A., and Rhomberg, P.: Thymustumor mit extremer Lymphopenie und Atrophie des Lymphatischen gewebes bei normaler Plasmazellzahl und mit Auftreten einer monoklonalen IGM (Lambda)-Vermehrung. *Schweizerische medizinische Wochenschrift*, 98:1188-1196, August 1968.

Brecher, G., Tanaka, Y., Malmgren, R. A., and Fahey, J. L.: Morphology and protein synthesis in multiple myeloma and macroglobulinemia. *Annals of the New York Academy of Sciences*, 113:642-653, February 28, 1964.

Broustet, A: *Étude cytogenetique et moleculaire de la macroglobulinemie de Waldenström*. Thesis. University of Bordeaux, Bordeaux, France, 1966, 117 pp.

Brown, A. K., Elves, M. W., Gunson, H. H., and Pell-Ilderton, R.: Waldenström's macroglobulinemia: A family study. *Acta haematologica*, 38:184-192, 1967.

Burnet, M.: *The Clonal Selection Theory of Acquired Immunity*. Nashville, Tennessee, Vanderbilt University Press, 1959, 209 pp.

Burtin, P., Hartmann, L., Heremans, J., Scheidegger, J. J., Westendorp-Boerma, F., Wieme,

MACROGLOBULINEMIA / 213

R., Wunderly, C., Fauvert, R., and Grabar, P.: Études immunochimiques et immuno-electrophoretiques des macroglobulinemies. *Revue Française d'Études Cliniques et Biologiques,* 2:161-177, February 1957.

Cass, R. M., Anderson, B. R., and Vaughan, J. H.: Waldenström's macroglobulinemia with increased serum IgG levels treated with low doses of cyclophosphamide. *Annals of Internal Medicine,* 71:971-977, November 1969.

Charlwood, P. A.: Ultracentrifugal studies on sera containing cold haemagglutinins. *British Journal of Haematology,* 3:273-275, July 1957.

Christenson, W. N., and Dacie, J. V.: Serum proteins in acquired haemolytic anaemia (auto-antibody type). *British Journal of Haematology,* 3:153-163, April 1957.

Clamp, J. R.: Some aspects of the first recorded case of multiple myeloma. *Lancet,* 2:1354-1356, December 23, 1967.

Clatanoff, D. V., and Meyer, O. O.: Response to chlorambucil in macroglobulinemia. *Journal of the American Medical Association,* 183:40-44, January 5, 1963.

Cline, M. J., Solomon, A., Berlin, N. I., and Fahey, J. L.: Anemia in macroglobulinemia. *American Journal of Medicine,* 34:213-220, February 1963.

Clubb, J. S., Posen, S., and Neale, F. C.: Disappearance of a serum paraprotein after parathyroidectomy. *Archives of Internal Medicine,* 114:616-620, November 1964.

Cohen, R. J., Bohannon, R. A., and Wallerstein, R. O.: Waldenström's macroglobulinemia. A study of ten cases. *American Journal of Medicine,* 41:274-284, August 1966.

Cohen, S., Solomon, A., Paronetto, F., and Popper, H.: Subacute hepatitis in Waldenström's macroglobulinemia. *American Journal of Medicine,* 34:256-263, February 1963.

Curtain, C. C., and O'Dea, J. F.: Possible sites of macroglobulin synthesis: A study made with fluorescent antibody. *Australasian Annals of Medicine,* 8:143-150, May 1959.

Dacie, J. V.: *The Haemolytic Anaemias: Congenital and Acquired. Part II—The Auto-Immune Haemolytic Anaemias.* 2nd edition. New York, New York, Grune & Stratton, Inc., 1962, pp. 341-718.

Dalloz, J. C., Castaing, N., Nezeloff, C., and Seligmann, M.: Paraproteinemie transitoire de type gamma. Observation chez un nourisson atteint du syndrome d'Aldrich. *La presse médicale,* 73:1541-1546, January 1965.

Dalrymple, J.: On the microscopical character of mollities ossium. *Dublin Journal of Medical Science,* 2:85-94, 1846.

Daniels, J. C., Cobb, E. K., Levin, W. C., and Ritzmann, S. E.: IV. Detection and differentiation of M-proteins by the acid-gel reaction: A re-evaluation. *Texas Reports on Biology and Medicine.* (In press.)

Daniels, J. C., Levin, W. C., and Ritzmann, S. E.: Hypertransferrinemia as cause of pseudo-M-proteinemia. *Texas Reports on Biology and Medicine.* (In press.)

Danon, F., Clauvel, J. P., and Seligmann, M.: Les "paraproteines" de type IgG et IgA en dehors de la maladie de Kahler. *Revue Française d'Études Cliniques et Biologiques,* 12:681-701, August-September 1967.

Derycke, C., Fine, J. M., and Boffa, G. A.: Dysglobulinemies "essentielles" chez les sujets ages. *Nouvelle Revue Française d'Hematologie,* 5:729-738, September-October 1965.

Deutsch, H. F., and Morton, J. I.: Dissociation of human serum macroglobulins. *Science,* 125:600, March 1957.

Dubi, A.: Idiopathische Paraproteinämien. *Schweizerische medizinische Wochenschrift,* 95:473, April 1965.

Dutcher, T. F., and Fahey, J. L.: Immunocytochemical demonstration of intranuclear localization of 18S gamma macroglobulin in macroglobulinemia of Waldenström. *Proceedings of the Society for Experimental Biology and Medicine,* 103:452-455, March 1960.

Elves, M. W., and Israëls, M. C. G.: Chromosomes and serum proteins: A linked abnormality. *British Medical Journal,* 2:1024-1027, October 26, 1963.

Engle, R. L., Jr., and Nachman, R. L.: Two Bence Jones proteins of different immunologic type in the same patient with multiple myeloma. *Blood, The Journal of Hematology,* 27:74-77, January 1966.

Eriksen, N.: Serum macroglobulin levels in relation to age, sex, and disease. *Journal of Laboratory and Clinical Medicine,* 51:521-529, April 1958.

Fahey, J. L.: Antibodies and immunoglobulins. *Journal of the American Medical Association,* 194:71-74, October 4, 1965.

———: Heterogeneity of γ-globulins. *Advances in Immunology,* 2:41-109, 1962.

———: Serum protein disorders causing clinical symptoms in malignant neoplastic disease. *Journal of Chronic Diseases,* 16:703-712, July 1963.

Fahey, J. L., Barth, W. F., and Solomon, A.: Serum hyperviscosity syndrome. *Journal of the American Medical Association,* 192:464-467, May 10, 1965.

Fahey, J. L., and Lawrence, M. E.: Quantitative determination of 6.6S γ-globulins, beta $_{2A}$-globulins and γ1-macroglobulins in human serum. *Journal of Immunology,* 91:597-603, November 1963.

Fahey, J. L., Scoggins, R., Utz, J. P., and Szwed, C. F.: Infections, antibody response and gamma globulin components in multiple myeloma and macroglobulinemia. *American Journal of Medicine,* 35:698-707, November 1963.

Fankhauser, S., Arnold, E., Schaub, F., and Lapp, R.: Hämolytisches Syndrome und Makroglobulinämie Waldenström. *Helvetica medica acta,* 23:645:648, March 1956.

Feizi, T.: A comparison of the structure of *Mycoplasma-pneumoniae*-induced cold agglutinins with those of the chronic cold agglutinin syndrome by a specific neutralisation technique. In *Proceedings of the Tenth Congress of the European Society of Haematology,* Strasbourg, France, 1965. Basel, Switzerland, and New York, New York, S. Karger, 1967, Vol. II (Part 2), pp. 1458-1461.

Felten, V. A. V., Regli, F., and Frick, P.: Sjögren-Syndrom mit Hypergammaglobulinämie, Kryoglobulinämie, Purpura und Raynaud-Phänomen. *Schweizerische medizinische Wochenschrift,* 93:1847-1851, December 1963.

Ferguson, J., and Mackay, I. R.: Macroglobulinaemia with chromosomal anomaly. *Australian Annals of Medicine,* 12:197-201, February 1963.

Filitti-Wurmser, S., Gentou, C., and Hartmann, L.: Existence de deux variétés 17 S ou 18,3 S de gamma-M-1 et d'une augmentation de globulines 6,6 S seriques dans la maladie de Waldenström. *Revue Française d'Études Cliniques et Biologiques,* 9:398-410, April 1964.

Franklin, E. C., Holman, H. R., Müller-Eberhard, H. J., and Kunkel, H. G.: An unusual protein component of high molecular weight in the serum of certain patients with rheumatoid arthritis. *Journal of Experimental Medicine,* 105:425-437, May 1, 1957.

Franklin, E. C., and Lowenstein, J.: Protein abnormalities associated with proliferative disorders of plasma cells and lymphocytes. *Seminars in Hematology,* 1:144-164, April 1964.

Fudenberg, H. H., and Kunkel, H. G.: Physical properties of the red cell agglutinins in acquired hemolytic anemia. *Journal of Experimental Medicine,* 106:689-702, November 1957.

Gabl, F., Pastner, D., Phomberg, H., Lederer, B., Braunsteiner, H., and Propst, A.: Thymustumor mit extremer Lymphopenie. In Heimpel, H., and Heilmeyer, L., Eds.: *Physiologie und Pathophysiologie der Erythropoese. Der heutige Stand der Behandlung der unreifzelligen Leukämie. Veränderungen des lymphozytären Systems und immunpathologische Reaktionen in der Mämatologie. Freie Vorträge* (Verhandlungen der 13, Tagung der Deutschen Gesellschaft für Hämatologie 16. bis 18. Mai 1968 in Ulm/Donau). Munich, West Germany, J. F. Lehmanns Verlag, 1969, pp. 211-214.

Gaté, J., and Papacostas, C.: Une nouvelle reaction des serums syphilitiques: Formol-gelification. *Revue Société Biologique,* 83:1432, 1920.

German, J. L., Biro, C. E., and Bearn, A. G.: Chromosomal abnormalities in Waldenström's macroglobulinaemia. *Lancet,* 2:48, July 1, 1961.

Gilbert, E. F., Harley, J. B., Anido, V., Mengoli, H. F., and Hughes, J. T.: Thymoma, plasma cell myeloma, red cell aplasia and malabsorption syndrome. *American Journal of Medicine,* 44:820-829, May 1968.

Glenchur, H., Zinneman, H. H., and Briggs, D. R.: Macroglobulinemia: Report of two cases. *Annals of Internal Medicine,* 48:1055-1069, May 1958.

Gordon, R.S.: The preparation and properties of the cold agglutinins. *The Journal of Immunology,* 71:220-225, October 1953.

Grabar, P., and Burtin, P.: *Immunoelectrophoretic Analysis. Applications to Human Biological Fluids.* Amsterdam, The Netherlands, London, England, and New York, New York, Elsevier Publishing Company, 1964, 302 pp.

Grubb, R., and Swahn, B.: Destruction of some agglutinins but not of others by two sulfhydryl compounds. *Acta pathologica et microbiologica scandinavica,* 43: 305-309, 1958.

Gutman, A. B.: The plasma proteins in disease. *Advances in Protein Chemistry,* 4:155-240, 1948.

Hällén, J.: Discrete gammaglobulin (M-) components in serum: Clinical study of 150 subjects without myelomatosis. *Acta medica scandinavica,* 179 (Suppl. 462):1-127, 1966.

Hällén, J.: Frequency of "abnormal" serum globulins (M-components) in the aged. *Acta medica scandinavica,* 173:737-744, 1963.

Hansen, P. F., and Faber, M.: Raynaud's syndrome originating from reversible precipitation of protein. *Acta medica scandinavica,* 129:81-100, 1947.

Harboe, M.: Biologically active "monoclonal" γM-globulins. *Series Haematologica,* 4 *(Gamma Globulins):* 65-75, 1965.

Harboe, M., and Deverill, J.: Immunochemical properties of cold haemagglutinins. *Scandinavian Journal of Haematology,* 1:223-237, 1964.

Harboe, M., van Furth, R., Schubothe, H., Lind, G., and Evans, R. S.: Exclusive occurrence of kappa chains in isolated cold haemagglutinins. *Scandinavian Journal of Haematology,* 2:259-266, 1965.

Harboe, M., Pande, H., Brandtzaeg, P., Tveter, K. T., and Hjort, R. F.: Synthesis of donor type-γG-globulin following thymus transplantation in hypo-γ-globulinaemia with severe lymphocytopenia. *Scandinavian Journal of Haematology,* 3:351-374, 1966.

Harley, J. B., Anido, V., and Gilbert, E. F.: Thymoma with red cell aplasia, multiple myeloma, and malabsorption syndrome. (Abstract) *Proceedings XI Congress International Society Haematology,* Sydney, Australia, 1966, p. 177.

Hemodynamic disturbances in macroglobulinemia and myeloma. (Editorial) *Journal of the American Medical Association,* 208:686, April 28, 1969.

Heni, V. F., and Siebner, H.: Chromosomenveränderungen bei der Makroglobulinaemia Waldenström. *Deutsche medizinische Wochenschrift,* 88:1781-1782, September 13, 1963.

Heremans, J.: *Les globulines sériques du système gamma. Leur nature et leur pathologie.* Brussels, Belgium, Editions Arscia S. A., and Paris, France, Masson et Cie, 1960, 340 pp.

_____: Proteins in myeloma and macroglobulinaemia. In Steffen, C., Ed.: *Methods of Immunohaematologic Research.* Basel, Switzerland, and New York, New York, S. Karger (published as *Bibliotheca Haematologica* Fasc. 14), 1963, pp. 159-163.

Hobbs, J. R.: Disturbances of the immunoglobulins. *Scientific Basis of Medicine: Annual Reviews,* pp. 106-127, 1966.

_____: Immunochemical classes of myelomatosis: Including data from a therapeutic trial conducted by a Medical Research Council Working Party. *British Journal of Haematology,* 16:599-606, June 1969.

Hochwald, G. M., and Thorbecke, G. J.: Occurrence of myeloma-like γ-globulin in C. S. F. of a four-month old infant with hydrocephalus. *Pediatrics.* 33:435-440, March 1964.

Hoffmann, L. S., and Ritzmann, S. E.: Plasmapheresis—application of modified technique in patients with monoclonal gammopathies. (Abstract) *Texas Reports on Biology and Medicine,* 23:651-652, Fall 1965.

Houston, E. W., Levin, W. C., and Ritzmann, S. E.: Endoreduplication in untreated and early leukemia. *Lancet,* 2:496, September 5, 1964.

Houston, E. W., Ritzmann, S. E., and Levin, W. C.: Chromosomal aberrations common to three types of monoclonal gammopathies. *Blood, The Journal of Hematology,* 29:214-232, February 1967a.

_____: Chromosomal aberrations common to three types of monoclonal gammopathies. In *Proceedings of the Tenth Congress of the European Society of Haematology,* Strasbourg, France, 1965. Basel, Switzerland, and New York, New York, S. Karger, 1967b, Vol. II (Part 1), pp. 563-568.

Huhnstock, K., and Grossman, H. D.: Critical evaluation of the serum acid gel reaction in multiple myeloma. *Clinica chimica acta,* 15:174, January 1967.

Imhof, J. W., Ballieux, R. E., and Mijnlieff, P. F.: Ultracentrifuge investigation of the serum proteins in Waldenström's macroglobulinemia. *Clinica Chimica Acta,* 5:801-811, 1960.

Imhof, J. W., Ballieux, R. E., Mul, N. A. J., and Poen, H.: Monoclonal and diclonal gammopathies. *Acta medica scandinavica,* Suppl. 445:102-114, 1966.

Jahnke, K., and Scholtan, W.: Die Bluteiweisskörper in der Ultrazentrifuge, Sedimentation-Flotation, Stuttgart, Germany, Georg Thieme Verlag, 1960, 207 pp.

Jeannet, V. M., and Hässig, A.: Uber die Beziehungen der Hämagglutination im kolliodalen Milieu zur Geldrollenbildung, Blutkörperchensenkung, und Sphärozytose. Blut, 10:297-305, November 1964.

Kahler, O.: Zur Symptomatologie des multiplem Myeloms; Beobachtung von Albumosurie. Prague medizinische Wochenschrift, 14:33, 1889.

Kahn, P.: Zur Paraprotein-Differenzierung mittels Rivanol. Klinische Wochenschrift, 45:101-103, January 1967.

Kaldor, G., Saifer, A., Terry, W., and Vecsler, F.: Physicochemical studies of a "purified" macrocryoglobulin (Waldenström). Journal of Laboratory and Clinical Medicine, 59:970-979, June 1962.

Kanner, O.: Nonspecific protein reactions: The quantitative formol-gel test. In Sunderman, F. W., and Sunderman, F. W., Jr., Eds.: Serum Proteins and the Dysproteinemias. Philadelphia, Pennsylvania, and Montreal, Canada, J. B. Lippincott Co., 1964, p. 197.

Kanzow, U.: Die Makroglobulinämie Waldenström. Klinische Wochenschrift, 32:154-159, February 1954.

Kappeler, R., Krebs, A., and Riva, G.: Klinik der Makroglobulinämie Waldenström, Beschreibung von 21 Fällen und Übersicht der Literatur. Helvetica medica acta, 25:54-101, April; 101-152, May 1958.

Klemm, D., Schubothe, H., and Hunstein, W.: Zytostatische Langzeitbehandlung makroglobulinämischer Erkrankkungen. (Abstract) 10th Congress of the International Society of Haematology, Stockholm, Sweden, 1964, p. D:31.

Knedel, M.: Die Doppel-Albuminämie, eine neue vererbliche Proteinanomalie. Blut, 3:129-134, May 1957.

Koning, J. de, van Bekkum, D. W., Dicke, K. A., Dooren, L. J., van Rood, J. J., and Radl, J.: Transplantation of bone-marrow cells and fetal thymus in an infant with lymphopenic immunological deficiency. Lancet, 1:1223-1227, June 21, 1969.

Kopp, W. L., Beirne, G. J., and Burns, R. O.: Hyperviscosity syndrome in multiple myeloma. American Journal of Medicine, 43:141-146, July 1967.

Kopp, W. L., MacKinney, A. A., Jr., and Wasson, G.: Blood volume and hematocrit in macroglobulinemia and myeloma. Archives of Internal Medicine, 123:394-396, April 1969.

Korngold, L.: Abnormal plasma components and their significance in disease. Annals of the New York Academy of Sciences, 94:110-130, August 31, 1961.

Kritzman, J., Fudenberg, H. H., and Liss, M.: A Bence Jones cryoglobulin: Chemical, physical and immunologic studies. (Abstract) Blood, The Journal of Hematology, 28:1002, December 1966.

Kritzman, J., Kunkel, H. G., McCarthy, J., and Mellors, R. C.: Studies of Waldenström-type macroglobulin with rheumatoid factor properties. Journal of Laboratory and Clinical Medicine, 57:905-917, June 1961.

Kunkel, H. G.: Macroglobulins and high molecular weight antibodies. In Putnam, F. W., Ed.: The Plasma Proteins. New York, New York, and London, England, Academic Press, 1960, Vol. I (Isolation, Characterization, and Function), 279 pp.

Kunkel, H. G., Müller-Eberhard, H. J., Fudenberg, H. H., and Tomasi, T. B.: Gamma globulin complexes in rheumatoid arthritis and certain other conditions. Journal of Clinical Investigation, 40:117-129, January 1961.

Kyle, R. A., and Bayrd, E. D.: "Benign" monoclonal gammopathy: A potentially malignant condition? American Journal of Medicine, 40:426-430, March 1966.

————: "Primary" systemic amyloidosis and myeloma: Discussion of relationship and review of 81 cases. Archives of Internal Medicine, 107:344-353, March 1961.

Laroche, C., Nenna, A., Seligmann, M., Richet, G., Caquet, R., and Bignon, J.: Dysprotéinémie pseudo-myélomateuse au cours de pyonéphroses. La presse médicale, 72:2833-2837, November 14, 1964.

Laurell, A. H. F.: Sera from patients with myeloma, macroglobulinemia, and related conditions as studied by ultracentrifugation. Acta medica scandinavica, Suppl. 367:69-86, 1961.

Laurell, C.-B., Laurell, H., and Waldenström, J.: Glycoprotein in serum from patients with myeloma, macroglobulinemia and related conditions. *American Journal of Medicine*, 22: 24-36, January 1957.

Leddy, J. P., Trabold, N. C., Vaughan, J. H., and Swisher, S. N.: The unitary nature of "complete" and "incomplete" pathologic cold hemagglutinins. *Blood, The Journal of Hematology*, 19:379-399, March 1962.

Leder, P.: Simple paper electrophoretic method for detecting macroglobulinaemia. *Nature*, 193:1087-1088, March 17, 1967.

Lerner, A. B., and Watson, C. J.: Studies of cryoglobulins: I. Unusual purpura associated with the presence of a high concentration of cryoglobulin (cold precipitable serum globulin). *American Journal of the Medical Sciences*, 214:410-415, October 1947.

Levin, W. C., and Ritzmann, S. E.: Relation of abnormal proteins to formed elements of blood: Cellular sources. *Annual Review of Medicine*, 16:187-200, 1965.

_____: Relation of abnormal proteins to formed elements of blood: Effects upon erythrocytes, leukocytes and platelets. *Annual Review of Medicine*, 17:323-336, 1966.

_____: Treatment of macroglobulinaemia. *British Medical Journal*, 1:1160, April 27, 1963.

Lewis, L. A., Ommen, R. A. V., and Page, I. H.: Association of cold-precipitability with beta-lipoprotein and cryoglobulin. *American Journal of Medicine*, 40:785-793, May 1966.

Lind, K , Mansa, B., and Olesen, H.: Penicillamine treatment in the cold-haemagglutinin syndrome. *Acta medica scandinavica*, 173:647-660, 1962.

Lindström, F. D., Williams, R. C., Jr., and Brunning, R. D.: Thymoma associated with multiple myeloma. *Archives of Internal Medicine*, 122:526-531, December 1968.

Loghem, J. J. van, Hart, M. van der, Veenhoven-van, Riesz E., Veer, M. van der, Engelsfriet, C. P., and Peetoom, F.: Cold auto-agglutinins and hemolysins of anti-I and anti-i specificity. *Vox Sanguinis*, 7:214-221, 1962.

London, R. E.: Multiple myeloma. Report of a case showing unusual remission lasting two years following severe hepatitis. *Annals of Internal Medicine*, 43:191-201, July 1955.

LoSpalluto, J., Dorward, B., Miller, W., Jr., and Ziff, M.: Cryoglobulinemia based on interaction between a gamma macroglobulin and 7S gamma globulin. *American Journal of Medicine*, 32:142-147, January 1962.

MacIntyre, W.: Mollities and fragilitas ossium. *Medical Chirurgical Transactions*, 33:211-232, 1850.

Mackay, I. R.: Macroglobulins and macroglobulinaemia. *Australasian Annals of Medicine*, 8:158-170, February 1959.

Märki, H. H., and Wuhrmann, F.: Häufigkeit und klinische Bedeutung der Paraproteinämie. *Klinische Wochenschrift*, 43:85-90, January 1965.

Marsh, W. L.: Anti-i-: A cold antibody defining the I:i relationship in human red cells. *British Journal of Haematology*, 7:200-209, April 1961.

Martin, N. H.: The immunoglobulins: A review. *Journal of Clinical Pathology*, 22:117-131, March 1969.

Martin, W. J., and Mathieson, D. R.: Pyroglobulinemia (heat-coagulable globulin in the blood). *Proceedings of the Staff Meetings of the Mayo Clinic*, 28:545-554, October 7, 1953.

Martin, W. J., Mathieson, D. R., and Eigler, J. O. C.: Pyroglobulinemia: Further observations and review of 20 cases. *Proceedings of the Staff Meetings of the Mayo Clinic*, 34:95-101, February 18, 1959.

Massari, K., Fine, J. M., and Metais, R.: Waldenström's macroglobulinaemia observed in two brothers. *Nature*, 196:176-178, October 13, 1962.

McCallister, B. D., Bayrd, E. D., Harrison, E. G., Jr., and McGuckian, W. F.: Primary macroglobulinemia. Review with a report on thirty-one cases and notes on the value of continuous chlorambucil therapy. *American Journal of Medicine*, 43:394-434, September 1967.

McKelvey, E. M., and Fahey, J. L.: Immunoglobulin changes in disease: Quantitation on the basis of heavy polypeptide chains, IgG (γG), IgA (γA), and IgM (γM), and of light polypeptide chains, type K (I) and type L (II). *Journal of Clinical Investigation*, 44:1778-1787, November 1965.

Mehrotra, T. N.: Immunological identification of the pathological cold auto-antibodies of acquired haemolytic anaemia as beta$_2$-M-globulin. *Immunology*, 3:265-271, July 1960.

Meltzer, M., and Franklin, E. C.: Cryoglobulinemia—a study of twenty-nine patients. I. IgG and IgM cryoglobulins and factors affecting cryoprecipitability. *American Journal of Medicine,* 40:828-836, June 1966.

Michaux, J. L., and Heremans, J. F.: Thirty cases of monoclonal immunoglobulin disorders other than myeloma or macroglobulinemia. A classification of diseases associated with the production of monoclonal-type immunoglobulins. *American Journal of Medicine,* 46:562-579, April 1969.

Miller, F., and Metzger, H.: Characterization of a human macroglobulin. I. The molecular weight of its subunit. *Journal of Biological Chemistry,* 240:3325-3333, August 1965.

————: Characterization of a human macroglobulin. III. The products of tryptic digestion. *Journal of Biological Chemistry,* 241:1732-1740, April 25, 1966.

Moretti, G., Hartmann, L., Staeffer, J., deGrouchy, J., Catanzano, G., and Broustet, A.: L'anomalie chromosomique de la maladie de Waldenström. *Annales de Genetique,* 8:55-59, 1965.

Nomenclature for human immunoglobulins. *Bulletin of the World Health Organization,* 30: 447-450, May 1964.

Norgaard, O.: Investigations into strongly anticomplementary human sera. *Acta pathologica et microbiologica scandinavica,* 40:445-452, 1957.

————: Recherches sur l'évolution préclinique du myélome multiple. *Acta medica scandinavica,* 176:137-146, 1964.

Nowell, P. C., and Hungerford, D. A.: Chromosome changes in human leukemia and a tentative assessment of their significance. *Annals of the New York Academy of Sciences,* 113:654-662, February 28, 1964.

Nutter, D. O., and Kramer, N. C.: Macroglobulinemia: Report of a case, with unusual spontaneous recovery. *American Journal of Medicine,* 38:462-469, March 1965.

Olesen, H.: Chlorambucil treatment in the cold agglutinin syndrome. *Scandinavian Journal of Haematology,* 1:116-128, May 1964.

Osserman, E. F.: Natural history of multiple myeloma before radiological evidence of disease. *Radiology,* 71:157-174, August 1958.

————: Plasma-cell myeloma. II. Clinical aspects (concluded). *The New England Journal of Medicine,* 261:1006-1014, November 12, 1959.

————: The plasmocytic dyscrasias. Plasma cell myeloma and primary macroglobulinemia. (Editorial) *American Journal of Medicine,* 31:671-675, November 1961.

Osserman, E. F., and Fahey, J. L.: Plasma cell dyscrasias. Current clinical and biochemical concepts. *American Journal of Medicine,* 44:256-269, February 1968.

Osserman, E. F., and Lawlor, D. P.: Abnormal serum and urine proteins in thirty-five cases of multiple myeloma, as studied by filter paper electrophoresis. *American Journal of Medicine,* 18:462-476, March 1955.

————: Immunoelectrophoretic characterization of the serum and urinary proteins in plasma cell myeloma and Waldenström's macroglobulinemia. *Annals of the New York Academy of Sciences,* 94:93-109, August 31, 1961.

————: Serum and urinary lysozyme (Muramidase) in monocytic and monomyelocytic leukemia. *Journal of Experimental Medicine,* 124:921-951, November 1966.

Osserman, E. F., and Takatsuki, K.: Considerations regarding the pathogenesis of the plasmacytic dyscrasias. *Series Haematologica,* 4(*Gamma Globulins*):28-49, 1965.

————: Plasma cell myeloma: Gamma globulin synthesis and structure. A review of biochemical and clinical data, with the description of a newly-recognized and related syndrone. "Hγ2-chain (Franklin's) Disease." *Medicine,* 42:357-384, November 1963.

Osserman, E. F., Takatsuki, K., and Talal, N.: The pathogenesis of "amyloidosis." Studies of the role of abnormal gamma globulins and gamma globulin fragments of the Bence Jones (L-polypeptide) type in the pathogenesis of "primary" and "secondary amyloidosis," and "amyloidosis" associated with plasma cell myeloma. *Seminars in Hematology,* 1:3-86, January 1964.

Ozer, F. L., and Chaplin, H., Jr.: Agglutination of stored erythrocytes by a human serum. Characterization of the serum factor and erythrocyte changes. *Journal of Clinical Investigation,* 42:1735-1752, November 1963.

Peetoom, F., and Loghem-Langereis, E. van: IgM-IgG (beta $_2$M-7S)-cryoglobulinaemia: An auto-immune phenomenon. *Vox Sanguinis,* 10:281-292, May-June 1965.

Pfeiffer, R. A., Kosenow, W., and Bäumer, A.: Chromosomenuntersuchungen an Blutzellen eines Patienten mit Makroglobulinämie Waldenström. *Klinische Wochenschrift*, 40:342-344, April 1962.

Rádl, V. J., and Masopust, J.: Idiopathische Paraproteinämie. *Schweizerische medizinische Wochenschrift*, 94:961-967, July 1964.

Ray, C.: Haemolytic test in kala-azar. *Indian Medical Gazette*, 66:9, 1921.

Reisner, C. A., and Franklin, E. C.: Studies on mercaptoethanol-dissociated normal human 19S γ-globulin and pathologic macroglobulins from patients with macroglobulinemia. *The Journal of Immunology*, 87:654-664, December 1961.

Rifkind, R. A., Osserman, E. F., Hsu, K. C., and Morgan, C.: The intracellular distribution of gamma globulin in a mouse plasma cell tumor (X5563) as revealed by fluorescence and electron microscopy. *Journal of Experimental Medicine*, 116:423-432, October 1, 1962.

Ritzmann, S. E., Cobb, E. K., and Levin, W. C.: III. Electrophoretic differentiation of myeloma and macroglobulinemia M-proteins: Effects of D, L-penicillamine and ephacridine lactate on M-proteins. *Texas Reports on Biology and Medicine*, 25:273-280, Summer 1967.

Ritzmann, S. E., Coleman, S. L., and Levin, W. C.: The effect of mercaptanes upon a macrocryogelglobulin; modifications induced by cysteamine, penicillamine, and penicillin. *Journal of Clinical Investigation*, 39:1320-1329, August 1960.

Ritzmann, S.E., Daniels, J. C., and Levin, W. C.: Unpublished data.

Ritzmann, S. E., and Levin, W. C.: Cold agglutinin disease: A type of primary macroglobulinemia: A new concept. *Texas Reports on Biology and Medicine*, 20:236-250, Summer 1962.

————: Cryopathies: A review. *Archives of Internal Medicine*, 107:754-772, May 1961.

————: Effects of mercaptanes in cold agglutinin disease. *Journal of Laboratory and Clinical Medicine*, 57:718-732, May 1961.

————: II. Polyclonal and monoclonal gammopathies. In Dettelbach, H. R., and Ritzmann, S. E., Eds.: *Lab Synopsis*. Kansas City, Missouri, Hoechst Pharmaceutical Company, Diagnostic Reagents Division, March 1967, Vol. 2, pp. 9-50.

————: II. Polyclonal and monoclonal gammopathies. In Dettelbach, H. R., and Ritzmann, S. E., Eds.: *Lab Synopsis*. 2nd revised edition. Woodbury, New York, Behring Diagnostics, Inc., November 1, 1969, pp. 9-38.

Ritzmann, S. E., Thurm, R. H., and Levin, W. C.: Alpha-2-myeloma—the fallibility of arbitrary classifications of myeloma proteins. *Texas Reports on Biology and Medicine*, 21: 74-92, Spring 1963.

Ritzmann, S. E., Thurm, R. H., Truax, W. E., and Levin, W. C.: The syndrome of macroglobulinemia. Review of the literature and a report of two cases of macrocryogelglobulinemia. *Archives of Internal Medicine*, 105:939-965, June 1960.

Ritzmann, S. E., Wolf, R. E., Lawrence, M. C., Hart, J. S., and Levin, W. C.: The Sia euglobulin test: A re-evaluation. *Journal of Laboratory and Clinical Medicine*, 73:698-705, April 1969.

Ritzmann, S. E., Wolf, R. E., Schrohenloher, R. E., Riedel, L. O., Houston, E. W., and Levin, W. C.: "Spontaneous" remission in macroglobulinemia (Waldenström). IgM-monoclonal gammopathy with hyperviscosity syndrome, infectious hepatitis and remission. (In preparation.)

Riva, G.: *Das Serumeiweissbild. Lehrbuch der Untersuchungsmethoden und der klinischen Smeiologie der Serum- und Plasmaeiweissveränderungen mit besonderer Berücksichtigung der Elektrophorese.* Bern, Switzerland, and Stuttgart, Germany, Verlag Hans Huber, 1957, 631 pp.

————: Idiopathische und Begleitparaproteinämien. *Helvetica medica acta*, 31:285-297, May 1964.

Roman, W., and Coles, M.: Paraproteins in folic-acid deficiency. *Lancet*, 1:211-212, January 22, 1966.

Rothfield, N. F., Frangione, B., and Franklin, E. C.: Slowly sedimenting mercaptoethanol-resistant antinuclear factors related antigenically to M immunoglobulins (γ_{1M}-globulin) in patients with systemic lupus erythematosus. *Journal of Clinical Investigation*, 44:62-72, January 1965.

Roulet, D. L. A., Spengler, G. A., Gugler, E., Butler, R., Ricci, C., Riva, G., and Hassig, A.:

Antigenanalytische Untersuchungen an Paraproteinen. *Helvetica medica acta*, 28:127-148, January 1961.

Saifer, A.: A simple chemical test for distinguishing myeloma globulins from macroglobulins. *Journal of Laboratory and Clinical Medicine*, 63:1054-1060, June 1964.

Saifer, A., and Gerstenfeld, S.: The photometric microdetermination of serum γ-globulin with a tryptophan reaction. *Clinica chimica acta*, 7:149-154, 1962.

Sandberg, A. A., Ishihara, T., Kikuchi, Y., and Crosswhite, L. H.: Chromosomal differences among the acute leukemias. *Annals of the New York Academy of Sciences*, 113:663-717, February 28, 1964.

Sanders, J. H., Fahey, J. L., Finegold, I., Ein, D., Reisfeld, R., and Berard, C.: Multiple anomalous immunoglobulins: Clinical, structural and cellular studies in three patients. *American Journal of Medicine*, 47:43-59, July 1969.

Schaller, J., Davis, S. T., Ching, Y.-C., Lagunoff, D., Williams, C. P. S., and Wedgewood, R. J.: Hypergammaglobulinaemia, antibody deficiency, autoimmune haemolytic anaemia and nephritis in an infant with familial lymphopenic immune defect. *Lancet*, 2:825-829, October 15, 1966.

Schaub, F.: Gleichzeitiges Vorkommen von Makroglobulinämie Waldenström und von malignen Tumoren. *Schweizerische medizinische Wochenschrift*, 83:1256-1257, 1953.

Scheurlen, P. G.: Über Serumeiweissveränderungen beim Diabetes Mellitus. *Klinische Wochenschrift*, 33:198-205, March 1955.

Schoen, I.: Comments on the acid gel reaction. *Clinica chimica acta*, 17:520, September 1967.

Schoen, I., Glover, S. N., and Labiner, G.: An acid gel reaction of serum in patients with multiple myeloma. *American Journal of Clinical Pathology*, 43:467-474, May 1965.

Schubothe, H.: The cold hemagglutinin disease. *Seminars in Hematology*, 3:27-47, January 1966.

Schubothe, H., Kitahama, K., Klemm, O., and Erpenbeck, J.: Quantitative und qualitative Untersuchungen der Makroglobuline in Seren von Patienten mit chromischer Kalteagglutinin Krankheit. (Abstract) In *Proceedings of the 10th Congress of the European Society of Haematology*, Strasbourg, France, 1965, Communication 292.

Schubothe, H., Klemm, D., and Conraths, H.: Macroglobulinämie mit gleichzeitigem Auftreten zweier verschiedener "biologisch aktiver" Serumkomponenten. *Klinische Wochenschrift*. 43:1340-1344, December 1965.

Schwab, P. J., and Fahey, J. L.: Treatment of Waldenström's macroglobulinemia by plasmapheresis. *The New England Journal of Medicine*, 263:574-579, September 22, 1960.

Schwab, P. J., Okun, E., and Fahey, J. L.: Reversal of retinopathy in Waldenström's macroglobulinemia by plasmapheresis: A report of two cases. *Archives of Ophthalmology*, 64:515-521, October 1960.

Seligmann, M.: A genetic predisposition to Waldenström's macroglobulinaemia. *Acta medica scandinavica*, 179 (Suppl. 445):140-146, 1966.

Seligmann, M., and Basch, A.: The clinical significance of pathological immunoglobulins. In *Plenary Session Papers*, XII Congress of the International Society of Hematology, New York, New York, 1968, pp. 21-31.

Seligmann, M., Danon, F., and Mihaesco, C.: Family studies in Waldenström's macroglobulinemia. *Series Haematologica, 4(Gamma Globulins)*:50-64, 1965.

Seligmann, M., Danon, F., Mihaesco, C., and Fudenberg, H. H.: Immunoglobulin abnormalities in families of patients with Waldenström's macroglobulinemia. *American Journal of Medicine*, 43:66-83, July 1967.

Shullenberger, C. C.: Personal communication.

Sia, R. G. P., and Wu, H.: Simple method for estimating quantitative differences in globulin precipitin test in kala-azar. *Chinese Medical Journal*, 35:527-532, 1924.

Siebner, V. H., Spengler, G. A., Butler, R., Heni, F., and Riva, G.: Chromosomenanomalien bei Paraproteinämie. *Schweizerische medizinische Wochenschrift*, 95:1767-1781, December 1965.

Skoog, W. A., Adams, W. S., and Coburn, J. W.: Metabolic balance study of plasmapheresis in case of Waldenström's macroglobulinemia. *Blood, The Journal of Hematology*, 19:425-438, April 1962.

Smith, E., Kochwa, S., and Wasserman, L. R.: Aggregation of IgG globulin in vivo. I. The hyperviscosity syndrome in multiple myeloma. *American Journal of Medicine,* 39:35-48, July 1965.

Solomon, A., and Fahey, J. L.: Plasmapheresis therapy in macroglobulinemia. *Annals of Internal Medicine,* 58:789-800, May 1963.

Solomon, A., Fahey, J. L., and Malmgren, R. A.: Immunohistologic localization of gamma-1-macroglobulins, beta-2A-myeloma proteins, 6.6 S gamma-myeloma proteins and Bence Jones proteins. *Blood, The Journal of Hematology,* 21:403-423, April 1963.

Solomon, A., and Kunkel, H. G.: A "monoclonal" type, low molecular weight protein related to γM-macroglobulins. *American Journal of Medicine,* 42:958-967, June 1967.

Solomon, J., and Steinfeld, J. L.: Pyroglobulinemia. Report of a case with protein turnover studies. *American Journal of Medicine,* 38:937-942, June 1965.

Somer, T.: The viscosity of blood, plasma and serum in dys- and paraproteinemias. *Acta medica scandinavica,* 180 (Suppl. 456):1-97, 1966.

Stats, D., Perlman, E., Bullowa, J. G. M., and Goodkind, R.: Electrophoresis and antibody nitrogen determination of a cold hemagglutinin. *Proceedings of the Society for Experimental Biology and Medicine,* 53:188-190, June 1943.

Stevens, A. R., Jr.: Evolution of multiple myeloma. *Archives of Internal Medicine,* 115:90-93, January 1965.

Stiehm, E. R., Vaerman, J.-P., and Fudenberg, H. H.: Plasma infusions in immunologic deficiency states: Metabolic and therapeutic studies. *Blood, The Journal of Hematology,* 28:918-937, December 1966.

Stobo, J. D., and Tomasi, T. B., Jr.: A low molecular weight immunoglobulin antigenically related to 19 S IgM. *Journal of Clinical Investigation,* 46:1329-1337, August 1967.

Stoop, J. W., Ballieux, R. E., and Weyers, H. A.: Paraproteinemia with secondary immune globulin deficiency in an infant. *Pediatrics,* 29:97-104, January 1962.

Stoop, J. W., Zegers, B. J. M., Heiden, C. van der, and Ballieux, R. E.: Monoclonal gammopathy in a child with leukemia. *Blood, The Journal of Hematology,* 32:774-786, November 1968.

Sunderman, F. W., Jr.: Studies of the serum proteins. VI. Recent advances in clinical interpretation of electrophoretic fractionations. *American Journal of Clinical Pathology,* 42:1-21, July 1964.

Tomasi, T. B., Jr.: Human gamma globulin. *Blood, The Journal of Hematology,* 25:382-403, March 1965.

Vannotti, A.: Etude clinique d'un cas de macroglobulinémie de Waldenström à caractère familial, associé à des troubles endocriniens. *Schweizerische medizinische Wochenschrift,* 93:1744-1746, December 1963.

Vasquez, J. J.: Immunocytochemical study of plasma cells in multiple myeloma. *Journal of Laboratory and Clinical Medicine,* 51:271-275, February 1958.

Wager, O., Mustakallio, K. K., and Räsänen, J. A.: Mixed IgA-IgG cryoglobulinemia: Immunological studies and case reports of three patients. *American Journal of Medicine,* 44:179-187, February 1968.

Waldenström, J.: Abnormal proteins in myeloma. *Advances in Internal Medicine,* 5:398-440, 1952.

_____: Die Frühdiagnose der Myelomatose. *Acta chirurgica scandinavica,* 87:365-379, 1942.

_____: Incipient myelomatosis or "essential" hyperglobulinemia with fibrinogenopenia—a new syndrome? *Acta medica scandinavica,* 117:216-247, 1944.

_____: Monoclonal and polyclonal gammopathies and the biological system of gamma globulins. In Kallos, P., and Waksman, B. H., Eds.: *Progress in Allergy.* Basel, Switzerland, and New York, New York, S. Karger, 1962, Vol. VI, pp. 320-348.

_____: The occurrence of benign, essential monoclonal (M type), non-macromolecular hyperglobulinemia and its differential diagnosis. IV. Studies in the gammopathies. *Acta medica scandinavica,* 176:345-365, 1964.

_____: Studies on conditions associated with disturbed gamma globulin formation (gammopathies). *The Harvey Lectures,* 56:211-231, 1961.

Waldenström, J. G.: *Monoclonal and Polyclonal Hypergammaglobulinemia.* Nashville, Tennessee, Vanderbilt University Press, and Cambridge, England, Cambridge University Press, 1968, 232 pp.

Waldmann, T. A.: Hereditary disorders of albumin synthesis, in serum proteins and the dysproteinemias. In Sunderman, F. W., and Sunderman, F. W., Jr., Eds.: *Serum Proteins and the Dysproteinemias.* Philadelphia, Pennsylvania, and Montreal, Canada, J. B. Lippincott Co., 1964, pp. 406-409.

Wallerstein, R. S.: Multiple myeloma without demonstrable bone lesions. *American Journal of Medicine,* 10:325-333, March 1951.

Wert, E. B.: Identification and measurement of thermoproteins (cryoglobulin, pyroglobulin, cryofibrinogen). In Sunderman, F. W., and Sunderman, F. W., Jr., Eds.: *Serum Proteins and the Dysproteinemias.* Philadelphia, Pennsylvania, and Montreal, Canada, J. B. Lippincott Co., 1964, pp. 217-222.

Wilde, H., and Hitzelberger, A. L.: Macroglobulinemia: Clinical features and differential diagnosis. *Blood, The Journal of Hematology,* 9:875-880, September 1954.

Williams, R. C., Jr.: Hyperviscosity syndromes. (Editorial) *Circulation,* 38:450-452, September 1968.

Wintrobe, M. M., and Buell, M. V.: Hyperproteinemia associated with multiple myeloma. With report of a case in which an extraordinary hyperproteinemia was associated with thrombosis of the retinal veins and symptoms suggesting Raynaud's disease. *Bulletin of the Johns Hopkins Hospital,* 52:156-165, February 1933.

Wright, J. H.: A case of multiple myeloma. *Transactions of the Association of American Physicians,* 15:137-145, 1900.

Wuhrmann, F.: Albumindoppelzacken als Vererbbare Bluteiweissanomalie. *Schweizerische medizinische Wochenschrift,* 89:150-152, January 1957.

———: Uber das Coma Paraproteinaemicum bei Myelomen und Makroglobulinaemien. *Schweizerische medizinische Wochenschrift,* 86:623-625, May 1956.

Wuhrmann, F., and Märki, H. H.: *Dysproteinämien und Paraproteinämien. Grundlagen, Klinik und Therapie.* 4th edition. Basal, Switzerland, and Stuttgart, Germany, Verlag Schwabe and Co., 1963, 851 pp.

Zawadzki, Z. A., and Edwards, G. A.: Hypertransferrinemia simulating paraproteinemia. (Abstract) *Proceedings of the 50th Annual Session of American College of Physicians,* Chicago, Illinois, 1969.

Zucker-Franklin, D., Franklin, E. C., and Cooper, N. S.: Production of macroglobulins in vitro and a study of their cellular origin. *Blood, The Journal of Hematology,* 20:56-64, July 1962.

Zucker-Franklin, D., and Mullaney, V.: Structural features of cells associated with the paraproteinemias. *Seminars in Hematology,* 1:165-198, April 1964.

Newer Radiodiagnostic Contributions to the Study of the Lymphoma Patient

SIDNEY WALLACE, M.D.

Department of Diagnostic Radiology, The University of Texas M. D. Anderson Hospital and Tumor Institute at Houston, Houston, Texas

THE COMPLETE GAMUT of diagnostic procedures is used in the evaluation of the patient with lymphoma. In recent years angiography, including arteriography, venography, lymphangiography, and transhepatic cholangiography, has substantially expanded the radiologists' capabilities.

Lymphangiography

Lymphangiography is now an essential step in the diagnosis and treatment of the patient with lymphoma. More than 50 per cent of the 600 lymphangiographic examinations performed each year at The University of Texas M. D. Anderson Hospital and Tumor Institute at Houston are for the purpose of determining the extent of involvement in patients with lymphomas.

Certain basic tenets must be reiterated and adhered to so that the maximum amount of information may be extracted from this procedure. These include:

1. Lymphangiography, as the name implies, is the opacification of lymphatic channels as well as lymph nodes. Important information can be derived from studying alterations of the lymphatics, especially in the presence of complete nodal replacement.

2. Lymphangiography is a macroscopic procedure. Only a positive study has any significance; a negative examination does not preclude microscopic disease or involvement of nonopacified nodes.

3. Only a portion of the total number of nodes are opacified in any one area. However, this represents substantially more than are presented to the pathologist for scrutiny.

223

4. Certain nodal patterns may be considered reasonably diagnostic since they consistently occur when definite histologic entities are present. The lymphangiographic patterns suggest certain differential diagnostic possibilities which must be evaluated in light of the clinical picture.

Normally, lymph nodes vary considerably in size and number, with an inverse relationship existing between size and number (*i.e.* the larger the size, the fewer the number). The afferent lymphatics lead to the marginal sinus which empties into the medullary sinusoids. The medullary sinusoids are incomplete endothelial-lined pathways which eventually reconstitute as efferent channels. The internal architecture is fairly homogeneous. Nodal defects are considered structurally normal or benign if lymphatic channels transverse without interruption.

During acute inflammatory diseases, lymph nodes are usually enlarged, but maintain their normal architecture, density, and configuration. However, chronic inflammatory processes such as collagen diseases may produce marked lymphoid hyperplasia which results in lymphangiographic patterns easily confused with those seen in patients with chronic lymphocytic leukemia. Chronic granulomatous diseases, such as Boeck's sarcoid, present a picture similar to that of nodular sclerosing Hodgkin's disease. Tuberculosis with caseation necrosis may simulate carcinomatous metastases. In any event, the differential diagnostic possibilities present valuable information which must be correlated with the clinical findings.

The importance of the lymphatic phase must be emphasized in the diagnosis of metastatic carcinoma. Carcinomatous foci occlude the peripheral sinus, thereby obstructing the lymphatic channels. This occurs early in metastatic carcinoma, but later in the course of lymphomatous disease. Lymphatic abnormalities also may occur with lymphoma and are especially significant in the presence of complete nodal replacement.

Lymphomatous diseases frequently are associated with an increase in the size and number of opacified nodes. Variations in the architectural patterns of the nodes are produced by the different histologic entities. For the most part, the marginal sinus of the node is preserved until late in the disease, whereas early changes are seen in the internal architectural pattern. Certain patterns which are seen frequently have excellent correlation with the presence of different histologic types of disease, allowing the radiologist to suggest a specific histologic diagnosis. This correlation depends on a close working relationship between the radiologist and the pathologist.

Hodgkin's Disease

Utilizing the Rye modification of the Lukes and Butler (1966) classification, Hodgkin's disease has been subdivided into the following four types: (1) lymphocytic predominance, (2) nodular sclerosis, (3) mixed cellularity, and (4) lymphocytic depletion.

This classification also uses the low-power microscopic assessment of the nodal architecture, which is more closely related to the lymphangiographic patterns. Wiljasalo (1969) has evaluated this relationship and with an accuracy of 74 per cent could differentiate Hodgkin's disease from other malignant lymphomas. Of the categories of Hodgkin's disease, an accuracy of 70 per cent was found in distinguishing nodular sclerosis from the other subgroups. The mean survival time as calculated from the time of lymphography to death was clearly longer (mean, 2.8 years) in patients who showed lymphographic filling defects, which are typical of nodular sclerosis in particular, than in patients with other lymphographic features (the mean survival time of patients with the other patterns was from 1 to 1.5 years).

The distribution most frequently seen in early nodular sclerosis is an admixture of normal and abnormal nodes (Bismuth, Bourdon, Desprez-Curely, and Markovits, 1967). These nodes may be normal in size or only slightly enlarged. The margins of the nodes are intact early in the disease. Lucent defects within the nodes are fairly well delineated in a relatively normal background pattern (Fig. 1*A* and *B*). As the disease progresses the nodes become more diffusely involved, the background coarse, the lucencies more irregular and larger, the margins interrupted, and at times only a "shell" or portion of the peripheral sinus is opacified (Fig. 1*C*).

Mixed cellularity Hodgkin's disease may still be recognizable as a variation of the pattern seen in nodular sclerosis. Lyphocytic predominance and lymphocytic depletion do not show as consistent a pattern, but can still be categorized as a lymphoma.

As total nodal replacement ensues, the lymphatic channels are displaced and/or obstructed. Once lymphatic channels are obstructed, those lymphatics that are present and patent serve as collateral pathways. These include endothelial-lined lymphatic pathways, the paralymphatic pathways (interstitial spaces, perineural and perivascular spaces, submucosal and subserosal spaces, and the body's potential cavities such as the pleural, pericardial, and peritoneal spaces, *etc.*) and lymphaticovenous anastomoses. In the presence of nodal replacement, lymphatic abnormalities should be confirmed by venography to demonstrate the abnormal masses. Patients with this manifestation must be differentiated from those who have little if any residual lymphoid tissue, as is seen following therapy, but the lymphatic channels usually maintain their normal distribution.

At times, the patient with Hodgkin's disease demonstrates a confusing picture as depicted by the presence of fragments of lymphoid tissue not completely diagnostic of nodal involvement. Close follow-up is essential until specific architectural changes can be appreciated.

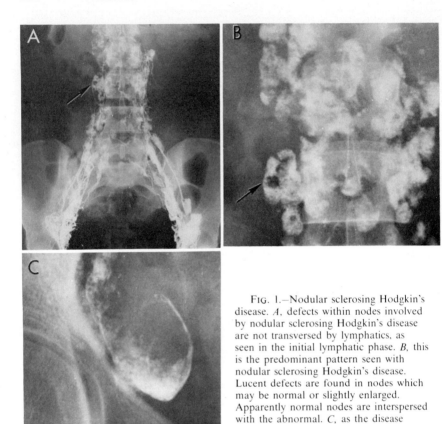

Fig. 1.—Nodular sclerosing Hodgkin's disease. *A*, defects within nodes involved by nodular sclerosing Hodgkin's disease are not transversed by lymphatics, as seen in the initial lymphatic phase. *B*, this is the predominant pattern seen with nodular sclerosing Hodgkin's disease. Lucent defects are found in nodes which may be normal or slightly enlarged. Apparently normal nodes are interspersed with the abnormal. *C*, as the disease progresses, the defects enlarge and almost totally replace the node.

In patients with Hodgkin's disease, the single most important application of lymphangiography is in staging by determining the extent of involvement. Restaging following lymphangiography has ranged from 16 per cent (Brickner, Boyer, and Perry, 1968) to 72 per cent (Wiljasalo, 1969). Approximately 35 per cent of stage I Hodgkin's disease patients show more advanced involvement as demonstrated by lymphangiographic findings (Davidson, Saini, and Peters, 1967; Schwarz, Lee, and Nelson, 1965). When presented with an equivocal picture or a "negative" examination, the following approach and philosophy may be considered:

1. A negative study is of no significance.
2. Opacification of the nodes will produce initial enlargement because of

the presence of the oil-based contrast material and the inflammatory reaction created. This subsides and the nodes regress in approximately two to four weeks without any therapy.

3. If there are clinical findings suggestive of more diffuse disease in the presence of normal or equivocal lymphangiographic findings, exploratory laparotomy is strongly recommended (Glatstein *et al.*, 1969). However, this approach is no panacea, for the surgeon may have considerable difficulty reaching and removing suspicious nodes in the retroperitoneal area. Some pathologists are still troubled by contrast-laden nodes, which undoubtedly create problems in the search for early changes. For this reason, suspicious nodes without contrast material might also be biopsied. Radiographs of the abdomen taken during the surgical procedure may be of assistance in the localization of specific lymph nodes.

4. An alternative to exploratory laparotomy is to follow the opacified nodes by repeat radiographs every two to three months until changes are noted. This is illustrated by a patient (Fig. 2*A*) with Hodgkin's disease, mixed cellularity, diagnosed by axillary node biopsy. One node in the right common iliac area was considered abnormal. The nodal configuration was more like that seen in carcinoma in that the defect was peripheral and lymphatics failed to transverse it. Nevertheless, this node is abnormal in a

Fig. 2.—Progression of mixed cellularity Hodgkin's disease. *A*, the initial study demonstrated a nodal defect which was not transversed by lymphatic channels. *B*, three months later, minimal residual contrast material was present and was displaced from its previous location, necessitating a repeat lymphangiogram. This study revealed extensive disease in the retroperitoneal lymph nodes.

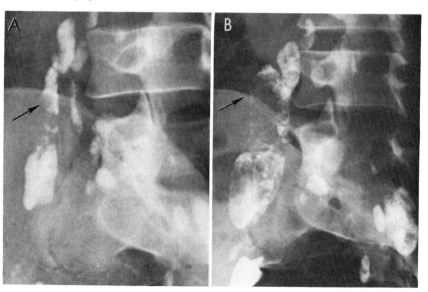

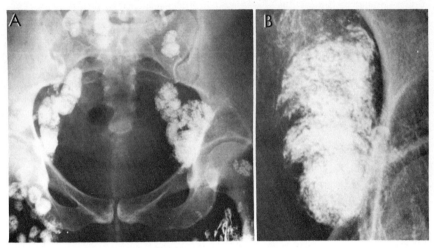

FIG. 3, *A* and *B.*—Nodular lymphoma. Coarse background pattern is a recognizable component of this entity.

patient with Hodgkin's disease. In three months, there was displacement of the minimal residual contrast material, which precipitated a repeat lymphangiogram. This time extensive changes were demonstrated in the retroperitoneal nodes (Fig. 2B). Subsequent follow-up examinations revealed the waxing and waning of disease while chemotherapy was being used. The longest period after which a single lymphangiogram was still diagnostically adequate was five years. Repeat lymphangiograms can be done when necessary for further clarification. We have repeated this examination as many as five times in one patient over a period of seven years with no obvious ill effects.

NODULAR LYMPHOMA

Nodular lymphoma (lymphoblastoma, follicular lymphoma, Brill-Symmer's disease) produces a lymphangiographic picture which is readily recognizable. The lymph nodes are usually enlarged, the margins for the most part are intact, and the internal architectural pattern is coarse (Fig. 3A and B). To illustrate the value of lymphangiography to visually chart the response of nodular lymphoma to therapy an examination one-and-a-half years after the initial study revealed marked regression of the disease (Fig. 4A and B).

LYMPHOCYTIC LYMPHOMA

Lymphocytic lymphoma (lymphosarcoma) has a much more delicate, lacy, or foamy background pattern (Fig. 5A). As the disease progresses, it

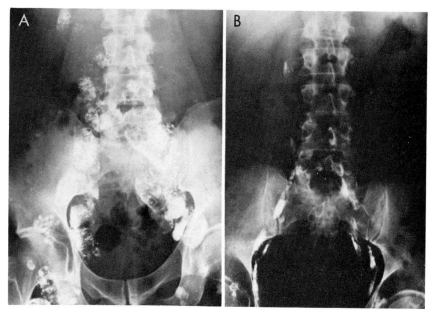

FIG. 4.—Evaluation of therapy. *A*, extensive involvement by nodular lymphoma as seen throughout the pelvic and para-aortic nodes. *B*, marked improvement following therapy is documented by the follow-up roentgen examination of the residual opacified nodes.

FIG. 5.—Lymphocytic lymphoma. *A*, these nodes have a more delicate, foamy, or lacy background pattern. The margins are usually intact. *B*, in more advanced disease, these nodes cannot be differentiated from chronic lymphocytic leukemia.

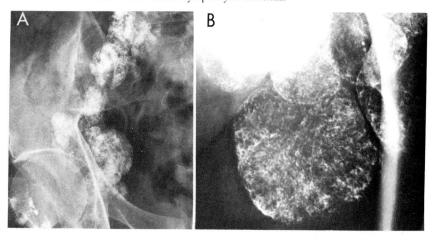

seems at times, to merge into patterns similar to those seen in chronic lymphocytic leukemia (Fig. 5B). Some pathologists have considerable difficulty in differentiating these two histologic entities.

Chronic Lymphocytic Leukemia

There is a fairly consistent lymphangiographic pattern early in the course of this disease. The contrast material clumps or flocculates in the node, producing a "salt and pepper" appearance. The margins of the nodes remain intact until late in the disease, in keeping with the lymphoma configuration (Fig. 6A and B). By the time the patient is first seen and the lymphangiogram performed, there is usually diffuse disease of approximately equal degree of involvement in all node groups.

Reticulum Cell Sarcoma

Reticulum cell sarcoma is difficult to describe. At times, it may have the lymphangiographic configuration of any of the aforementioned patterns or of patterns seen in carcinomatous involvement (Fig. 7). Perhaps our confusion is a reflection of the pathologist's difficulty in diagnosing this entity.

Fig. 6.—Chronic lymphocytic leukemia. A, there is usually an increase in size and number of nodes with a "salt and pepper" appearance. Almost all of the nodes opacified are involved to a fairly similar extent. B, extensive involvement of the axillary lymph nodes.

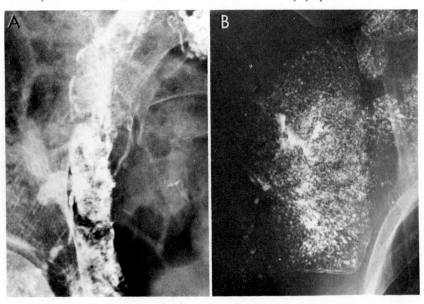

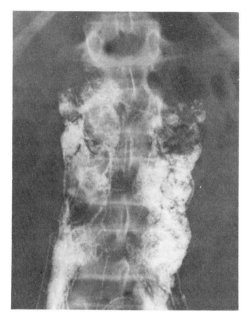

FIG. 7.—Reticulum cell sarcoma. The pattern illustrated is one of many seen with reticulum cell sarcoma.

In summary, lymphangiography will be of tremendous assistance in staging the disease only if it is positive. If negative, the study is of no value for the patient still may have the disease. Exploratory laparotomy and lymph node biopsy may supply essential information. The patient could also be followed by repeat radiographs of the opacified lymph nodes. Re-examination can be done when there is insufficient residual contrast material to be of diagnostic value.

Transhepatic Cholangiography

Percutaneous transhepatic cholangiography is a well-established procedure and has been utilized in the Diagnostic Radiology Department of Anderson Hospital for the demonstration of the etiologic agent in the production of obstructive jaundice in approximately 200 patients (Dodd, Greening, and Wallace, 1965). Jaundice in patients with lymphoma has also been investigated by this approach.

At present in our department, percutaneous transhepatic cholangiography is performed by percutaneous puncture in the right midaxillary line at the midportion of percussible liver dullness. The catheter-sheathed needle is directed toward the liver hilum usually in the line of projection of the twelfth thoracic vertebral body. The needle obturator is removed, leaving the Teflon catheter in place. Gradual withdrawal of the catheter is done

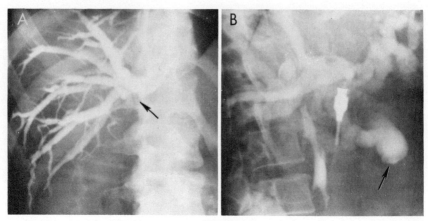

FIG. 8.—*A*, Hodgkin's disease involving the nodes at the hilum of the liver and producing complete obstruction. *B*, obstruction of the common bile duct by reticulum cell sarcoma.

until bile is aspirated, designating a biliary duct. Following maximal decompression of the bile duct, water-based radiopaque contrast material is injected. Opacification is readily accomplished when the ducts are dilated and only occasionally when they are of normal caliber. As much of the contrast medium is removed as is possible once the obstruction is demonstrated. The catheter is left in place until the operation is performed. The patient must be scheduled and prepared for surgical therapy to immediately follow the procedure. If for some reason the operation is postponed, drainage can be accomplished via the percutaneous catheter. This sequence is essential in order to diminish complications.

Both patients depicted in Figure 8 have lymphoma producing obstructive jaundice. Complete obstruction at the hilum of the liver by nodes involved with Hodgkin's disease is seen in Figure 8*A;* the other patient had a mass in the right upper quadrant caused by reticulum cell sarcoma producing obstruction of the common duct (Fig. 8*B*).

Arteriography and Venography

Inferior venacavography has been discussed previously as a complementary procedure to lymphangiography to be utilized in the presence of abnormal channels and nodal replacement. In patients with pulmonary disease which negates the performance of lymphangiography, inferior venacavography may be used to determine the existence of retroperitoneal nodal disease. This technique is of limited value, however, because only masses on the right side of the retroperitoneal space and large enough to impinge upon the inferior vena cava can be appreciated. Arteriography has

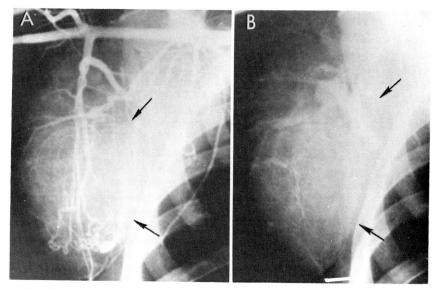

FIG. 9, *A* and *B*.—Nodular sclerosing Hodgkin's disease. There is an increased vascularity to an enlarged node involved by Hodgkin's disease.

been used sparingly in the diagnosis of lymphomatous diseases. Arterial catheterization by means of the Seldinger technique can be used to advantage as illustrated by the following cases.

A 15-year-old male was seen because of a large, freely movable mass in the right axilla which had been present for at least one year. A bruit was heard at the base of the neck on the right. Arteriography was performed to delineate the vascular supply to this mass, which eventually proved to be a huge node involved with nodular sclerosing Hodgkin's disease. There was an increase in vascularity in the axillary mass and in a smaller mass in the base of the neck. The configuration of these vessels was unusual (Fig. 9). This suggests the potential application of this procedure to evaluate mesenteric nodes, which usually escape detection, by selective superior and inferior mesenteric arteriography.

Arteriography in combination with lymphangiography was used to determine the etiologic agent for the next patient's complaint of abdominal and back pain. A retroperitoneal mass was opacified by arteriography (Fig. 10*A* and *B*). This was diagnosed more specifically by lymphangiography as retroperitoneal nodes involved by reticulum cell sarcoma (Fig. 10*C* and *D*). Obstruction of the lumbar lymphatic trunks and opacification of the liver portal venous capillaries were seen. These collateral pathways via lymphaticoportal vein anastomoses were accompanied by inferior vena caval occlusion.

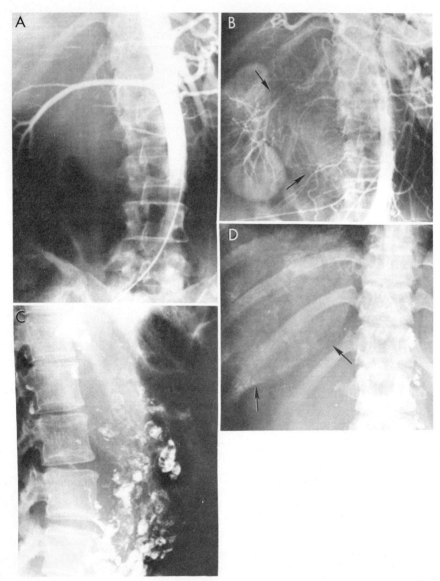

FIG. 10.—Reticulum cell sarcoma involving the retroperitoneal nodes. *A*, the right renal artery is displaced by the retroperitoneal mass. *B*, the abnormal vasculature delineated a mass in the retroperitoneal space displacing the right kidney. *C*, lymphomatous involvement of the lumbar lymph nodes was demonstrated by lymphangiography. *D*, oil-based contrast material seen in the liver as a manifestation of obstruction of the lumbar lymphatic trunks and inferior vena cava with collateral flow through lymphaticoportal vein anastomoses.

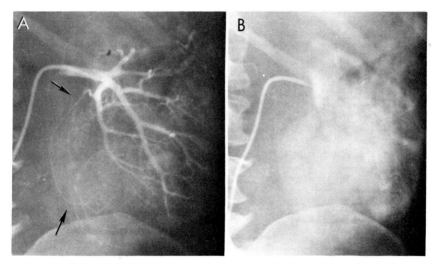

Fig. 11.—Perirenal Hodgkin's disease. *A,* the kidney is displaced laterally. *B,* abnormal vasculature is seen originating from the capsular and pelvic branches of the left renal artery. The Hodgkin's mass encased the kidney. (Courtesy of Dr. A. F. Barrett, Heights Hospital, Houston, Texas.)

Perhaps the most promising use of arteriography is the demonstration of involvement by lymphoma of solid organs, the liver, spleen, and kidneys (Fig. 11). This also is illustrated by a patient (Fig. 12) who was examined by arteriography for the intra- vs. extrahepatic localization of a right upper quadrant mass. The mass, which contained abnormal vessels, was supplied by the right hepatic artery and, therefore, was within the anterior inferior segment of the right lobe of the liver. Another patient (Fig. 13*A*) with known reticulum cell sarcoma had a precipitous onset of ascites and lower extremity edema. Liver biopsy revealed venous engorgement and, combined with the clinical findings, suggested hepatic vein obstruction, as in a Budd-Chiari syndrome. The arteriogram revealed diffuse abnormal liver vasculature with wide separation of the vessels to the left lateral lobe of the liver. The tract produced by the liver biopsy was opacified. The patient had had a splenectomy previously accounting for the configuration of the splenic artery. Partial occlusion of the inferior vena cava by a mass in the liver was considered confirmation of hepatic vein obstruction (Fig. 13*B*). Following chemotherapy, there was considerable improvement in the caliber of the inferior vena cava and hepatic veins.

The increased utilization of these procedures can provide essential information in determining the extent of the disease and in assisting in the treatment of these patients.

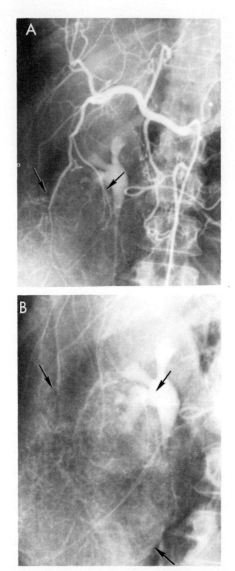

FIG. 12.—*A*, malignant lymphoma manifested as a localized mass in the anterior-inferior segment of the right lobe of the liver. The anterior branches of the right hepatic artery are displaced. *B*, abnormal vasculature is noted in the lymphomatous mass.

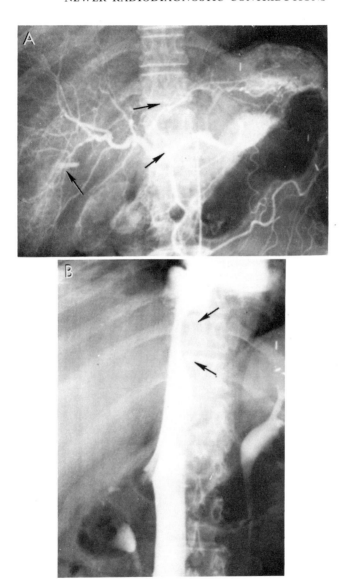

FIG. 13.—Reticulum cell sarcoma producing a Budd-Chiari syndrome. *A*, the celiac arteriogram revealed abnormal vasculature in the liver. The left hepatic branches are displaced by a mass. The tract (arrows) depicted the site of the previous needle biopsy. *B*, the inferior vena cava is partially obstructed by the mass in the liver.

238 / WALLACE

REFERENCES

Bismuth, V., Bourdon, R., Desprez-Curely, J. P., and Markovits, P.: Lymphography in malignant lymphoma: Panel-discussion IV. In Ruttimann, A., Ed.: *Progress in Lymphology, Proceedings of the International Symposium on Lymphology,* Zurich, Switzerland, July 19-23, 1966. Stuttgart, West Germany, Georg Thieme Verlag, and New York, New York, Hafner Publishing Co., 1967, p. 160.

Bourdon, R., Desprez-Curely, J. P., Bismuth, V., Dana, M., and Markovits, P.: Incidences de la lymphographie sur la classification clinique de la maladie de Hodgkin. *Nouvelle Revue Française d'Hématologie,* 6(1):32-46, 1966.

Brickner, T. J., Jr., Boyer, C. W., Jr., and Perry, R. H.: Limited value of lymphangiography in Hodgkin's disease. *Radiology,* 90:52-56, January 1968.

Davidson, J. W.: Lymphography in malignant disease: Radiological aspects. *Canadian Medical Association Journal,* 97:1283-1289, November 18, 1967.

Davidson, J. W., Saini, M., and Peters, M. V.: Lymphography in lymphoma. With particular reference to Hodgkin's disease. *Radiology,* 88:281-286, February 1967.

Dodd, G. D., Greening, R. R., and Wallace, S.: The radiologic diagnosis of cancer. In Nealson, T. F., Jr., Ed.: *Management of the Patient with Cancer.* Philadelphia, Pennsylvania, and London, England, W. B. Saunders Co., 1965, pp. 72-113.

Fuchs, W. A.: In Panel-Discussion IV. In Ruttimann, A., Ed.: *Progress in Lymphology, Proceedings of the International Symposium on Lymphology,* Zurich, Switzerland, July 19-23, 1966. Stuttgart, West Germany, Georg Thieme Verlag, and New York, New York, Hafner Publishing Co., 1967, p. 158.

Fuchs, W. A., and Hartel, M.: Prognosis of Hodgkin's disease according to radiographic pattern of lymph nodes. In Ruttimann, A., Ed.: *Progress in Lymphology, Proceedings of the II International Symposium on Lymphology,* Miami Beach, Florida, 1968. Stuttgart, West Germany, Georg Thieme Verlag, and New York, New York, Hafner Publishing Co. (In press.)

Glatstein, E., Guernsey, J. M., Rosenberg, S. A., and Kaplan, H. S.: The value of laparotomy and splenectomy in the staging of Hodgkin's disease. *Cancer,* 24:709-718, October 1969.

Jing, B.-S., and McGraw, J. P.: Lymphangiography in diagnosis and management of lymphomas. *Cancer,* 19:565-572, April 1966.

Kaplan, H. S., and Rosenberg, S. A.: The cure of malignant lymphomas. *Hospital Practice,* 3:29-33, March 1968.

Lee, B. J.: Correlation between lymphangiography and clinical status of patients with lymphoma. *Cancer Chemotherapy Reports,* 52:205-211, January 1968.

———: Evaluation of the patient with lymphoma by means of lymphangiography; comments on importance and complications. In Ruttimann, A., Ed.: *Progress in Lymphology, Proceedings of the International Symposium on Lymphology,* Zurich, Switzerland, July 19-23, 1966. Stuttgart, West Germany, Georg Thieme Verlag, and New York, New York, Hafner Publishing Co., 1967, p. 127.

Lukes, R. J., and Butler, J. J.: The pathology and nomenclature of Hodgkin's disease. *Cancer Research,* 26:1063-1081, June 1966.

Myo, K., and Koehler, R. P.: Renal and perirenal lymphoma: Arteriographic findings. *Radiology,* 93:1055-1058, November 1969.

Peters, M. V., Brown, T. C., Davidson, J. W., Saxena, V. S., and Saini, M.: The value of locating occult disease in the treatment of Hodgkin's disease. In Ruttimann, A., Ed.: *Progress in Lymphology, Proceedings of the International Symposium on Lymphology,* Zurich, Switzerland, July 19-23, 1966. Stuttgart, West Germany, Georg Thieme Verlag, and New York, New York, Hafner Publishing Co., 1967, p. 119.

Rosenberg, S. A.: Contribution of lymphangiography to our understanding of lymphoma. *Cancer Chemotherapy Reports,* 52:213-228, January 1968.

Rosenberg, S. A., and Kaplan, H. S.: Evidence for orderly progression in the spread of Hodgkin's disease. *Cancer Research,* 26:1225-1231, June 1966.

Schwarz, G., Lee, B. J., and Nelson, J. H.: Lymphography, cavography, and urography in the evaluation of malignant lymphomas: A study of 100 consecutive lymphoma cases. *Acta radiologica (Diagnosis)*, 3:138-144, March 1965.

Seltzer, R. A., and Wenlund, D. E.: Renal lymphoma: Arteriographic studies. *The American Journal of Roentgenology, Radium Therapy and Nuclear Medicine*, 101:692-695, November 1967.

Viamonte, M., Jr., Altman, D., Parks, R., Blum, E., Bevillacqua, M., and Recher, L.: Radiographic-pathologic correlation in the interpretation of lymphangioadenograms. *Radiology*, 80:903-916, June 1963.

Wallace, S., and Jackson, L.: Diagnostic criteria for lymphangiographic interpretation of malignant neoplasia. *Cancer Chemotherapy Reports*, 52:125-145, January 1968.

Wiljasalo, M.: Lymphographic differential diagnosis of neoplastic diseases. *Acta radiologica*, (Suppl. 247): 1-143, 1965.

Wiljasalo, S.: Lymphographic polymorphism in Hodgkin's disease. *Acta radiologica*, (Suppl. 289):1-89, 1969.

Williams, L. H., Anastopulos, H. P., and Presant, C. A.: Selective renal arteriography in Hodgkin's disease of the kidney. A case report. *Radiology*, 93:1059-1060, November 1969.

Results of Definitive Radiotherapy in Localized Hodgkin's Disease, as Related to both Clinical Presentation and Pathological Classification*

LILLIAN M. FULLER, M.D.,
JESS F. GAMBLE, M.D., AND
JAMES J. BUTLER, M.D.

*Departments of Radiotherapy, Medicine, and Pathology, The University of Texas
M. D. Anderson Hospital and Tumor Institute at Houston, Houston, Texas*

RADIOTHERAPEUTIC RESULTS in the treatment of Hodgkin's disease have only recently been recognized as being dependent not only on the stage of disease, treatment fields, and tumor dose, but also on the site of origin and the specific pathology (Keller, Kaplan, Lukes, and Rappaport, 1968). Although Kaplan's four-stage system for classifying extent of disease originating in lymph nodes generally has been accepted (Kaplan, 1966), unanimity has not been achieved on a classification for disease originating in extranodal sites. Our method, exemplified in Figure 1, is a four-stage system based on Peters' (1950) original classification, which included disease originating in extranodal sites, more common in the lymphomas, as well as disease of lymph node origin. Conventionally, the letters A and B were retained to designate constitutional status; A represents no constitutional symptoms, and B represents systemic symptomatology, *i.e.* fever, night sweats, pruritis, or profound weight loss.

Although Jackson and Parker (1947) were able to correlate prognosis with two histological extremes, Hodgkin's paragranuloma and Hodgkin's

---

*This investigation was supported in part by Public Health Service Grants No. CA 06294 and No. CA 05654.

241

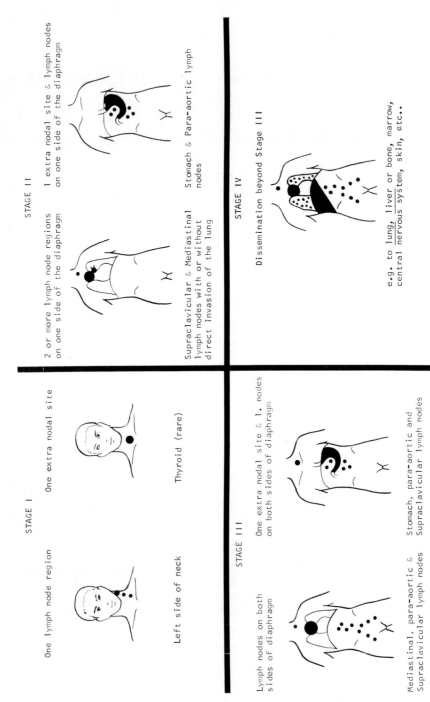

STAGE I

One lymph node region   One extra nodal site

Left side of neck   Thyroid (rare)

STAGE II

2 or more lymph node regions   1 extra nodal site & lymph nodes
on one side of the diaphragm   on one side of the diaphragm

Supraclavicular & Mediastinal   Stomach & Para-aortic lymph
lymph nodes with or without   nodes
direct invasion of the lung

STAGE III

One extra nodal site & l. nodes
on both sides of diaphragm

Lymph nodes on both
sides of diaphragm

Mediastinal, para-aortic &   Stomach, para-aortic and
Supraclavicular lymph nodes   Supraclavicular lymph nodes

STAGE IV

Dissemination beyond Stage III

e.g. to lung, liver or bone, marrow,
central nervous system, skin, etc..

Fig. 1.—*Stage I.* The disease is limited to one lymphatic system, or one extranodal site exclusive of liver, bone marrow, or diffuse involvement of the skin, *etc.* Stages I through IV are further subdivided according to constitutional symptoms; *e.g.*, in stage IA there are no constitutional symptoms; whereas in stage IB, constitutional symptoms are present.

Stage II. The disease is limited to one side of the diaphragm, *i.e.*, to two or more lymphatic systems, with or without involvement of a single organ other than liver, *etc.* Since direct invasion of adjacent structures is potentially curable with radiotherapy (as opposed to diffuse involvement), this is considered stage II, as per example, and not stage IV.

Stage III. The disease has progressed beyond stage II to involve the lymphatic systems on both sides of the diaphragm. See description of stage II.

Stage IV. The disease has generalized beyond stage III to diffusely involve lung, liver, bone, bone marrow, skin, central nervous system, *etc.*

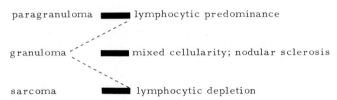

Fig. 2.—Relation of the Jackson and Parker system of classification to the Rye modification of the Lukes and Butler system.

sarcoma, their method of classification was not refined sufficiently to be of value in the Hodgkin's granuloma group. Recognizing that a more refined classification might permit better correlation of histological type with prognosis, Lukes and Butler developed a classification based on predominant cell types. A simplified version of their original classification (Lukes and Butler, 1966) known as the Rye modification (Lukes *et al.*, 1966) is shown in relation to the Jackson and Parker system in Figure 2.

In a retrospective analysis of a large series of patients with Hodgkin's disease of all stages treated in a variety of ways, Lukes (1963) concluded that the prognosis was better for nodular sclerosing Hodgkin's disease than for the mixed cellularity type, particularly when the disease involved the mediastinum as part of a localized process. This observation was confirmed subsequently by Butler for a more homogeneous group of our patients treated with intensive, large-volume irradiation for localized Hodgkin's disease involving the mediastinum (Fuller, Jing, Shullenberger, and Butler, 1967). In an attempt to correlate specific pathology with other sites of origin, a recent review was undertaken of patients with stages I and II Hodgkin's disease admitted to The University of Texas M. D. Anderson Hospital and Tumor Institute at Houston from 1947 through 1963, the majority of whom were treated intensively with large-volume radiotherapy.

Material

As of August 1968, 164 patients with a diagnosis of localized Hodgkin's disease had been analyzed. A pathological review was undertaken in 153 of the 164 cases for purposes of reclassification according to the method of Lukes and Butler (1966) and of eliminating patients with disease other than Hodgkin's disease. Of 136 patients in whom the diagnosis of Hodgkin's disease was reconfirmed, the breakdown was as follows: lymphocytic predominance, 13; nodular sclerosing, 71; mixed cellularity, 43; lymphocytic

TABLE 1.—DISTRIBUTION OF HODGKIN'S DISEASE ACCORDING
TO SPECIFIC PATHOLOGY*

	TOTAL	LYMPHOCYTIC PREDOMINANCE	NODULAR SCLEROSING	MIXED CELLULAR	LYMPHOCYTIC DEPLETION
	132 (74)†	13 (8)	71 (42)	43 (23)	5 (1)
Male	81 (40)	11 (7)	33 (17)	33 (15)	4 (1)
Female	51 (34)	2 (1)	38 (25)	10 (8)	1 (0)

*Fifteen cases are not included in this table. The slides were not available for review in 11 cases diagnosed initially as Hodgkin's disease in our institution. In four others, the biopsy specimen was too small for subclassification.
†Figures in parentheses indicate number of patients living.

depletion, 5; unclassifiable because the biopsy specimen was too small, 4 (Table 1, Fig. 3). Of 28 not confirmed as Hodgkin's disease, 13 were considered to be malignant lymphomas other than Hodgkin's disease. In three others, the diagnosis was uncertain. Only one case was considered to be definitely benign. In the 11 others, the slides were unavailable for review, but since their clinical course supported our original diagnosis of Hodgkin's disease, these cases were included in this study.

On the basis of our previous observation (Fuller, Jing, Shullenberger, and Butler, 1967) that localized Hodgkin's disease involving the mediastinum is predominantly nodular sclerosing, an analysis of the 132 cases of Hodgkin's disease, subclassified by specific histological type, was undertaken to determine differences in incidence and prognosis by apparent site of origin, or major area of involvement when two or more adjacent areas were affected (Fig. 3). Assignment to major areas, i.e. neck, mediastinum, abdomen, etc., was based on the probability of adjacent spread. For example, involvement of the mediastinum, neck, and axillae was plotted under mediastinum, the mediastinum being the most important region from the standpoint of subsequent spread of disease. Involvement of the axilla and ipsilateral supraclavicular fossa was carried under axilla. The head and neck region was subdivided according to whether disease was limited to Waldeyer's ring, one side of the neck (the upper and lower portions of the neck being considered separately), or both sides of the neck. Although the majority of the patients were young males, the age and sex distribution was affected by site of origin when correlated with histological type. Whereas Hodgkin's disease in the mediastinum was predominantly nodular sclerosing and affected young females (Fuller, Jing, Shullenberger, and Butler, 1967), Hodgkin's disease of one side of the upper neck was limited almost exclusively to young males, the specific histology being mixed cellularity (Fig. 3, Table 2).

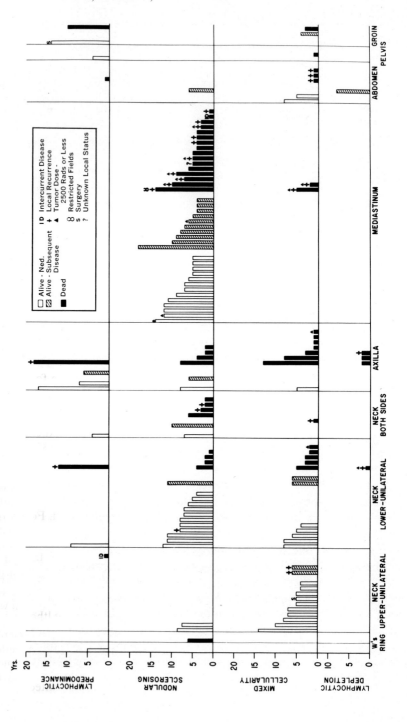

FIG. 3.—The relative incidence and prognosis can be determined for the four histological types by major site of involvement by comparing the bar graphs on the individual survival status of 132 stages I and II patients, reclassified according to the method of Lukes and Butler. With the exception of two patients treated successfully by radical dissection, all the patients were treated with irradiation therapy. Two patients, surviving 18 years and four years, who were treated for nodular sclerosing Hodgkin's disease of the mediastinum (stage II), developed an axillary node as a single new area. These extensions were considered minor. Note the low incidence of involvement of Waldeyer's (W's) ring.

TABLE 2.—DISTRIBUTION BY AGE OF PATIENTS WITH CANCER OF THE HEAD AND NECK: STAGES I AND II*

SITE	AGE	LYMPHOCYTIC PREDOMINANCE				NODULAR SCLEROSING				MIXED CELLULAR				LYMPHOCYTIC DEPLETION				TOTALS			
		T	M	A	F	T	M	A	F	T	M	A	F	T	M	A	F	T	M	A	F
W's ring	Under 40	1	1 (1)		0	1	1 (0)		0	0				0				2 (1)	2 (1)		0
	Over 40		0				0														
Upper neck	Under 40	1	1 (0)		0	2	2 (2)		0	12 (12)	7 (7)		1 (1)	0				15 (14)	12 (11)		3 (3)
	Over 40		0								2 (2)		2 (2)								
Lower neck	Under 40	2	2 (1)		0	16 (12)	3 (3)		7 (6)	12 (7)	8 (5)		2 (2)	1	1 (0)		0	31 (20)	19 (10)		12 (10)
	Over 40		0				3 (1)		3 (2)		2 (0)		0		0						
Both neck	Under 40	1	1 (1)		0	6 (2)	4 (1)		1 (1)	1	1 (0)		0	0				8 (3)	6 (2)		2 (1)
	Over 40		0				0		1		0										
Totals		5 (3)	5 (3)		0	25 (16)	13 (7)		12 (9)	25 (19)	20 (14)		5 (5)	1 (0)	1 (0)		0	56 (38)	39 (24)		17 (14)

*In this series, the histological type of Hodgkin's disease of the neck was related to the site of origin. For example, disease limited to one side of the upper neck was almost exclusively of the mixed cellular variety. Despite the fact that the sex incidence was predominantly male, the prognosis was excellent (Fig. 3. Table 7).
Abbreviations: A, alive; F, female; M, male; T, total.

Treatment

In keeping with the present-day approach to the treatment of localized Hodgkin's disease, our policy has been to administer intensive radiotherapy to the involved region or regions. During the earlier years, however, a few patients were treated less intensively because their disease was considered too extensive for kilovoltage techniques. These patients and two who had radical surgical procedures for stage I disease (Fig. 2) have been included for comparison. Whether or not prophylactic irradiation was administered in conjunction with definitive treatment was dependent upon the proximity of the adjacent regions. For example, patients treated definitively to the supraclavicular fossa received prophylaxis to the mediastinum, whereas prophylaxis was not administered to the para-aortic nodes in patients treated for disease involving the upper mediastinum.

The optimum tumor dose in terms of local control and freedom of complications was somewhat dependent on the site of origin, specific histological diagnosis, volume of tumor, and the dose rate.

NECK

For involvement of the neck, doses of 3,000 to 4,000 rads, delivered at a rate of 750 or, preferably, 1,000 rads per week generally were sufficient, provided additional treatment was given for residual disease (Table 3).

The over-all value of prophylactic irradiation to the mediastinum has yet to be determined on the basis of a randomized series of cases. However, our policy has been to irradiate the mediastinum prophylactically for patients with disease localized to the neck, with one exception. Of 15 patients with involvement of one side of the upper part of the neck, treatment was limited to the affected region in eight, and the other seven received prophylaxis to the mediastinum. During the kilovoltage era, the mediastinum, neck, and axillae generally were treated in series. Prophylactic irradiation to the mediastinum tended to be prolonged. Judging by the recurrences for tumor doses of 2,500 rads delivered in a period of more than three weeks, this dose rate was too slow. However, 2,500 rads delivered at a rate of 1,000 rads per week was apparently adequate.

With the introduction of megavoltage and the resultant improvement in local and systemic tolerance, the mediastinum and axillae were prophylactically irradiated concurrent with treatment to the neck via a single anterior "mantle" field (Fig. 4) opposed by separate posterior fields covering the mediastinum, axillae, and neck, but not the supraclavicular fossae, where the lymph nodes are anterior. By using a differential loading of approximately 3:2 in favor of the anterior field, a uniform daily dose to the neck, mediastinum, and axillae was achieved. When the mediastinum

TABLE 3.—Relationship of Dose to Local Control of Hodgkin's Disease of the Neck: Stages I and II*

Dose† (Rads)		Supplement to Residual Disease					Local Control	Local Recurrence
		None	250	500	1,000	1,500		
<3,000	2	2 (C 2)					2	
3,000	1	1 (C 1)					1	
3,500	20	11 (C 9, R 2)	2 (C 2)	2 (C 2)	5 (C 5)	2 (C 2)	17	3
4,000	7	4 (C 2, R 2)			2 (C 2)	1 (C 1)	5	2
4,500	25	12 (C 10, R 2)		5 (C 4, R 1)	5 (C 5)	1 (C 1)	22	3
5,000	4	1 (R 1)		2 (C 1, R 1)		1 (C 1)	2	2
Total	59	31 (C 24, R 7)	2 (C 2)	9 (C 7, R 2)	12 (C12)	5 (C 5)	49	10

*Not included was one patient treated by radical neck dissection and one patient with disease confined to Waldeyer's ring. (One patient with involvement of Waldeyer's ring metastatic to the ipsilateral neck is included.)

Although tumor doses of 3,000 to 4,000 rads delivered at a rate of 750 to 1,000 rads per week were effective in the majority of patients with Hodgkin's disease of the neck, the best results were obtained when supplementary doses of 1,000 to 1,500 rads were administered for residual disease.

†Approximate dose in rads.

Abbreviations: C, disease controlled; R, disease recurrent.

and axillae reached a prophylactic tumor dose of 2,500 to 3,000 rads, treatment to these regions was discontinued. Thereafter treatment to the neck was carried to definitive dose levels.

MEDIASTINUM

The definitive dose range for Hodgkin's disease of the mediastinum was the same as for the neck, except that additional treatment for residual disease seldom was used. Although tumor doses of 3,000 rads will permanently control mediastinal disease in the majority of cases, our preference was to irradiate the mediastinum to tolerance, i.e. 4,000 rads, because of

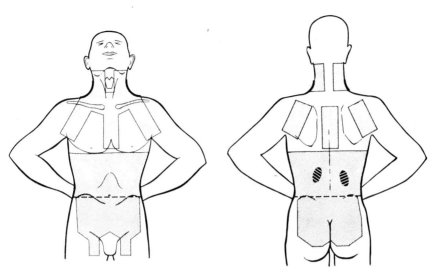

Fig. 4.—*Upper torso.* An anterior "mantle" supplemented by posterior mediastinal, axillary, and cervical fields is commonly used for combinations of definitive and prophylactic treatment. *Lower torso.* The abdomen and pelvis may be treated with fields extending from the dome of the diaphragm to the symphysis pubis. An alternative is to treat the abdomen and pelvis in two courses, the separation of the treatment fields being drawn at the iliac crest *(dotted line).* A discussion of irradiation techniques and tumor doses is presented in the text.

the risk of such serious complications as pericarditis and paraplegia encountered with retreatment for recurrent disease. However, in irradiating the mediastinum to tumor doses of 4,000 rads in four to five weeks, the treatment fields were reduced with reduction in the tumor mass to avoid excessive paramediastinal fibrosis (Fig. 5).

ABDOMEN

Our approach to the treatment of frank abdominal disease differs from most centers in that we do not use the inverted T- or Y-shaped fields; instead, we include the entire abdomen and pelvis, our rationale being to treat the liver and spleen prophylactically. Our opinion that these organs should be treated prophylactically is based on the fact that the majority of patients eventually develop involvement of the liver and spleen. Whether treatment to the abdomen was administered in one or two courses depended upon the extent of involvement, the age of the patient, the white blood cell and platelet counts, *etc.* For whole-abdomen irradiation administered with the cobalt-60 unit, the treatment fields extended from the dome of the diaphragm to the midsymphysis anteriorly and posteriorly (Fig. 4*A* and *B*). The kidneys were shielded posteriorly with two half-value layers of lead

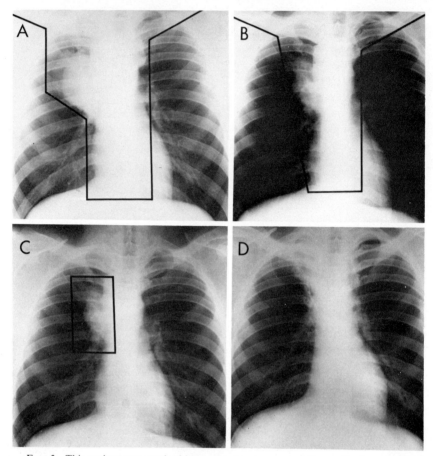

FIG. 5.—This patient presented with massive involvement of the mediastinum and right neck secondary to nodular sclerosing Hodgkin's disease. To spare normal lung, the treatment fields (^{60}Co) were initially shaped as shown in A. With loss of tumor volume, the fields were narrowed appropriately (B). Following a tumor dose of 4,000 rads, additional treatment was administered for residual disease (500 rads tumor dose) through very reduced fields (C). Follow-up films (D) demonstrated minimal paramediastinal fibrosis. (Courtesy of Fuller, Jing, Shullenberger, and Butler, 1967.)

from the onset of treatment to reduce the over-all dose to tolerable levels. Treatment was administered at a rate of 750 rads tumor dose for a total of 3,000 rads, the dose to the kidneys being approximately 2,000 rads. Additional treatment was given for residual disease when possible.

When treatment was given in two courses, the more involved or symptomatic area was treated initially. For example, if the upper two thirds of the abdomen were treated preliminarily, a rest period of six to eight weeks would be allowed before initiating treatment to the pelvis.

TABLE 4.—ABSOLUTE FIVE-YEAR SURVIVAL BY SPECIFIC PATHOLOGY:
PATIENTS ADMITTED 1947-1963 FOLLOWED TO AUGUST 1968:
STAGES I AND II

	STAGE		STAGE		
Lymphocytic	I A	83.3 % (5/6)	II A	100.0% (2/2)	
Predominance	I B	100.0 % (1/1)	II B	— (0/0)	
Total Stages I & II					88.9 % (8/9)
Nodular	I A	72.2 % (13/18)	II A	75.9 % (22/29)	
Sclerosing	I B	50.0 % (1/2)	II B	72.7 % (8/11)	
Total Stages I & II					73.3 % (44/60)
Mixed	I A	70.8 % (17/24)	II A	33.3 % (1/3)	
Cellularity	I B	50.0 % (1/2)	II B	33.3 % (1/3)	
Total Stages I & II					
Lymphocytic	I A	— (0/1)	II A	— (0/3)	
Depletion	I B	— (0/0)	II B	100.0 % (1/1)	
Total Stages I & II					20.0 % (1/5)
Grand Total Stages I & II					66.9 % (75/112)

A—No constitutional symptoms Stages I A and II A
B—Constitutional symptoms Stages I B and II B

The effect of constitutional symptoms on the survival figures was dependent on the stage of disease. Although the results for Stage I A were better than for I B, the reverse was true for Stages II A and II B. The majority of the patients with Stage II B had mediastinal involvement with associated fever which responded promptly to irradiation therapy, suggesting that fever associated with mediastinal disease does not have the same prognostic significance as constitutional symptoms associated with other sites of involvement such as the abdomen.

Patients presenting with disease limited to the inguinal or femoral nodes, who received prophylaxis to the iliac and para-aortic chains, were treated through the inverted T- or Y-shaped fields.

Results

At the time of this study, 100 per cent follow-up had been obtained on the 147 patients admitted with clinically localized Hodgkin's disease from 1947 through 1963. The absolute five- and 10-year survival figures for the entire group were 66 and 43 per cent (Table 5). Contrary to the findings in most series, the results for a small group of stages IB and IIB patients who presented with constitutional symptoms did not differ significantly from the results for patients with no constitutional symptoms. Although the results for stage IA were better than for stage IB, the reverse was true for stages IIA and IIB (Table 4). A plausible explanation for this apparent discrepancy is that fever, which disappears on instituting radiotherapy for mediastinal involvement, has little or no apparent effect on prognosis.

TABLE 5.—ABSOLUTE SURVIVAL BY REGION: PATIENTS
ADMITTED 1947 THROUGH 1963 AND FOLLOWED TO AUGUST 1968: STAGES I AND II*

SITE	1 YEAR		3 YEARS		5 YEARS		7 YEARS		10 YEARS	
Head and neck	58/61	95.1%	48/61	78.7%	37/53	69.8%	21/38	55.3%	6/16	37.5%
Mediastinum	46/57	97.9%	43/47	91.5%	29/40	72.5%	20/33	60.6%	11/20	55.0%
Axilla	22/24	91.7%	13/24	54.2%	10/21	47.6%	8/17	47.1%	3/11	27.3%
Abdomen	7/9	77.8%	5/9	55.6%	5/8	62.5%	2/3	66.7%	-	-
Pelvis	2/2	100.0%	1/2	50.0%	0/1	0.0%	0/1	0.0%	0/1	0.0%
Inguinal	4/4	100.0%	4/4	100.0%	2/3	66.7%	2/3	66.7%	2/3	66.7%
Total†	139/147	94.6%	114/147	77.6%	83/126	65.9%	53/95	55.8%	22/51	43.1%

*Table includes 11 cases whose slides were not available for review.
†The survival figures for the 136 patients in whom a diagnosis of Hodgkin's disease was confirmed are essentially the same by region. Note the comparatively poor results for Hodgkin's disease presenting in the axilla as compared with the results for the other major regions. See Table 6 for a detailed analysis of the results of treatment for Hodgkin's disease of the head and neck by specific subregion.

TABLE 6.—ABSOLUTE SURVIVAL OF PATIENTS WITH CANCER OF THE HEAD AND NECK:
PATIENTS ADMITTED 1947 THROUGH 1963 AND FOLLOWED TO AUGUST 1968: STAGES I AND II*

SITE†	1 YEAR		3 YEARS		5 YEARS		7 YEARS		10 YEARS	
Unilateral upper neck	14/15	93.3%	14/15	93.3%	12/13	92.3%	6/7	85.7%	1/1	100.0%
Unilateral lower neck	35/36	97.2%	28/36	77.8%	21/33	63.6%	14/26	53.8%	5/13	38.5%
Both sides of neck	7/8	87.5%	4/8	50.0%	3/6	50.0%	1/4	25.0%	0/2	0.0%
Waldeyer's ring	2/2	100.0%	2/2	100.0%	1/1	100.0%	0/1	0.0%	-	-
Total	58/61	95.1%	48/61	78.7%	37/53	69.8%	21/38	55.3%	6/16	37.5%

*Table includes four cases whose slides were not available for pathology review.
†When analyzed by site of origin, the results at five years for the head and neck ranged from 92 per cent for patients with involvement of the ipsilateral side of the upper neck only to 50 per cent for patients with involvement of both sides of the neck.

When analyzed by histological type, the five-year survival figures confirmed other reports on the natural history of the lymphocytic predominant and lymphocytic depletion varieties; the difference in the absolute survival at five years was 89 per cent as opposed to 20 per cent, respectively (Table 4). A considerable difference also was demonstrated between the nodular sclerosing (73 per cent) and mixed cellularity (58 per cent) groups. However, a graphic presentation (Fig. 3) of the incidence and survival status for the specific histological types by major areas of involvement indicates that the results for mixed cellularity depend on the apparent site of origin. For the most common presentations, i.e. one side of the upper and lower portions of the neck, the survival status of patients with mixed cellularity and nodular sclerosing Hodgkin's disease were comparable. Since the survival figures for patients presenting with involvement of the axilla were inferior regardless of histology (Table 5), the most likely explanation for the better over-all results in nodular sclerosing Hodgkin's disease of the mediastinum is that the survival of patients irradiated for this disease tended to be prolonged regardless of the final outcome (Fig. 3).

Although the numbers involved were too small for statistical analysis of each histological type by site of origin, a relative impression can be obtained by comparing the information provided in Figure 3 with the over-all results for each of the major areas (Table 5). Except for the axilla, the five-year survival figures were very similar, the range being between 67 per cent for the inguinal areas and 73 per cent for the mediastinum. Although the over-all results for the head and neck region were in the same range (70 per cent), a further breakdown revealed differences for one side of the upper part of the neck (92 per cent), the ipsilateral lower part of the neck (64 per cent), and both sides of the neck (50 per cent) (Table 6).

Contrary to the five-year survival figures, the 10-year results for the major areas varied considerably. Other than for the persistently inferior results for the axilla, the most notable differences were 38 per cent for the head and neck and 55 per cent for the mediastinum. Although the results for one side of the lower neck dropped precipitously from 64 per cent at five years to 38 per cent at 10 years, the results for the ipsilateral upper part of the neck remained stable.

The development of differences in results for the major areas of involvement during the five- and 10-year period suggests such possibilities as: (1) differences in biological behavior associated with specific pathology and apparent site of origin and (2) differences in patterns of initial involvement including occult disease or in patterns of spread. The influence of specific histological type on survival status as related to major areas of involvement is shown in Figure 3. The incidence of the first important clinical manifes-

TABLE 7.—HODGKIN'S DISEASE—STAGES I AND II
MEDIASTINUM: FIRST AREA OF NEW DISEASE*

TOTAL	LUNG—DIRECT EXTENSION	ABDOMEN	ABDOMEN INCLUDING LIVER STAGE IV	WIDESPREAD DISSEMINATION	UNKNOWN
27/47	3	14	3	6	1

*Mediastinal recurrence occurred additionally in 12, the majority of whom received inadequate treatment.

tation of new disease as related to initial site of involvement is provided in Tables 7, 8, and 9 for the most commonly involved sites of origin (stage I) or major areas of involvement (stage II), namely the head and neck, mediastinum, and axilla. As anticipated, the abdomen was the most common major area affected secondarily in patients presenting with involvement of the mediastinum and associated supraclavicular fossae or neck (Table 7). Whether patients presenting with Hodgkin's disease of the head and neck developed subsequent new disease depended on the site of initial involvement. For example, only two of 15 patients with Hodgkin's disease involving one side of the upper part of the neck developed subsequent new disease, whereas the incidence was 18 of 36 for initial involvement of the lower part of the neck and six of eight for involvement of both sides of the neck. Of a total group of 27 patients whose disease eventually generalized, the abdomen was secondarily affected in 18, including 10 with evidence of liver involvement (Table 8). Although subsequent mediastinal involvement may have been prevented by previous prophylactic irradiation, the possibility is that the mediastinum was bypassed by the thoracic duct.

TABLE 8.—HODGKIN'S DISEASE—STAGES I AND II
HEAD AND NECK: FIRST AREA OF NEW DISEASE*

	TOTAL	MEDIASTINUM	ABDOMEN	ABDOMEN INCLUDING LIVER	WIDESPREAD DISSEMINATION
Grand total	27/61	4	8	10	5
Upper neck (one side)	2/15		1	1	
Lower neck (one side)	18/36	3	6	7	2
Both sides	6/8	1		2	3
Waldeyer's ring	1/2		1		

*The majority of patients received prophylaxis to the mediastinum.

TABLE 9.—HODGKIN'S DISEASE—STAGES I AND II
AXILLA: FIRST AREA OF NEW DISEASE*

TOTAL	MEDIASTINUM	ABDOMEN	ABDOMEN INCLUDING LIVER (STAGE IV)	DISSEMINATED STAGE IV
19/24	1	4	3	11

*New disease under five years—15; new disease five years or over—four.

In contrast to the results for the other major sites of initial involvement, the absolute survival figures for the axilla were inferior at both five and 10 years, being 48 and 27 per cent. Such relatively early poor results would suggest that in a majority of instances, axillary involvement was merely a manifestation of a more generalized disease process which probably included involvement of the upper abdomen. In support of this theory, the distribution of the second clinical manifestation of new disease in 19 of 24 patients with initial axillary involvement was widespread dissemination in 11 and abdominal disease in seven with associated liver involvement in three. Only one patient developed a mediastinal mass (Table 9).

Discussion

Since Peters published her first paper on Hodgkin's disease in 1950, many papers have been written confirming her initial observation that localized Hodgkin's disease managed with intensive regional irradiation is potentially curable. Today, the two most controversial issues in the management of localized disease are: (1) the significance of constitutional symptoms and (2) the areas at risk as related to the initial site of involvement.

Despite opinions to the contrary, our experience has been that the usual constitutional symptoms, *i.e.* fever and sweats, commonly associated with mediastinal involvement, categorically were not indicative of more generalized disease. Rather than to consider all such cases as generalized from the standpoint of appropriate treatment, our current approach would be to base our decision as to future investigation and management on the initial effect of local radiotherapy on constitutional symptoms.

Until recently, regions immediately adjacent to the primary site have logically been considered to be the areas at greatest risk for direct spread of disease. However, a study of actual patterns of spread for each of the major sites of clinical presentation (Tables 7, 8, and 9) would suggest that the common lymphatic pathways frequently bypass immediately adjacent regions, as exemplified by the high incidence of associated involvement of abdominal and cervical lymph nodes. Undoubtedly, the percentage of patients developing extension to the abdomen would have been lower had all the patients in this series been studied initially by lymphangiography. However, our experience in 29 patients who were staged following lymphangiography was that more than 50 per cent eventually developed abdominal involvement.

The answer to whether Hodgkin's disease originates in the neck or in the abdomen is important. Spread to the para-aortic nodes from the neck via the thoracic duct would suggest early extension suitable for treatment with para-aortic or inverted Y fields. Judging by the direction of flow of lymph in the thoracic duct, the reverse hypothesis of extension is more apt to be correct. Eventually, information garnered from a number of sources such as retrospective studies, ongoing randomized clinical trials in radiotherapy, and abdominal exploration may provide the answer to both the incidence and extent of abdominal involvement and, finally, the solution to the question of prophylactic irradiation to the abdomen.

Similarly, although the high incidence of nodular sclerosing Hodgkin's disease occurring in the supraclavicular fossae and mediastinum would suggest that prophylaxis to the mediastinum may be of value in nodular sclerosing Hodkgin's disease of the lower part of the neck, the advisability of administering prophylactic irradiation to the mediastinum regardless of cell type is questionable. Whether the indications for prophylactic irradiation will be changed as a result of randomized clinical trials remains to be seen.

Summary

In the past, our approach to the management of clinically localized Hodgkin's disease has been to irradiate the involved regions intensively. Whether prophylactic irradiation was administered depended on the proximity of the adjacent areas. Our results for patients treated for stages I and II disease between 1947 and 1963 have been reviewed in terms of stage of disease and constitutional symptoms as related to specific pathology classified according to the Rye modification and the Lukes and Butler method (Lukes *et al.*, 1966). The relative incidence and survival status of the four histological types have been compared by major areas of involvement. Finally, the incidence of subsequent new areas of disease has been shown in relation to the initial major areas of involvement.

REFERENCES

Fuller, L. M., Jing, B. S., Shullenberger, C. C., and Butler, J. J.: Radiotherapeutic management of localised Hodgkin's disease involving the mediastinum. *British Journal of Radiology*, 40:913-925, December 1967.

Jackson, H., Jr., and Parker, F., Jr.: *Hodgkin's Disease and Allied Disorders.* New York, New York, Oxford University Press, 1947, 177 pp.

Kaplan, H. S.: Role of intensive radiotherapy in the management of Hodgkin's disease. *Cancer,* 19:356-367, March 1966.

Keller, A. R., Kaplan, H. S., Lukes, R. J., and Rappaport, H.: Correlation of histopathology with other prognostic indicators in Hodgkin's disease. *Cancer,* 22:487-499, September 1968.

Lukes, R. J.: Relationship of histologic features to clinical stages in Hodgkin's disease. *The American Journal of Roentgenology, Radium Therapy and Nuclear Medicine,* 90:944-955, November 1963.

Lukes, R. J., and Butler, J. J.: The pathology and nomenclature of Hodgkin's disease. *Cancer Research,* 26:1063-1081, June 1966.

Lukes, R. J., Craver, L. F., Hall, T. C., Rappaport, H., and Ruben, P.: Report of the nomenclature committee. *Cancer Research,* 26:1311, June 1966.

Peters, M. V.: A study of survivals in Hodgkin's disease treated radiologically. *The American Journal of Roentgenology, Radium Therapy and Nuclear Medicine,* 53:299-311, March 1950.

Changing Concepts in Radiotherapy for the Lymphomas

M. VERA PETERS, M.D.

The Ontario Cancer Institute, The Princess Margaret Hospital,
Toronto, Ontario, Canada

THE CHANGING CONCEPTS in radiotherapy for lymphomas reflect the changing concepts about the natural course of these diseases. Before the discovery of radiotherapy, surgical extirpation was the treatment of choice for patients with lymphoma, but its usefulness was limited. The arsenical preparations proposed by Billroth in 1871 also were employed, but were disappointing.

The history of radiotherapy for the lymphomas prior to 1960 can be divided into three 20-year periods. In the period after 1900, the first responses to radiation were reported by Pusey (1902), by Senn (1903), and by Williams (1903), all American radiotherapists. Single cutaneous erythema doses were delivered at repeated intervals to sites of involvement using weak radiation sources. A few radiotherapists recommended full-trunk radiation in small dosages, but their recommendations found little support. It was Schwarz (1925), a European, who first advised against using single large doses in 1914. He was the first to recommend fractionated irradiation and advised the use of small daily doses over a period of two to three weeks to involved lymph nodes. In 1923, Desjardins and Ford reported a 9.8 per cent five-year survival rate using the methods which were developed during the first 20-year period of radiotherapy.

During the next 20 years (1920 to 1940), some of the mysteries of radiation were solved, reports on depth-dose distributions appeared, and methods of measuring radiation were described. In 1934, Leucutia also described the importance of a high depth dosage and the distribution of radiation. In 1932, Hummel reported a 17.7 per cent five-year survival rate in 45 cases of Hodgkin's disease. Gilbert (1939) recommended segmental irradiation for patients with lymphoma and standardized a method of treating all the main lymph node regions in succession: each region of involvement would receive 500 to 1,500 R in 15 days and the remaining regions would receive 500 R. Gilbert reported a 34.2 per cent five-year survival rate in 46 cases.

The early experience at the Ontario Cancer Institute (Peters, 1950) belongs in the third 20-year period. Although many radiotherapists continued to prescribe radiation only to sites of involvement, our director, the late Dr. Richards, followed Gilbert's lead in prescribing segmental radiation. In 1937, the installation of 400-kv equipment at our institute allowed fractionation at higher total depth dosages to sites of involvement. In 1953, the addition of ^{60}Co therapy allowed even higher tumor doses. Approximately one half of all lymphoma patients received additional low-dose prophylactic treatment to uninvolved lymphatic regions. In a previous study, the extra treatment was shown to improve the five-year salvage rate, but did not appear to affect the 10-year survival rate in patients with Hodgkin's disease. Such prophylactic treatment appeared to be effective only in Hodgkin's disease. Until 1960, our five-year survival rate in patients with Hodgkin's disease remained around 40 per cent. Comparable survival rates were reported by Nice and Stenstrom (1954) and Smithers (1959). Chemotherapy for the lymphomas originated during this period, and the responses to such treatment were promising.

About 1960, the mounting interest in the lymphomas led to an explosion of studies on their etiology, pathology, clinical course, and management. Much more interest centered around Hodgkin's disease than lymphosarcoma or reticulum cell sarcoma. Consequently, this paper will focus chiefly on studies of Hodgkin's disease.

In 1962, Kaplan of Stanford reported a technical advance in the radiotherapy for lymphomas. His proposal was inspired by the earlier suggestions that prophylactic radiation was worthwhile and his plan of treatment was made feasible by megavoltage radiation equipment. In Kaplan's technique, all the main lymphatics and spleen received a high radiation dose in two courses of treatment, one to the chest "mantle" and one to the abdominal "inverted Y," with an extension of the field to include the spleen.

About the same time, lymphography and inferior venacavography began to have importance in delineating retroperitoneal disease sites which were not detectable otherwise.

Many studies on Hodgkin's disease were carried out by eminent pathologists (Rappaport, Winter, and Hicks, 1956; Lukes and Butler, 1966). In 1963, Lukes published a modification of the former Jackson and Parker pathological classification of Hodgkin's disease and brought to our attention the "nodular sclerosing" histological variant which so often affects the mediastinum. Consequently, histological factors became much more significant in the assessment of disease in the individual patient.

Variations in host resistance have always been recognized clinically, both in the course of Hodgkin's disease and in the peculiar systemic effects which sometimes accompany the disease. Immunologists now suggest that host factors may, in time, be measured by antigen tests. The field of immunology also offers possibilities in the measurement of responses, especially when there is no physical parameter to assess response to treatment.

The more precise clinical assessment of the new patient during the present period has stimulated a number of studies on the anatomical distribution and natural course of each histological type of Hodgkin's disease. This led to speculations on the primary focus and direction and mode of spread of the disease. For example, in a recent study of all the histological types of lymphoma, only patients presenting with nodular sclerosing Hodgkin's disease which included disease in the mediastinum appeared to be potentially curable. For all other histological types of Hodgkin's disease and for the other lymphomas, mediastinal and, particularly, hilar involvement appeared to represent a late stage of the disease. Thus, in most instances, this newly identified histological type of Hodgkin's disease probably starts in the mediastinum. In contrast, most curable patients with lymphomas other than nodular sclerosing Hodgkin's disease presented with early, but sometimes massive, disease below the diaphragm.

In 1967, I submitted a report on the remarkable differences among the natural courses of disease in the three major types of lymphomas (Peters, Hasselback, and Brown, 1968).

Prophylactic treatment, as formerly practiced for all lymphoma patients presenting with lymph node involvement, had not increased the five-year survival rate of patients with lymphosarcoma and reticulum cell sarcoma as it had for those with Hodgkin's disease (Peters, 1963). The reason for this failure became apparent during the preparation of the report: the hope for a gain in survival rate by prophylactic treatment during the early stages of lymphosarcoma and reticulum cell sarcoma necessitates radiation far beyond the main lymph node regions, particularly in abdominal sites. Jenkin *et al.* (1969), in his study of primary gastrointestinal tract lymphomas in children, furnished an example of this finding. This conclusion agrees with the reported high rate of positive lymphograms from patients with these two diseases. Also, necropsy findings from patients with lymphomas other than Hodgkin's disease demonstrate that 70 per cent have widespread involvement of the intestinal tract and mesenteric nodes. In contrast to the other lymphomas, only one third of patients with Hodgkin's disease show involvement of these sites at autopsy. Thus, curative prophylactic treatment can be limited to the main trunk lymphatic chains in patients with early stages of Hodgkin's disease, but not in those with other lymphomas.

In radiotherapy for Hodgkin's disease, a greater degree of standardization of treatment evolved after Kaplan's (1962) first description of irradiation of the chest "mantle" for the upper lymph chains and of the abdominal "inverted Y" for the lower trunk lymphatics with an extension of this field to include the spleen; the tumor dose ranged from 3,000 to 4,000 rads, depending on the extent of disease.

Some radiotherapists now advise using both fields, or "total lymphoid" radiation, at a high dosage for all patients with stages I, II, and III Hodgkin's disease. However, is it necessary to radiate more than the primary presenting site and the immediate continuous regions? At present, I do not see the need for total lymphoid radiation in patients with stages I, IIA, or IIB nodular sclerosing Hodgkin's disease who present with mediastinal disease. Also, local and regional radiation appear to be adequate treatment for patients with retroperitoneal Hodgkin's disease. Patients with lymphocyte-predominant disease presenting in submandibular or parotid nodes appear to be cured by local radiation without any other treatment (but is this condition benign?). Doctor Fuller (personal communication) has gone a step further with local radiation only; she includes the mixed cellularity cases with involvement of the upper half of neck in this group.

For late Hodgkin's disease (*i.e.*, stages IIIB and IV), however, the standard radiotherapy methods prescribed for the earlier stages are usually inadequate to achieve remissions. Many controlled studies are in progress dealing with these two late stages.

For the other lymphomas, classified in the diffuse histological group (lymphocytic or reticular), the primary focus appears to be intra-abdominal in most patients with early disease, and the whole abdomen should be irradiated (total dose ± 2,000 rads) to achieve longer survivals. Radiation to all the peripheral lymph node regions also may be indicated, but this decision depends on the sites of presentation. For nodular, lymphocytic, and reticular lymphomas (formerly called Brill-Symmers disease), the advantage of active treatment of the asymptomatic patient is not clear. We have watched patients in this category for as long as 10 years or more before the disease became aggressive and symptomatic. When treatment is indicated, radiotherapy is useful. Local radiation in patients with stage I disease is worthwhile because the disease in many such patients appears to be controlled for indefinite periods. For stages II and III disease, treatment should encompass all sites of suspected disease, which usually include all the peripheral lymph node regions and the abdomen. However, if intrathoracic disease is identified or if there is involvement of other systems such as skin or skeleton, radiation is used only for local palliation, when necessary, while administering chemotherapy.

Thus, for all the lymphomas, the radiotherapeutic approach has changed dramatically during the past 10 years. The histological assessment and the anatomical sites of presentation are equally as important as the clinical stage in determining the plan of management.

The newest approach in the assessment of lymphomas is laparotomy investigation. This usually is more helpful in patients with Hodgkin's disease than in those with other lymphomas. Kaplan and Rosenberg pioneered this endeavor and recently published their initial findings (Glatstein, Guernsey, Rosenberg, and Kaplan, 1969). Equivocal findings from lymphograms and other studies triggered this form of investigation, but the importance of laparotomy reaches far beyond the realm of clarifying equivocal reports. More information on the probabilities of extension of the disease has been obtained. Eventually, these laparotomy investigations will assist in determining the forms of oxygenation and the mode of spread so necessary to clarify the concept of the natural course of the disease and thereby improve the methods of treatment in the future.

At our institute, we have performed only one third of the number of laparotomy investigations reported by the Stanford group, but already we have gleaned valuable information. After each operation, the value to the patient is assessed critically. Points of discrimination in choosing suitable candidates for this procedure have become apparent. I would refrain from advising laparotomy for most patients over 50 years of age. As a group, the older patients usually have more disease than suspected; such a discovery at laparotomy is discouraging and may require more radical treatment than often is advisable. Conversely, in younger patients with Hodgkin's disease, particularly those under 30 years of age, it often is vital to verify the extent of disease before prescribing radical radiation to sites which might entail distressing complications in the future. For the young woman faced with the possibility of castration by radiation for suspected disease below the diaphragm, laparotomy is of special importance. Recently, we have advised laparotomy for three young patients for whom suspected disease below the diaphragm was disproved by the procedure and for others who had early retroperitoneal disease, but who had ovarian transplants to avoid sterilization. One of the case histories in the former group deserves recording because it demonstrates an unusual indication for a laparotomy.

CASE HISTORY.—Mrs. J.T., 27-year-old married graduate nurse with two children, consulted her physician in August 1969 because of an unusual distress in her chest. A chest x-ray film revealed a superior anterior mediastinal mass. Findings from cervical sentinel node biopsies were negative, as were other cursory findings. Thoracotomy was performed, and the mass was shelled out completely. Pathologically, this was a classical case of nodular sclerosing Hodgkin's disease. There was no history of systemic effects.

The patient was referred to The Princess Margaret Hospital in October 1969. Lymphogram, intravenous pyelogram, I.C.C.G. studies and an upper gastrointestinal series were done, as were baseline peripheral blood studies and liver and spleen scans. The lymphogram findings were positive in the para-aortic region, and scans revealed that the spleen was twice the normal size. Other tests were negative.

Because this patient had had a severe episode of infectious mononucleosis 10 years previously and because she was anxious to have more children, I elected to advise a laparotomy. The enlarged spleen and many enlarged lymph nodes were removed, and a wedge biopsy of the liver was performed. Careful sectioning of all material by the pathologist did not reveal any evidence of Hodgkin's disease or any focal areas which were suspect.

Prior to the laparotomy, opinions about the management of this patient's disease varied from a close-watch policy to radical radiotherapy or chemotherapy because the disease was so advanced. However, the close connection between infectious mononucleosis and Hodgkin's disease demanded histological proof before beginning unnecessary treatment.

This preamble brings us up to date in the evolution of concepts of radiotherapy for the lymphomas; these changing concepts have related to improvements in our understanding of each disease, particularly Hodgkin's disease, and the increasing efficiency of radiotherapy equipment and techniques. However, the rapid changes in concept since 1960 invoke certain questions, and some fears arise periodically. What does the future offer? Complete clinical assessment is becoming more and more complete. Radical treatment for all stages of Hodgkin's disease is becoming more and more radical.

What late sequelae can be expected when high-dose, total node irradiation is done in patients with stages I and II Hodgkin's disease, most of whom are young patients? Some of our patients who have survived more than 20 years after even less radical treatment are now dying of atherosclerotic heart disease. Does the improved state of knowledge of the course of the disease according to histologic type and sites of presentation allow more discriminative therapy? These are questions which need to be answered in future reports.

Present Study

The study which I shall now report to illustrate the changing concept involves all new patients with Hodgkin's disease registered in the years 1966 and 1967 at The Princess Margaret Hospital in Toronto. A comparable study of a recent experience in managing the other lymphomas is not available. Relationships of clinical influences such as age, sex, and clinical stage to the histological types were studied. Of the 150 new cases registered during these two years, 108 had lymphographic studies as part of the initial assessment. Prior to January 1966, very few lymphograms were done in new patients. A few comparisons will be made with the previous experience

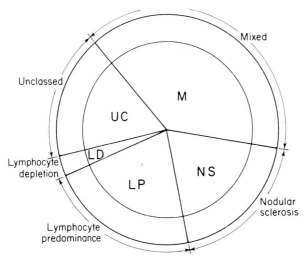

FIG. 1.—Histological distribution of 150 new cases of Hodgkin's disease diagnosed in 1966 and 1967.

from 1961 through 1965. Naturally, in the 1966 and 1967 study, only two-year survivals can be reported. The year 1967, although slightly premature from a statistical standpoint, is included to demonstrate the influence of the more intensive investigation prior to treatment. Only six patients considered free of disease have not quite reached the two-year mark.

It is chiefly the histological type which appears to govern the chronicity and the pattern of the natural course of Hodgkin's disease. Therefore, the histological characteristic has been chosen as the common denominator, and all studies will be related to it. The histological patterns of the 150 new cases admitted in 1966 and 1967 are shown in Figure 1.

Figure 2 shows the age distribution (in terms of younger than or older than 40 years) within each histological group. In the lymphocyte-predominant group, the disease is evenly distributed between all age groups, whereas in the group with nodular sclerosing Hodgkin's disease, the majority are 20 to 40 years of age. All ages appear in the mixed cell type group with the majority under 40 years of age.

In sex distribution (Fig. 3), the only irregularity appeared in the mixed cell type group, in which there were more males than females in the younger age group.

The relationship of clinical stage to the histological type is shown in Figure 4. In the groups with nodular sclerosing and lymphocyte-predominant disease, only 22 per cent presented with stages IIIB and IV disease, whereas in the remaining histological groups, 43 per cent presented with late stages of the disease.

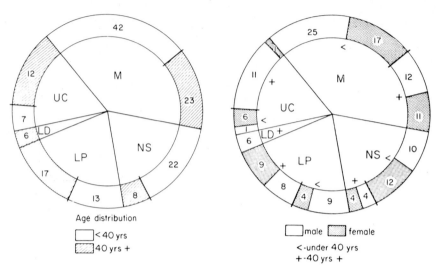

FIG. 2. (left)—Relationship of age to histological type in 150 cases of Hodgkin's disease. Abbreviations: *LD*, lymphocyte depletion; *LP*, lymphocyte predominance; *M*, mixed; *NS*, nodular sclerosing; *UC*, unclassified.

FIG. 3. (right)—Relationship of sex to age and histological type in 150 new cases of Hodgkin's disease. Abbreviations: *LD*, lymphocyte depletion; *LP*, lymphocyte predominance; *M*, mixed; *NS*, nodular sclerosing; *UC*, unclassified.

FIG. 4. (left)—Relationship of clinical stage to histological type in 150 new patients (109 of whom had lymphograms) with Hodgkin's disease. Abbreviations: *LD*, lymphocyte depletion; *LP*, lymphocyte predominance; *M*, mixed; *NS*, nodular sclerosing; *UC*, unclassified.

FIG. 5. (right)—Relationship of lymphographic findings to histologic type in 109 of 150 new cases of Hodgkin's disease. Lymphograms were not done in 41 patients. Abbreviations: *LD*, lymphocyte depletion; *LP*, lymphocyte predominance; *M*, mixed; *NS*, nodular sclerosing; *UC*, unclassified.

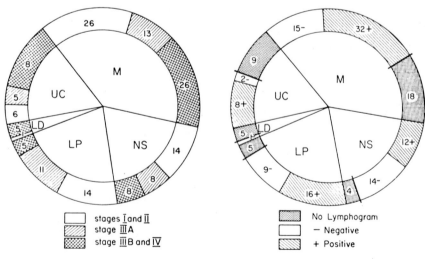

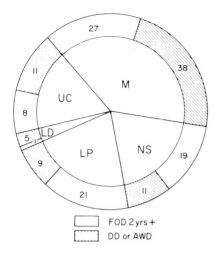

FOD 2 yrs +

DD or AWD

FIG. 6.—Present status of 150 patients who presented with Hodgkin's disease in 1966 and 1967, Abbreviations: *AWD*, alive with disease; *DD*, dead from disease; *FOD*, free of disease; *LD*, lymphocyte depletion; *LP*, lymphocyte predominance; *M*, mixed; *NS*, nodular sclerosing; *UC*, unclassified.

Lymphographic studies were carried out in 109 of the 150 new patients. Approximately two thirds of those in the mixed type group, less than two thirds in the lymphocyte-predominant group, and less than one half in the nodular sclerosing group had positive lymphograms. The proportions are shown in Figure 5.

Figure 6 represents an attempt to show the two-year free-of-disease survival rate. Approximately less than half of those with mixed disease are free of disease at two years. In contrast, two thirds in the lymphocyte-predominant and nodular sclerosing groups are still free of disease. However, all clinical stages are included and there is an uneven distribution of clinical stages within the histological groups.

The tables present a few comparisons with the experience from 1961 through 1965 to demonstrate the recent transition. Table 1 shows redistribution by clinical stage, which appears to have been a direct result of the inclusion of lymphographic and other investigations in the preliminary assessment of disease. The proportion of those with stages I and II disease

TABLE 1.—HODGKIN'S DISEASE 1961 THROUGH 1967:
DISTRIBUTION BY STAGE

STUDY	I + II	IIIA	IIIB + IV
1961-1965 (246 patients)	66%	7%	27%
1966-1967 (150 patients)	41%	17%	42%

TABLE 2.—HODGKIN'S DISEASE: TWO-YEAR SURVIVAL RATE
FREE OF DISEASE* BY STAGE GROUPING

YEAR	I + II	IIIA	IIIB + IV
1961-1965	54%	28%	15%
	(162)	(18)	(66)
1966-1967	74%	70%	10%
	(61)	(37)	(52)

*Clinically.

has decreased from two thirds of the total number to a little more than one third. The proportion of patients presenting with stage IIIA disease has increased 10 per cent and the number with stages IIIB and IV disease has increased from 27 to 42 per cent.

Table 2 compares the new two-year free-of-disease survival rate by stage grouping in the new and the older experience groups. One notes the 20 per cent improvement in survival rate in patients with stages I and II disease, which is chiefly the result of the advancement to stage IIIB of most of the cases which would have been considered stage IIB before lymphography was used. The corresponding 42 per cent improvement in survival rate of those in stage IIIA is more remarkable, but this stage now includes cases which were formerly considered stages I and IIA. For patients in stages IIIB and IV, the difference in survival is not significant in spite of the fact that these stages now include cases which were formerly thought to be early

TABLE 3.—HODGKIN'S DISEASE: PREDICTED IMPROVEMENT IN
FIVE-YEAR SURVIVAL (NEW CASES ONLY)

STUDY	ALIVE 2 YEARS	F.O.D. 2 YEARS	ALIVE 5 YEARS	F.O.D. 5 YEARS
1961-1963				
(127 patients)	66%	40%	46%	32%
1964-1965				
(119 patients)	71%	45%	51%	36%
1966-1967			Prediction	
(150 patients)	73%	51%	56%	40%
1966-1967				
(108 patients) Lymphogram series	82%	62%	67%	54%

Abbreviation: F.O.D., free of disease.

TABLE 4.–HODGKIN'S DISEASE 1966 THROUGH 1967:
TWO-YEAR SURVIVAL FREE OF DISEASE BY HISTOLOGY AND STAGE

CLASSIFICATION	I AND II	IIIA	IIIB AND IV
Lymphocyte predominence (30)	79%	81%	1/5
Nodular sclerosis (30)	79%	87%	1/8
Mixed (65)	70%	46%	12%
Lymphocyte depletion (6)	1/1	-	0/5
Unclassified (19)	4/6	4/5	0/8
Total	74%	70%	10%
(150)	(61)	(37)	(52)

disease. For patients with these two stages of disease, the more recent radical chemotherapy approach offers promise for better survival rates.

Table 3 shows an attempt to predict the over-all five-year survival rate and five-year free-of-disease survival rate in this group of patients which have been followed only two to three years. An over-all improvement of 10 per cent in the five-year survival rates is possible. If one excludes the cases which did not have specialized investigation, an improvement of 20 per cent in the five-year survival rates could be predicted. However, several of the patients who did not have lymphograms were known to have late disease; thus, this prediction might be too optimistic.

Table 4 shows two important findings: (1) that the two-year free-of-disease survival rate is equally as good in patients with stage IIIA disease as in those with stages I and II disease and (2) that the survival rates, even at two years, of patients in stages I, II, and IIIA are better for those with the lymphocyte-predominant and nodular sclerosing types than for those with the mixed cell histological type.

Discussion

The study described emphasizes the value of a complete histological and clinical assessment of the patient with Hodgkin's disease. In the years 1966 and 1967, almost all the patients with stages I, II, and III disease (including the B category) had radiation therapy initially, but none of those with stages I and II disease had total lymphoid radiation initially. A few patients presenting with stage IIIB disease had chemotherapy initially; since 1967, a radical chemotherapy approach has been employed primarily for this stage of disease, and an improvement is anticipated. Most of the stage IV patients had chemotherapy initially; some received palliative radiation to troublesome sites of involvement.

For stages I and II disease, both A and B categories, a very few centers, commendably, are attempting total lymphoid radiation for stages I and II disease. Nevertheless, the survival rates following less radical radiation therapy for stages I and II disease are excellent, especially in lymphocyte-predominant and nodular sclerosing disease. Although one does not hesitate to treat all the main lymphatics in patients with stage IIIA disease, the two-year survival rate for patients in this stage is almost the same as for those in stages I and II. However, we still do not know whether the long-term response rate in the stage IIIA cases detected by lymphography will be better than if the para-aortic disease had not been detected as early. Some patients in this group were formerly classified as stages I and II cases, which, historically, have achieved a satisfactory proportion of long survivals. For the present, the treatment of choice for stage IIIA disease is still radiotherapy.

The early and late complications of radiation observed from time to time demand a constant critical analysis of therapeutic techniques. Should the mediastinum be treated when the patient presents without detectable disease in the mediastinum on hilar regions? This is a very important consideration because the hazards entailed might prove to outweigh the longer survival time. The late high-dose radiation effect on the respiratory system, heart, and major vessels cannot be assessed for a few years. However, in the early period after radiation, the danger lies chiefly in the confusion surrounding the interpretation of the chest radiographic findings (radiation pneumonitis, infection, or new disease). For all the lymphomas except nodular sclerosing Hodgkin's disease, I would prefer to leave the mediastinum untreated until disease becomes evident. Studies on the natural course of the disease suggest that involvement of the mediastinum is a late manifestation of the disease in all but those who present with nodular sclerosing mediastinal disease.

Likewise, caution is necessary when radiating areas close to the kidneys, especially when there is a past history of urinary tract disease. The practice of kidney shielding has helped to overcome this hazard.

There are other complications such as transverse myelitis which can occur if overlap between fields is allowed or if the tumor dose at any points along the spinal cord exceeds the maximum tolerance dose (approximately 3,500 rads). The radiotherapist should be continually aware of normal structures as well as of the sites of disease during any course of irradiation.

A close surveillance of findings of peripheral blood studies during and after treatment is equally as important as other precautions, but this topic will not be discussed in this paper.

The proposal to investigate by laparotomy those with early disease deserves attention. We have benefited by the Stanford experience and have had enough personal experience to find a few guidelines in the selection of cases for this investigation. In patients under 50 years of age, a laparotomy seems to be worthwhile, particularly if disease in the spleen is suspected clinically or if the added information is necessary to plan the course of treatment. A laparotomy, including transplantation of the ovaries, is of special importance for the young, potentially curable female patient who might look forward to subsequent pregnancies.

The revelation of many important clinicopathological relationships, particularly in patients with Hodgkin's disease, and the adoption of more adequate therapy for this disease have highlighted the era since 1960. Both of these advances have been made possible by a more precise clinical assessment of the untreated patient. Megavoltage radiotherapy has allowed technical improvements in the management of all the lymphomas, and more aggressive chemotherapy is beginning to have an important place in the management of advanced disease.

We are extemely grateful for the progress in the methods of investigation which has allowed a better delineation of the extent of disease before treating the patient and for the progress in chemotherapy and in the techniques of radiation therapy. However, it is still premature to judge the effectiveness and hazards of the more radical approaches conceived during this decade. Let us hope that the next 10 years will become an era of discrimination, with more individualized radiotherapy and chemotherapy.

Acknowledgments

The study reported in this paper represents the work of several members of the radiotherapy and chemotherapy staff of The Princess Margaret Hospital, all of whom deserve recognition. In addition, I am indebted to Miss Sandra Innes (secretary), Mrs. Marianne Gaettens (photographer), Mr. Douglas McCourt (artist), and Miss Adele Curry (librarian) for their assistance in preparing this paper.

REFERENCES

Desjardins, A. U., and Ford, F. A.: Hodgkin's disease and lymphosarcoma: A clinical and statistical study. *Journal of the American Medical Association,* 81:925-927, September 15, 1923.

Fuller, L. M.: Personal communication.

Gilbert, R.: Radiotherapy in Hodgkin's disease (malignant granulomatosis): Anatomic and clinical foundations; governing principles; results. *American Journal of Roentgenology, Radium Therapy and Nuclear Medicine,* 41:198-241, February 1939.

Glatstein, E., Guernsey, J. M., Rosenberg, S. A., and Kaplan, H. S.: The value of laparotomy and splenectomy in the staging of Hodgkin's disease. *Cancer,* 24:709-718, October 1969.

Hummel, R.: Zur Behandlung der Lymphogranulomatose. *Röntgenpraxis,* 4:781-787, September 1932.

Jenkin, R. D. T., Sonley, M. J., Stephens, C. A., Darte, J. M. M., and Peters, M. V.: Primary gastrointestinal tract lymphoma in childhood. *Radiology*, 92:763-767, March 1969.

Kaplan, H. S.: The radical radiotherapy of regionally localized Hodgkin's disease. *Radiology*, 78:553-561, April 1962.

Leucutia, T.: Irradiation in lymphosarcoma, Hodgkin's disease and leukemia. *American Journal of the Medical Sciences*, 188:612-623, 1934.

Lukes, R. J.: Relationship of histologic features to clinical stages in Hodgkin's disease. *American Journal of Roentgenology, Radium Therapy and Nuclear Medicine*, 90:944-955, November 1963.

Lukes, R. J., and Butler, J. J.: The pathology and nomenclature of Hodgkin's disease. *Cancer Research*, 26:1063-1083, June 1966.

Nice, C. M., and Stenstrom, D. W.: Irradiation therapy in Hodgkin's disease. *Radiology*, 62:641-652, May 1954.

Peters, M. V.: A study of survivals in Hodgkin's disease treated radiologically. *American Journal of Roentgenology, Radium Therapy and Nuclear Medicine*, 63:299-311, March 1950.

_____: The contribution of radiation therapy in the control of early lymphomas. *American Journal of Roentgenology, Radium Therapy and Nuclear Medicine*, 90:956-967, November 1963.

Peters, M. V., Hasselback, R., and Brown, T. C.: The natural history of lymphomas related to the clinical classification. In Zarafonetis, C. J. D., Ed.: *Proceedings of the International Conference on Leukemia-Lymphoma*, The University of Michigan, Ann Arbor, Michigan, 1967. Philadelphia, Pennsylvania, Lea & Febiger, 1968, pp. 357-370.

Pusey, W. A.: Cases of sarcoma and of Hodgkin's disease treated by exposures to X-rays: A preliminary report. *Journal of the American Medical Association*, 28:166-169, January 18, 1902.

Rappaport, H., Winter, W. J., and Hicks, E. B.: Follicular lymphoma: A re-evaluation of its position in the scheme of malignant lymphoma, based on a survey of 253 cases. *Cancer*, 9:792-821, 1956.

Schwarz, G.: Die forgesetzte Kleindosis und deren biologische Begründung. *Strahlentherapie*, 19:325-332, 1925.

Senn, N.: The therapeutic value of the röntgen ray in the treatment of pseudoleucaemia. *New York State Medical Journal*, 77:665-668, April 18, 1903.

Smithers, D. W.: Tumours of the thyroid gland in relation to some general concepts of neoplasia. *Journal of the Faculty of Radiologists*, 10:3-16, January 1959.

Williams, F. H.: *The Rontgen Rays in Medicine and Surgery*. Third Edition. New York, New York, The Macmillan Company, 1903.

Supportive Therapeutic Measures for Patients under Treatment for Leukemia or Lymphoma

EMIL J FREIREICH, M.D.,
GERALD P. BODEY, M.D.,
DAVID S. DE JONGH, M.D.,
JOHN E. CURTIS, M.D., AND
EVAN M. HERSH, M.D.

*Departments of Developmental Therapeutics and Clinical Pathology,
The University of Texas M. D. Anderson Hospital and Tumor Institute at
Houston, Houston, Texas*

THERAPEUTIC MEASURES directed at complications of the diseases leukemia and lymphoma are commonly referred to as supportive therapy. However, this type of therapy is more than supportive. Rather, it constitutes an integral part of the treatment for leukemia and lymphoma. The major cause of failure to induce a complete remission or complete regression of leukemic and lymphomatous disease is still the occurrence of complications of these diseases, represented overwhelmingly by the complications of infection and hemorrhage. The therapy designed to control these complications, to decrease morbidity, and to avoid mortality are specific measures which allow for the chemotherapeutic agents directed against the diseases to demonstrate their effectiveness. It has been shown repeatedly that improvement in supportive therapy can be associated with improvement in responsiveness to a given chemotherapeutic agent by diminishing the mortality resulting from complications, particularly in the first four to six weeks of therapy. Shortly after Dr. Sidney Farber described the induction of remissions in children with acute leukemia, he clearly enunciated the concept of total care (Farber, Toch, Sears, and Pinkel, 1956). This term actually is preferable to the concept of supportive therapy since it indicates that the therapy for hemorrhage, infection, and other complications is part of the total therapy directed at the control of these diseases.

Treatment for Hemorrhage

The major cause of hemorrhage in a patient with leukemia or lymphoma is thrombocytopenia. Recently, the great importance of disseminated intravascular coagulation as a cause of hemorrhagic diathesis, particularly in patients with acute granulocytic leukemia, has been emphasized, as has the potential for its control by heparin therapy. However, these and other coagulation disturbances are relatively uncommon; the overwhelmingly significant cause is thrombocytopenia. The risk of bleeding for a patient can be quantitatively evaluated by measuring the concentration of platelets in the peripheral blood by an adequate method. The widespread use of the electronic particle-counting instruments for estimating platelet concentrations has represented a major advance for the management of hemorrhage (Bull, Schneiderman, and Brecher, 1965). The risk of hemorrhage is quantitatively related to the degree of thrombocytopenia (Gaydos, Freireich, and Mantel, 1962). Grossly visible, life-threatening hemorrhage rarely occurs at platelet levels above 20,000 and the risk of hemorrhage is high at levels below 10,000. Thus, the presence of thrombocytopenia provides a clear indication for prophylactic therapy and the effectiveness of that therapy can be evaluated by the change in platelet count. At the present time, the only effective way to elevate the platelet count is by the transfusion of allogeneic platelets. The optimal product is freshly drawn platelets transfused within six hours of donation. Platelet transfusion from allogeneic donors became a practical reality with the introduction of simplified, closed-system, plastic equipment which would allow the donation of two units of platelet-rich plasma with the red cells being returned, a technique which greatly increases the availability of platelets for donation (Kliman, Gaydos, Schroeder, and Freireich, 1961). Optimal platelet replacement procedures recently have been summarized by a Subcommittee of the Acute Leukemia Task Force, E. J Freireich, Chairman (Platelet Transfusion Subcommittee of the Acute Leukemia Task Force, 1968). In general, to achieve an increase in circulating platelets of $25,000/mm^3$ in a child of average size (1 m^2 body surface area) requires the platelets from two whole units of blood (2×10^{11} platelets); for the adult of average size (2 m^2 body surface area), approximately twice this quantity would be required. Because the average platelet half-life is three to five days, these treatments need to be repeated approximately two to three times weekly (Freireich *et al.*, 1963). It has recently been reported that platelets can be stored for 24 hours provided that the platelets are not chilled, but are maintained at or above room temperature.

This should provide a valuable tool for blood banks for increasing the availability of platelets (Murphy and Gardner, 1969). The development of an effective panel of volunteer donors, the extensive application of plasmapheresis as a technique for the donation of platelets, and the transfusion in adequate doses to patients with leukemia or lymphoma who have thrombocytopenia can greatly reduce and virtually eliminate the morbidity and mortality resulting from hemorrhage.

Treatment for Infections

The major morbidity associated with the leukemias and lymphomas is infection, and as with hemorrhage, the risk of infection can be estimated by measurements of the concentration of circulating granulocytes (Fig. 1). When the circulating granulocyte concentration is below 1,000/mm³, infections are observed with regularity. The most powerful tool for the control of infectious complications is, of course, prompt recognition of infection, prompt identification of the infecting organism, and the application of specific chemotherapy as indicated, if available (Bodey, Buckley, Sathe,

FIG. 1.—Relation between granulocyte count and infection.

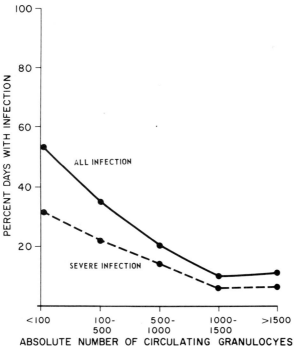

ABSOLUTE NUMBER OF CIRCULATING GRANULOCYES

TABLE 1.—Organisms Causing Septicemia
in Leukemia Patients

Organism	No. of Episodes	% of Episodes
Gram-positive cocci	1	2
Gram-negative bacilli	47	96
Pseudomonas	20	41
E. coli	9	18
Klebsiella-Enterobacter	15	31
Total episodes*	49	100

*More than one causative organism could be involved in an episode.

and Freireich, 1966). The major tool for the recognition of infection is fever. In patients with acute leukemia, for instance, over 70 per cent of the febrile episodes are shown to be caused by proved infection. Thus, the occurrence of fever is an indication for obtaining the necessary blood cultures, but should be followed by the prompt institution of antibiotic chemotherapy (Bodey, Rodriguez, and Whitecar, in press). Virtually all gram-positive organisms can be controlled easily with available antibiotics. The major cause of serious infection in leukemic and lymphoma patients is, therefore, the result of gram-negative rod infections (Table 1). A major cause of fatal infection in this population is *Pseudomonas aeruginosa*. The recent discovery of a new drug, carbenicillin, a semisynthetic penicillin which has proved activity against the pseudomonas organisms (Bodey, Rodriguez, and Luce, 1969), has altered this picture (Table 2). This drug is highly effective against pseudomonas infection and has a low frequency of side effects. Nonetheless, other gram-negative organisms such as the *Serratia* species and fungi remain major causes of morbidity and mortality in patients undergoing chemotherapy.

TABLE 2.—Effect of Carbenicillin Against
Pseudomonas Infections

Type of Infection	Episodes	Response		
		Complete	Partial	Relapse
Pneumonia	3	2	1	0
Cellulitis	6	3	1	2
Septicemia alone	3	3	0	0
Miscellaneous	3	2	1	0
Total	15	10	3	2
All septicemia	9	8	1	0

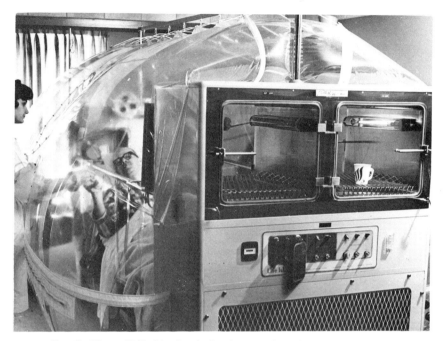

FIG. 2.—View of Life Island unit showing console and pass-through locks.

Another approach to the control of infectious complications, is through the prevention of such infections by control of environmental contamination to which the patient is exposed. Studies of a "Life-Island" patient-isolator type of environment (Bodey, Hart, Freireich, and Frei, 1968) (Fig. 2) were undertaken in an effort to protect the patient from environmental organisms. The plastic tent provides a positive barrier between the patient and the outside environment and all the air within the tent is filtered and relatively sterile. All food, water, and medications which enter the patient's environment are presterilized. To further reduce the exposure to bacterial organisms (Bodey, Loftis, and Bowen, 1968), nonabsorbable antibiotics can be given orally and applied topically to the skin to reduce the patient's own population of bacteria. This type of environment greatly reduces the risk of infectious complications, but provides an abnormal and relatively limited environment for the patient.

More recently, studies of hospital rooms which are equipped with laminar air flow to provide sterilized air for the patient have been initiated (Bodey, 1969; Bodey, Freireich, and Frei, in press) (Fig. 3). Figure 3 shows two such units under study at The University of Texas M. D. Anderson Hospital and Tumor Institute at Houston. The entire head of the room

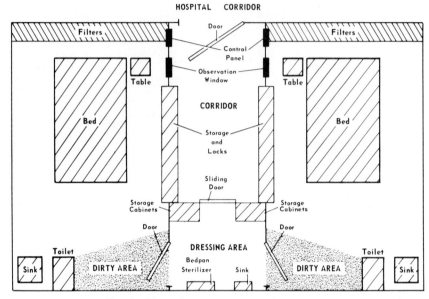

FIG. 3.—Floor plan of the laminar air flow unit.

contains filters through which air passes from the head of the room to the foot of the room in a horizontal laminar, nonturbulent pattern. The air moves at a velocity of 90 ft./minute, providing over 350 air exchanges per hour. As a result, individuals entering at the foot of the room cannot pass organisms against the flow of air toward the patient. Manipulations and examinations on the patient are conducted by individuals who are thoroughly gowned and masked. This type of environment (Fig. 4) provides a relatively normal hospital bedroom environment for the patient. These studies of the control of environmental organisms in an effort to prevent infection have been promising to date. They have indicated that the morbidity and mortality from infection can be greatly reduced by such prophylactic measures.

Another approach to the control of infectious complications is the replacement of white cells by transfusion (Freireich *et al.*, 1964). Unfortunately, the intravascular life span of leukocytes is extremely short (a half-life of approximately six hours) and the space occupied by transfused leukocytes is approximately 20 times the circulating blood volume. To achieve an increase in circulating granulocytes of $1,500/mm^3$ requires, therefore, the transfusion of 10^{11} granulocytes. This is twice the number of granulocytes in the entire circulating blood volume of an adult of average size. The only way such quantities of granulocytes can be collected is from multiple units

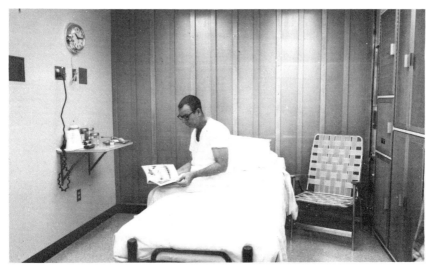

FIG. 4.—Appearance of the laminar air flow room showing filter wall, storage cabinets, and furnishings.

FIG. 5.—The in vivo blood cell separator during a leukapheresis procedure. The donor needle is located in the right arm, in which the blood pressure cuff is inflated to obstruct the vein and increase the rate of bleeding. The blood is passed through the centrifuge at the head of the bed and then reinjected into the recipient through the left arm.

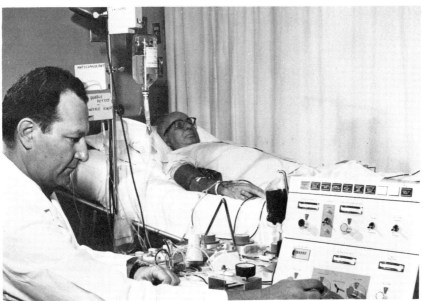

of whole blood. However, by collecting granulocytes from patients with chronic granulocytic leukemia, it has been demonstrated that increases of circulating granulocytes in the recipients can be observed and that such increases can be associated with the control of established septicemia.

To develop equipment which would produce large quantities of leukocytes for the purpose of transfusion, we initiated work on a continuous flow, in vivo, blood cell separator (Freireich, Judson, and Levin, 1965). This instrument, which is known as the NCI-IBM blood cell separator, now has come to a state of development in which significant quantities of leukocytes can be collected in vitro from a single donor (Figs. 5 and 6). This instrument is capable of processing blood at the rate of 50 ml./minute or three liters in an hour, and several blood volumes can be processed continuously from a single donor. In hematologically normal donors, the instrument can recover 30 per cent of the white cells in a single pass through the instrument at 50 ml./minute (Freireich, Curtis, and Hersh, in press). It collects lymphocytes with a higher efficiency than polymorphonuclear granulocytes; however, it is capable of returning over 90 per cent of the platelets and more than 98 per cent of the red cells to the donor, allowing such a procedure (leukocyte donation) to be done frequently.

The capability for the collection of more than 10 billion leukocytes from a single donor has greatly expanded the horizons for research on leukocytes. These include studies of abnormal or leukemic leukocytes by collection of

FIG. 6.—Operator's view of the continuous flow, blood cell separator in operation during a leukapheresis procedure on a patient.

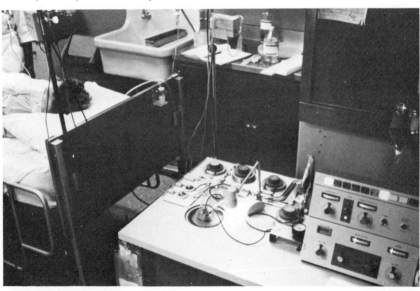

cells from leukemic donors. In addition, with improvements in the technique of collection, the studies of transfusion of granulocytes from single donors into leukopenic recipients should be greatly improved. Recent studies in our institution have demonstrated that the transfusion of lymphocytes collected with the blood cell separator can result in the transfer of primary immunity from donor to recipient (Curtis, Hersh, and Freireich, 1969). The possibility of the use of such an instrument for the transfer of specific immunological information for the control of fungal and viral infections seems attractive. Immunotherapy of malignant disease is another potential application.

Finally, it has been demonstrated that peripheral blood in animals contains stem cells which are capable of repopulating the bone marrow in irradiated or chemotherapy-treated recipients. The ideal form of supportive therapy would be the ability to regularly create bone marrow homografts from allogeneic donors which would temporarily produce the formed elements of the blood needed by the recipient undergoing chemotherapy and would subsequently be rejected by the host when his immunological system recovered with decrease in the chemotherapy.

Summary

Supportive therapy is an integral part of the therapy for leukemia and lymphoma. Protection from the morbidity and mortality resulting directly from the disease and from the therapy is an essential tool for extending the therapeutic index of the agents available for the control and potential eradication of the malignant cells in leukemia and lymphoma.

REFERENCES

Bodey, G. P.: Studies of a patient laminar air flow facility. *Advances in Instrumentation*, 24 (Part IV), paper 655, October 1969.

Bodey, G. P., Buckley, M., Sathe, Y. S., and Freireich, E. J: Quantitative relationships between circulating leukocytes and infection in patients with acute leukemia. *Annals of Internal Medicine*, 64:328-340, February 1966.

Bodey, G. P., Freireich, E. J, and Frei, E., III: Studies of patients in a laminar air flow unit. *Cancer*. (In press.)

Bodey, G. P., Hart, H., Freireich, E. J, and Frei, E., III: Studies of a patient isolator unit and prophylactic antibiotics in cancer chemotherapy. General techniques and preliminary results. *Cancer*, 22:1018-1026, November 1968.

Bodey, G. P., Loftis, J., and Bowen, E.: Protected environment for cancer patients. Effect of a prophylactic antibiotic regimen on the microbial flora of patients undergoing cancer chemotherapy. *Archives of Internal Medicine*, 122:23-30, July 1968.

Bodey, G. P., Rodriguez, V., and Luce, J. K.: Carbenicillin therapy of gram-negative bacilli infections. *American Journal of the Medical Sciences*, 257:408-414, June 1969.

Bodey, G. P., Rodriguez, V., and Whitecar, J. P.: Severe infections in leukemic patients. An approach to antibiotic therapy. *Excerpta Medica*. (In press.)

Bull, B. S., Scheiderman, M. A., and Brecher, G.: Platelet counts with the Coulter counter. *American Journal of Clinical Pathology*, 44:678-688, December 1965.

Curtis, J. E., Hersh, E. M., and Freireich E. J: Transfer of immunity in man with peripheral blood leukocytes (PBL). (Abstract) *Proceedings of the American Association for Cancer Research,* 10:17, March 1969.

Farber, S., Toch, R., Sears, E. M., and Pinkel, D.: Advances in chemotherapy of cancer in man. *Advances in Cancer Research,* 4:1-72, 1956.

Freireich, E. J, Curtis, J. E., and Hersh, E. M.: Use of the blood cell separator to collect lymphocytes: Characteristics of the collection and effects on the donor. In *Proceedings of the International Symposium of the Centre National de la Recherche Scientifique on White Cell Transfusion,* Paris, France, 1969. (In press.)

Freireich, E. J, Judson, G., and Levin, R. H.: Separation and collection of leukocytes. *Cancer Research,* 25:1516-1520, October 1965.

Freireich, E. J, Kliman, A., Gaydos, L. A., Mantel, N., and Frei, E., III: Response to repeated platelet transfusion from the same donor. *Annals of Internal Medicine,* 59:277-287, September 1963.

Freireich, E. J, Levin, R. H., Whang, J., Carbone, P. P., Bronson, W., and Morse, E. E.: The function and fate of transfused leukocytes from donors with chronic myelocytic leukemia in leukopenic recipients. *Annals of the New York Academy of Sciences,* 113:1081-1089, February 1964.

Gaydos, L. A., Freireich, E. J, and Mantel, N.: The quantitative relationship between platelet count and hemorrhage in patients with acute leukemia. *New England Journal of Medicine,* 266:905-909, May 3, 1962.

Kliman, A., Gaydos, L. A., Schroeder, L. R., and Freireich, E. J: Repeated plasmapheresis of blood donors as a source of platelets. *Blood, The Journal of Hematology,* 18:303-309, September 1961.

Murphy, S., and Gardner, F. H.: Platelet preservation. Effect of storage temperature on maintenance of platelet viability—deleterious effect of refrigerated storage. *New England Journal of Medicine,* 280:1094-1098, May 5, 1969.

Platelet Transfusion Subcommittee of the Acute Leukemia Task Force (Cohen, E., Djerassi, I., Freireich, E. J [Chairman], Gilchrist, G. S., Kliman, A., Schmidt, P. J., and Shively, J. A.): Platelet transfusion procedures. *Cancer Chemotherapy Reports,* 1:1-12, December 1968.

Combined Use of Chemotherapy and Radiation Therapy in the Treatment for Generalized Hodgkin's Disease

JESS F. GAMBLE, M.D.,
LILLIAN M. FULLER, M.D., AND
C. C. SHULLENBERGER, M.D.

Departments of Medicine and Radiotherapy, The University of Texas M. D. Anderson Hospital and Tumor Institute at Houston, Houston, Texas

IT HAS BECOME EVIDENT that a significant proportion of patients with stages I and II Hodgkin's disease have prolonged remissions and possibly are cured when adequately treated with x-ray therapy. Even when less sophisticated irradiation equipment and staging techniques were available, a small percentage of patients with a stage III classification of Hodgkin's disease had prolonged survivals.

As shown in Table 1, Dr. Vera Peters (1950) recorded a 17 per cent five-year survival rate in patients who received irradiation to involved plus proximal nodes; there were no survivals in patients who received treatment to involved nodes only. Easson (1966) also has reported long survivals in patients who probably had stage III Hodgkin's disease.

With the development of ^{60}Co and other megavoltage units, it has become possible to treat the entire abdomen with intensive x-ray therapy (Fuller, 1966). As a result of this advancement and some improvement in our ability to stage patients, programs are being developed to attempt to duplicate in stage III Hodgkin's disease the results obtained in less advanced disease.

One treatment plan that has evolved uses as a basis the premise that all involved areas should be treated in a segmental manner. In 1968, Dr. Henry Kaplan reported his results with radical extended-field therapy in patients

TABLE 1.—INFLUENCE OF PROPHYLACTIC IRRADIATION ON
FIVE-YEAR SURVIVAL OF PATIENTS WITH STAGE III
HODGKIN'S DISEASE, 1924-1942*

GROUP	STAGE III	
	No. of Cases	% 5-Year Survival
A. Irradiation to involved nodes plus proximal nodes	24	17
B. Irradiation to involved nodes only	20	0
C. Improvement in cure rate by prophylactic irradiation		17

*Adapted from Peters, 1950.

with stage III Hodgkin's disease (Table 2). Four of five patients with stage IIIA disease have had good remissions. Seven (41 per cent) of 17 patients with stage IIIB disease were reported as being continuously free of disease from 15 to 51 months. The patient who lived 51 months died of a central nervous system (CNS) hemorrhage; no Hodgkin's disease was found at autopsy. Dr. Kaplan pointed out (Fig. 1) that there are very few relapses in Hodgkin's disease in treated fields receiving a radiation tumor dose of 4,000 rads. In his series, there were four recurrences in 91 fields.

In addition to these advances made in x-ray therapy, there has been a parallel improvement in chemotherapy. Dr. Luce (personal communication) has permitted me to use the following unpublished data (Table 3). The complete remission rate in advanced Hodgkin's disease managed with vinblastine was 20 per cent, with a total objective remission rate of 61 per cent. The lower part of the table shows the improvement with combination chemotherapy programs. The MOPP treatment plan (combined use of mechlorethamine, vincristine, procarbazine, and prednisone) seems to be especially effective in Hodgkin's disease. The Southwest Cancer Chemotherapy Study Group (SWCCSG) reports a complete remission rate of 72 per cent and a total objective remission rate of 89 per cent. As Dr. Burchenal reported in this conference (1970, see pages 93-104, this volume) of the 81 per cent of Dr. DeVita's patients who achieved complete remission with MOPP treatment, 28 per cent were in complete remission more than two years later. The duration of these remissions remains to be determined.

In the present pilot study, we are attempting a combination chemotherapy-irradiation approach to the problem of curing or at least obtaining prolonged remissions in patients with stage III Hodgkin's disease. It is difficult to give x-ray therapy doses in a range of 4,000 rads to all of the

TABLE 2.—Results of X-ray Therapy in Hodgkin's Disease, Stage III*†

X-ray Therapy	Total Patients	Follow-up Period		No. of Deaths		Patients Continuously Free of Disease	
		Range (Months)	Median (Months)	With Disease	Without Disease	No.	Duration (Months)
Stage IIIA:							
Palliative—1,500 R (limited fields)	6	30-62	41	2(33%)	0	3(50%)	30,39,43
Radical—3,500-4,000 R (extended fields)	5	14-47	24	1(20%)	0	4(80%)	14,24,43, 47
Stage IIIB:							
Palliative—1,500 R (limited fields)	9‡	29-53	36	5‡(56%)	0	0	
Radical—3,500-4,000 R (extended fields)	17§	8-57	16	7(41%)	1#	7(41%)	15,15,15, 22,23,25, 51#

*After Kaplan, 1968.
†Eight or more at risk.
‡One patient had presumptive liver involvement.
§One patient had documented liver involvement.
#Patient died of cerebrovascular accident 51 months after initiation of treatment for stage IIIB disease; no Hodgkin's disease found at autopsy.

major bone marrow areas of the body without severe and lasting bone marrow depression. Too, the prolonged use of intensive chemotherapy is not without immunological impairment and other hazards. By combining effective chemotherapy and irradiation, some of the risks might be diminished. Repeated injections of chemotherapy and a piecemeal irradiation program would be avoided. Other factors that might be important are listed in Table 4.

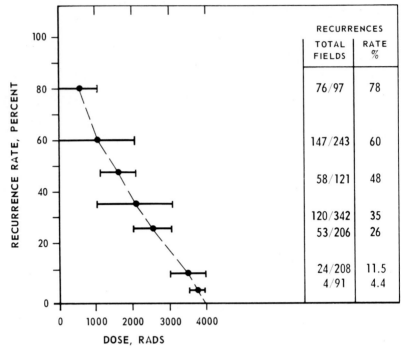

FIG. 1. Composite data on recurrence rate of Hodgkin's disease as a function of the dose. (Courtesy of Kaplan, 1966.)

TABLE 3.—REMISSION INDUCTION IN HODGKIN'S DISEASE*

RESULTS OF CHEMOTHERAPY BY DIFFERENT GROUPS	NO. OF PATIENTS	OBJECTIVE REMISSION RATE (%) Total	Complete Remission
Single agent chemotherapy			
Cyclophosphamide			
Leukemia B - EST	86	54	14
collected series	389	56.1	11
Vinblastine			
Leukemia B - EST	88	61	20
Combination chemotherapy			
COP	107	77	36
MOPP (HN₂, Vcr, Procarb, Pred)			
NCI	43	-	81
SWCCSG	110	89	72

*Luce, personal communication.
Abbreviations: COP, Cytoxan, vincristine, and prednisone; EST, Eastern Solid Tumor Group B; MOPP, nitrogen mustard, vincristine, procarbazine, and prednisone; NCI, National Cancer Institute; SWCCSG, Southwest Cancer Chemotherapy Study Group.

TABLE 4.—Reasons for Intensive Chemotherapy and
X-ray Therapy in Stage III Hodgkin's Disease

1. Maximum therapy as early as possible after the diagnosis and stage have been established
2. Reduction in node size—perhaps of special importance in regard to mediastinal involvement
3. Early control of symptoms
4. The initial chemotherapy may delay tumor growth during the period of prolonged x-ray therapy
5. Possible cure or long-term control of disease

We have approached this treatment program with caution since we wanted to avoid irreversible bone marrow damage that might accompany combination chemotherapy and intensive irradiation to most of the axial skeleton. We chose to start with cyclophosphamide 20 mg./kg. of body weight and 2 mg. of vincristine, both given intravenously. X-ray treatment was started about two weeks later. The most critical region was treated first, the choice being dependent on the size of the tumor masses, local symptomatology, and surrounding vital structures. The tumor doses ranged between 3,000 and 4,000 rads with additional treatment for residual disease. None of these patients had received prior treatment. All of the patients had lymphangiograms, chest x-ray films, and liver function tests. Patients were staged as Dr. Fuller (1970, see pages 241-259, this volume) has discussed. The stage IV patients that were included had grossly abnormal liver function test results.

Our results are shown in Table 5. We have treated a total of 12 Hodgkin's disease patients with this treatment plan. There were eight stage IIIB, one IIIA, and three IVB patients. The living patients are considered to be in complete remission. As outlined, all of the IIIB patients with a nodular sclerosing classification are living with remissions. One patient with a diagnosis of mixed cellularity died 28 weeks from the onset of treatment; the postmortem diagnosis was viral pneumonia. Patients with IVB disease had poor responses. One patient of this group with a diagnosis of granuloma has now been reclassified as having Hodgkin's disease with mixed cellularity. Originally, we did not plan to include this patient in the study since an exploratory operation had shown abdominal Hodgkin's disease with direct invasion of the liver. Later the patient developed neck nodes and treatment was given to the neck. The patient is living and in apparent remission.

Figure 2 shows the x-ray treatment received by stage IV patients. The solid area indicates treatment was completed and the dotted area means that the radiotherapist was unable to complete treatment of the area

TABLE 5.—HODGKIN'S DISEASE TREATED WITH CHEMOTHERAPY
FOLLOWED BY X-RAY THERAPY

HISTOLOGICAL CLASSIFICATION	NO. OF PATIENTS		WEEKS FROM ONSET OF TREATMENT	STAGING	NO. OF PATIENTS
Nodular sclerosing	7	Living 6	20,28,99,100,132,140	IIIB	6
		Dead 1	28	IVB	1
Mixed cellularity	3	Living 2	18,32	IIIA	1
				IIIB	1
		Dead 1	28	IIIB	1
Lymphoid depletion	1 - Dead		10	IVB	1
Granuloma	1 - Living		100	IVB	1

marked. Treatment fields are listed at the top of the figure. Rest periods between treatment periods averaged six weeks. The word skip means that the chest x-ray film was negative for mediastinal disease.

The first patient completed treatment to the upper two thirds of his abdomen, but died six months later of progressive disease; he had received one course of MOPP. The second patient was unable to complete treatment but died with progressive disease and liver failure. The third patient has been discussed previously. He had direct involvement of the liver. His chest x-ray film was negative with no evidence of disease.

Figure 3 lists patients with a diagnosis of mixed cellularity Hodgkin's disease and a stage III classification. The first patient, with IIIA Hodgkin's disease, developed herpes zoster and treatment had to be stopped. He has now recovered, and treatment will be given to the mediastinum and axillary

FIG. 2.—Chemotherapy x-ray treatment received by patients with stage IVB Hodgkin's disease. Dark areas mean treatment to that site was completed; dots indicate treatment not completed.

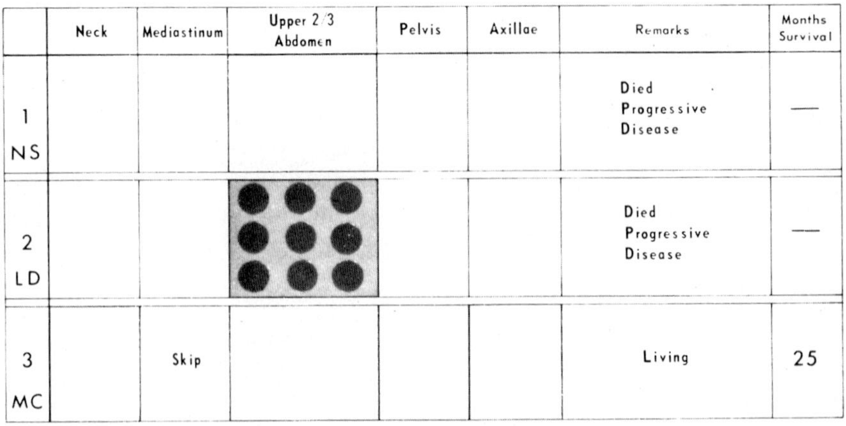

	Neck	Mediastinum	Upper 2/3 Abdomen	Pelvis	Axillae	Remarks	Months Survival
1 NS						Died Progressive Disease	——
2 LD			●●● ●●● ●●●			Died Progressive Disease	——
3 MC		Skip				Living	25

Pat. No.	Neck	Mediastinum	Upper 2 3 Abdomen	Pelvis	Axillae	Remarks	Months Survival
1		Skip				Herpes Zoster Day 133, Day 182 Thrombocytopenia	8
2						Day 140 Died Day 192 Viral Pneumonia	8
3		Skip			Treatment Started		4 1/2

FIG. 3.—Chemotherapy and x-ray treatment received by stage III and mixed cellularity Hodgkin's disease patients. Darkened areas indicate that treatment to these sites was completed.

areas. The second patient completed treatment but died of viral pneumonia. The third patient will receive treatment to the mediastinum and axillary areas.

Figure 4 shows results in patients with stage IIIB nodular sclerosing Hodgkin's disease. The second patient received 2,200 rads to the pelvis; further treatment was not given because of leukopenia. Early in his course of treatment, a second dose of 1,000 mg. of Cytoxan was necessary to control symptoms. The third patient also required additional chemotherapy on day 6 to control his symptoms. The patient developed a solitary pulmonary nodule 391 days from the start of treatment; this was treated. The fifth patient received treatment to the neck and pelvis at the same time but did not tolerate this dose of radiotherapy. Treatment now is being resumed. The sixth patient is under treatment.

Figure 5 summarizes the results in two patients who received more intensive chemotherapy. These patients received four courses of cyclophosphamide and vincristine followed by intensive irradiation (time is given in months). Each patient received similar courses of treatment with each dose consisting of about 1,000 mg. of cyclophosphamide and 2 mg. of vincristine.

The tumor dose and area treated is given for each patient. Ten months after therapy was started, the first patient developed pneumonia and what we thought was an aspirin gastritis; however, treatment was completed. The patient now shows no evidence of disease. The second patient relapsed with a rib lesion and pleural effusion 12 months from the start of treatment. The patient may have had bone marrow involvement with stage IV disease even

Pat. No.	Neck	Mediastinum	Upper 2/3 Abdomen	Pelvis	Axillae	Remarks	Months Survival
1						Day 229	35
2				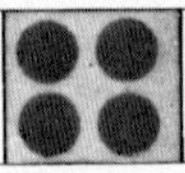 ●● ●●		Day 211 Leukopenia	33
3						Day 191, Velban Day 6 Relapse Day 391, 4000 Rads Solitary Lung Nodule	29
4						Day 107 Leukopenia	24
5	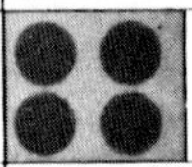 ●● ●●	Skip		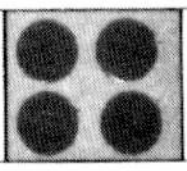 ●● ●●		Day 108 Leukopenia Thrombocytopenia	7
6				Under Treatment		Day 153 Leukopenia Thrombocytopenia	5

FIG. 4.—Chemotherapy and x-ray treatment received by patients with stage IIIB nodular sclerosing Hodgkin's disease. Dark areas mean treatment to that site was completed; dots indicate treatment not completed.

FIG. 5.—Results of two patients who received four courses of cyclophosphamide and vincristine followed by intensive irradiation. Time is given in months.

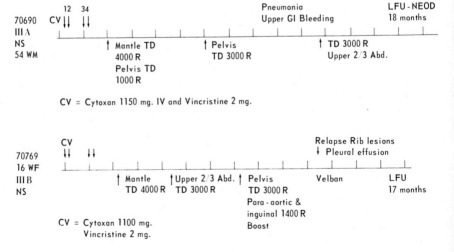

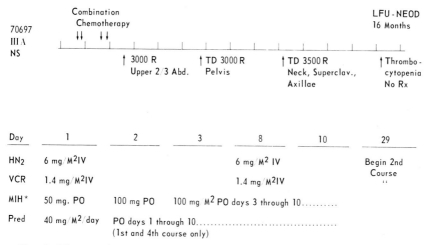

FIG. 6.—Therapy of one patient with two courses of MOPP. Listed at the bottom are the chemicals and the dose schedules for the MOPP treatment plan.

when first seen. This emphasizes the difficulty in bone marrow evaluation.

Dr. Frei (personal communication) has treated one patient with two courses of MOPP with good results (Fig. 6). The patient developed thrombocytopenia, and treatment to the mediastinum has been delayed. However, there has now been complete recovery of the peripheral blood values. Listed at the bottom of the figure are the chemicals and dose schedule for the MOPP treatment plan. Nitrogen mustard and vincristine are injected intravenously on days 1 and 8 of each course. The patient receives oral procarbazine and prednisone for 10 days. A second course is given 29 days after the start of the first course of treatment.

Because of the good results obtained with the MOPP treatment program, we have decided to treat a series of Hodgkin's disease patients with stage IIIA or IIIB classification with two courses of one-half MOPP. This means that the nitrogen mustard will be reduced to 3 mg./m² of the patient's surface area; there is a similar reduction in procarbazine. Intensive irradiation will be started one month after the two courses of chemotherapy have been completed.

In conclusion, this reported pilot study has offered encouraging results, especially in stage IIIB Hodgkin's disease, and there have been no irreversible bone marrow depressions as a result of this treatment plan. However, a longer period of follow-up will be necessary before conclusions can be made as to the merit of this program. It is evident that even with a limited dose of chemotherapy, it is sometimes difficult to complete the planned irradiation therapy program.

REFERENCES

Burchenal, J. H.: Features suggesting curability in leukemia and lymphoma. In *Leukemia-Lymphoma*, A Collection of Papers Presented at the 14th Annual Clinical Conference on Cancer, 1969, at The University of Texas M. D. Anderson Hospital and Tumor Institute at Houston. Chicago, Illinois, Year Book Medical Publishers, Inc., 1970, pp. 93-104.

Easson, E. C.: Long-term results of radical radiotherapy in Hodgkin's disease. *Cancer Research*, 26:1244-1247, June 1966.

Frei, E., III: Personal communication.

Fuller, L. M.: Results of large volume irradiation in the management of Hodgkin's disease and malignant lymphomas originating in the abdomen. *Radiology*, 87:1058-1064, December 1966.

Fuller, L. M., Gamble, J. F., and Butler, J. J.: Results of definitive radiotherapy in localized Hodgkin's disease, as related to both clinical presentation and pathological classification. In *Leukemia-Lymphoma*, A Collection of Papers Presented at the 14th Annual Clinical Conference on Cancer, 1969, at the University of Texas M. D. Anderson Hospital and Tumor Institute at Houston. Chicago, Illinois, Year Book Medical Publishers, Inc., 1970, pp. 241-259.

Kaplan, H. S.: Clinical evaluation and radiotherapeutic management of Hodgkin's disease and the malignant lymphomas. *New England Journal of Medicine*, 278:892-899, April 18, 1968.

Kaplan, H. S.: Evidence for tumoricidal dose level in the radiotherapy of Hodgkin's disease. *Cancer Research*, 26:1221-1224, June 1966.

Luce, J. K.: Personal communication.

Peters, M. V.: A study of survivals in Hodgkin's disease treated radiologically. *The American Journal of Roentgenology, Radium Therapy and Nuclear Medicine*, 63:299-311, March 1950.

Chemotherapy for Lymphomas: Current Status

JAMES K. LUCE, M.D.

Department of Developmental Therapeutics, The University of Texas M. D. Anderson Hospital and Tumor Institute at Houston, Houston, Texas

SINGLE CANCER CHEMOTHERAPEUTIC DRUGS can produce a 70 per cent rate of remission in patients with Hodgkin's disease and a 50 to 80 per cent remission in patients with lymphosarcoma and reticulum cell sarcoma. These rates of remission include patients who show a greater than 50 per cent reduction in tumor or organ size, that is, both partial and complete remissions. Ten to 20 per cent of these patients will have complete clinical remission (defined as the absence of disease as measured by currently available techniques). Drugs which can produce this degree of remission in patients with Hodgkin's disease include the alkylating agents (*i.e.*, nitrogen mustard, cyclophosphamide, and chlorambucil), the vinca alkaloids (vincristine and Velban), and the methylhydrazine derivative, procarbazine, which is now marketed as Matulane. The most effective agents in patients with lymphosarcoma and reticulum cell sarcoma are cyclophosphamide, chlorambucil, and vincristine. The adrenal corticosteroids such as prednisone also produce an antitumor effect by actual cell lysis; although they have a lower order of activity than other agents, they are useful in certain clinical situations, as will be outlined.

Current chemotherapeutic regimens have increased not only the total remission rate but particularly the rate of complete clinical disappearance of tumor(s). Furthermore, with some programs, the duration of complete remission following completion of treatment averages over two years.

At this point, it may be well to examine the concepts of cell kill worked out by Skipper and his associates (1970, see pages 27 to 36, this volume) and to seriously consider the concept of cure as described by Burchenal (1970, see pages 93 to 104, this volume). A complete clinical remission means that the clinician can find no visible or laboratory or radiological evidence of disease. However, this clinical situation can occur when therapy reduces the tumor load to only about 10 per cent of its kinetic pretreatment size. Thus, in a patient with 1×10^{11} tumor cells initially, or about 100 g. of tumor, a 90 per cent reduction in tumor size would result in 10 g. of tumor remaining. If this 10 g. of remaining tumor is spread diffusely throughout the node-bearing area, it probably cannot be detected clinically. A 90 per cent reduction in number of tumor cells will result in only a 1 log reduction, *i.e.*, the patient will still have 1×10^{10} tumor cells remaining. A given therapeutic maneuver results in about the same proportion of cells killed regardless of the total number of cells present. Therefore, a repeat of this maneuver would again reduce the tumor load 90 per cent, leaving 1×10^9 cells. It is apparent, then, that 10 such maneuvers would be required to reduce the cell population to one cell or 10^0 cells.

It is clear that a clinically complete remission may be far from complete eradication of malignant cells. If we have one or more effective agents, how will we be able to remove the total disease burden? Two choices of action are apparent: (1) to use a bigger dose of drug or drugs to effect a greater cell kill and (2) to give enough treatment courses to eliminate the last remaining cell, *i.e.*, many courses of treatment beyond the point at which the tumor has disappeared clinically. We and other investigators have proceeded with these concepts in mind.

With most antitumor agents, there is a rough parallel between the dose administered and magnitude of antitumor response; therefore, the maximum dosage of an agent consistent with tolerable toxicity should be used. With the myelosuppressive agents, this usually means producing moderate myelosuppression with each course of treatment. A second way of increasing the effective dose is to utilize two or more drugs concurrently.

Combination chemotherapy was used initially in patients with acute leukemia (Freireich, Karon, and Frei, 1964). It was demonstrated that agents with different dose-limiting toxicities can be combined at full dosage and that agents with different mechanisms of action but with myelosuppression as a common toxicity can be combined using somewhat greater than half the dose of each drug to produce myelosuppression equal to that of the single agents used alone. Untreated patients with acute leukemia die from the disease on an average of approximately three months after diagnosis. This disease serves as a good model for testing the concept of amount of cell kill. Thus, if survival is lengthened and the rate of division of the cells is known, one can extrapolate to determine what proportion of the malignant cells was killed by a particular therapeutic regimen. The situation is somewhat more difficult in patients with lymphoma because the rate of tumor growth is ordinarily slower than that in patients with acute leukemia and because there is a great range in rate of cell division between patients with a similar histologic type of tumor. The concept which usually is appl. d in determining the efficacy of treatment in patients with lymphoma .s how much shrinkage of tumor mass is produced by a given therapeutic program. It is apparent, however, that if an objective remission is produced by such a program but measurable tumor still remains, very little actual progress has been made against the disease. Now that a higher rate of complete remission can be achieved, a more useful concept is to measure the length of time from cessation of a treatment program until the patient again shows evidence of tumor(s). The longer this period of time, the greater the cell kill and the closer the patient comes to cure.

Based on the experience in acute leukemia studies, in 1965, Lacher and Durant initiated combination chemotherapy for patients with lymphoma using vinblastine and chlorambucil. This combination produced complete remission in 10 of 16 patients with Hodgkin's disease.

During the past three years, a multitude of combination chemotherapeutic regimens have been devised for and applied to patients with lymphoma.

Rather than attempt to discuss the results of all of the many studies which have been and are being done, I will describe a pilot study done at the National Institutes of Health (NIH) and two studies we have performed at The University of Texas M. D. Anderson Hospital and Tumor Institute at Houston in cooperation with the Southwest Cancer Chemotherapy Study Group (SWCCSG).

Three years ago, investigators at the National Institutes of Health initiated a study on a four-drug regimen for patients with previously untreated stages III and IV Hodgkin's disease (DeVita, Serpick, and Carbone, 1969). The regimen consisted of monthly courses of four drugs, Mustargen, Oncovin, procarbazine, and prednisone, and was called MOPP. Nitrogen mustard (Mustargen) was given on days 1 and 8, vincristine (Oncovin) was given on days 1 and 8, procarbazine (Matulane) was given as a 10-day course, and high doses of prednisone were given for 10 days. Treatment was given mostly to outpatients; the patients tolerated the drugs well. Myelosuppression was moderate with an average white blood cell count depression to 2,000-3,000/mm^3 following each course of drugs. Of the first 30 patients treated, 27 (90 per cent) achieved complete clinical remission. Patients were given six complete courses of drug and, if they had achieved a complete remission, treatment was stopped and they were watched for evidence of relapse. The most striking aspect of this program was that the majority of patients tended to stay in remission even with no treatment. At 27 months after the end of treatment, 50 per cent of the patients are still in complete remission. It is apparent that the total cell kill achieved by this regimen is considerably greater than that with other treatment regimens.

Because these patients were carefully selected and were treated in a specialized institution, it seemed to us that the regimen should be tested in

TABLE 1.—COMBINATION TREATMENT (MOPP)
FOR HODGKIN'S DISEASE BY THE SWCCSG

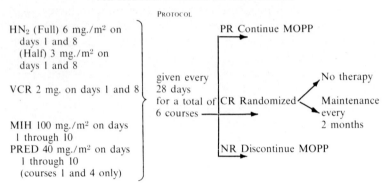

Abbreviations: CR, complete remission; HN$_2$, nitrogen mustard; MIH, procarbazine; MOPP, combination treatment consisting of Mustargen, Oncovin, procarbazine, and prednisone; NR, no remission; PR, partial remission; PRED, prednisone; VCR, vincristine.

patients with various degrees of prior treatment by therapists at a number of different institutions. In November 1967, we started a similar protocol which was sponsored by the SWCCSG (Table 1). We made two major changes in the protocol: (1) we selected patients who had had considerable prior treatment and (2) if the marrow reserve was low, we lowered the initial doses of nitrogen mustard and procarbazine. Since half of the patients given the NIH regimen relapsed with no maintenance after having achieved a complete remission, we randomly allocated our patients in complete remission to two groups: maintenance and nonmaintenance after their initial six courses. The patients on maintenance received additional courses of treatment every two months.

In a preliminary analysis of 110 patients, we divided the patients into four categories in relation to prior treatment (Tables 2 and 3). Category A included 68 patients who had had little or no prior chemotherapy or radiotherapy. Of these 68 patients, 53 (78 per cent) achieved complete remission and another five achieved nearly complete remission with only questionable evidence of remaining disease. Category B included patients who had little prior radiotherapy but major prior chemotherapy with at least one type of alkylating agent. Of the 27 patients in this category, 12 (44 per cent) achieved complete remission. Category C (Table 3) included patients with major prior radiotherapy to the mediastinum, abdomen, or pelvis. Seven of the eight patients in this group achieved complete remission. Category D included patients who had had both prior radiotherapy

TABLE 2.—COMBINATION TREATMENT (MOPP)
FOR HODGKIN'S DISEASE BY THE SWCCSG

PREVIOUS TREATMENT	NO. OF PATIENTS	CR	NEARLY CR	TOTAL NO. RESPONDING
Category A (little or no prior chemotherapy or irradiation therapy)	68	53 (78%)	5	65 (95%)
Category B (little prior radiotherapy; major prior chemotherapy)	27	12 (44%)	2	21 (79%)

Abbreviations: CR, complete remission; MOPP, combination treatment consisting of Mustargen, Oncovin, procarbazine, and prednisone.

TABLE 3.—COMBINATION TREATMENT (MOPP)
FOR HODGKIN'S DISEASE BY THE SWCCSG

RESPONSE	NO. OF PATIENTS	COMPLETE REMISSION	TOTAL NO. RESPONDING
Category C (major prior radiotherapy; little prior chemotherapy)	8	7	8
Category D (major prior radiotherapy and chemotherapy)	7	1	4

Abbreviation: MOPP, combination treatment consisting of Mustargen, Oncovin, procarbazine, and prednisone.

and chemotherapy: one patient of the seven achieved a complete remission, and four of the seven had at least 50 per cent shrinkage of tumor(s). It is clear, then, that in relation to response, this four-drug regimen is indeed superior to other chemotherapeutic regimens, even in a broad trial with many investigators.

It is still too early to evaluate the duration of remission produced with this regimen by members of the SWCCSG. However, of 41 patients who achieved complete remission and were randomly selected for either maintenance treatment or no maintenance therapy, a greater than 10-week duration of complete remission has been obtained in the maintained group and a greater than 19-week median duration of remission has been achieved in

TABLE 4.—COMBINATION TREATMENT (MOPP)
FOR HODGKIN'S DISEASE BY THE SWCCSG
(DURATION OF COMPLETE REMISSION IN WEEKS
AFTER RANDOMIZATION; CATEGORY A PATIENTS ONLY)

	NO. OF PATIENTS*	MEDIAN	RANGE
Maintained	20	10+	0–31+
Unmaintained	21	19+	0–37+

*Only two patients, one in each group, have relapsed.
Abbreviation: MOPP, combination treatment consisting of Mustargen, Oncovin, procarbazine, and prednisone.

the unmaintained group (Table 4). Only two patients, one in each group, have relapsed.

In 1966, we initiated a combination chemotherapy program (COP) consisting of cyclophosphamide, vincristine (Oncovin), and prednisone for patients with all types of lymphomas, including Hodgkin's disease. The treatment was given as "pulses" every two weeks. The two-week interval was chosen because myelosuppression caused by cyclophosphamide begins to show recovery at this time and we wished to apply courses as frequently as possible to prevent regrowth of tumor between administration of the chemotherapeutic drugs. Again, patients were divided into two categories in relation to an estimate of bone marrow reserve. Patients with good marrow reserve were given 800 mg./m^2 or approximately 25 mg./kg. of cyclophosphamide as a single intravenous injection. They were also given 2 mg. total dose of vincristine and 100 mg. of prednisone daily for five days, followed by a three-day tapering-off period. Patients were treated for a minimum of 10 courses and, if they had achieved a complete remission, they were randomly selected for maintenance treatment every month or for no maintenance therapy.

Toxicity was tolerable. Of the 250 patients treated, only four died, in part

TABLE 5.—COMBINATION TREATMENT (COP) FOR PATIENTS
WITH HODGKIN'S DISEASE BY THE SWCCSG

AMOUNT OF DRUGS RECEIVED	NO. OF PATIENTS	COMPLETE RESPONSE	NEARLY COMPLETE RESPONSE	ALL RESPONDERS
Full dose	55	38%	2%	76%
Half dose	51	22%	10%	77%

Abbreviation: COP, cyclophosphamide, Oncovin, prednisone.

TABLE 6.—COMBINATION TREATMENT (COP) FOR PATIENTS
WITH LYMPHOSARCOMA BY THE SWCCSG

AMOUNT OF DRUGS RECEIVED	NO. OF PATIENTS	COMPLETE RESPONSE	NEARLY COMPLETE RESPONSE	ALL RESPONDERS
Full dose	42	40%	10%	86%
Half dose	30	43%	3%	89%

Abbreviation: COP, cyclophosphamide, Oncovin, prednisone.

or totally caused by toxic effects of drugs. Two of these four patients died from severe myelosuppression, but the dose of the drug was not appropriately lowered from a previous course of treatment. This points to the necessity of closely watching patients who undergo multiple drug chemotherapy and of regulating the dosage of drugs to achieve moderate, but not severe or life-threatening myelosuppression. The dose of vincristine chosen was satisfactory. In patients who lost their deep-tendon reflexes and developed some paresthesia, the dose was not lowered. A few developed severe obstipation or muscle weakness requiring a lowering of the dose. The most severe side effect of prednisone was peptic ulceration, which usually was easily controlled with an appropriate antacid regimen.

Tables 5, 6, and 7 show the results of treatment for each disease. Fifty-five patients with Hodgkin's disease were started on the full-dose Cytoxan regimen, and 51 were started on the half-dose Cytoxan regimen. The complete response rate was 38 per cent for the full-dose and 22 per cent for the half-dose Cytoxan regimen. This response rate is significantly better than that which can be achieved with single agents, but is not as good as that which can be achieved with the MOPP four-drug regimen.

The complete remission response rates to COP in patients with lymphosarcoma were 40 per cent in patients who were started on treatment with full doses of cyclophosphamide and 43 per cent in patients who were started on

TABLE 7.—COMBINATION TREATMENT (COP) FOR PATIENTS
WITH RETICULUM CELL SARCOMA BY THE SWCCSG

AMOUNT OF DRUGS RECEIVED	NO. OF PATIENTS	COMPLETE RESPONSE	NEARLY COMPLETE RESPONSE	ALL RESPONDERS
Full dose	37	35%	3%	78%
Half dose	28	32%	11%	79%

Abbreviation: COP, cyclophosphamide, Oncovin, prednisone.

the half dose of cyclophosphamide. Similarly, of 37 patients with reticulum cell sarcoma who were started on full doses of cyclophosphamide, 35 per cent achieved complete remission and 32 per cent of 28 patients with the same disease who were started on half-dose cyclophosphamide achieved complete remission. It has been the clinical impression of many therapists that patients with reticulum cell sarcoma do not respond well to chemotherapeutic agents; however, the response rate to the COP regimen was on a par with the response rate of patients with lymphosarcoma and Hodgkin's disease. Almost 80 per cent of patients with reticulum cell sarcoma showed at least a 50 per cent reduction in tumor mass.

Again, the best test of actual cell kill produced by this combination of drugs is the duration of unmaintained complete remission (Table 8). Patients with Hodgkin's disease who were not given maintenance therapy had a median duration of remission of 18 weeks; this is superior to the 10-week duration of remission produced by single agents, but not as good as that obtained with the four-drug regimen (MOPP). A 21-week unmaintained remission was seen in patients with lymphosarcoma, and a 25-week remission was seen in patients with reticulum cell sarcoma. The duration of maintained remissions in patients with reticulum cell sarcoma was as good as that for those receiving no maintenance therapy, suggesting that these patients developed resistance to the drugs more rapidly than patients with the other lymphomas and that extra courses of treatment with the same drugs do not prolong the duration of remission.

It is clear, then, that multiple-agent regimens produce a higher rate of remission and a longer duration of remission than single drugs. The effect of these regimens on survival is not known at this time; however, there is every reason to believe that survival will be prolonged since patients whose disease is in complete remission are essentially well and would not be expected to suddenly relapse and die.

This is the current status of treatment for patients with lymphoma. What

TABLE 8.—DURATION OF UNMAINTAINED COMPLETE REMISSION
IN LYMPHOMA PATIENTS RECEIVING
COMBINATION TREATMENT (COP) BY THE SWCCSG*

Type of Lymphoma	Maintained		Not Maintained	
	No. of Patients	Median Weeks to Relapse	No. of Patients	Median Weeks to Relapse
Hodgkin's disease	11	42	20	18
Lymphosarcoma	17	47	15	21
Reticulum cell sarcoma	11	24	8	25

*Length of complete remission in weeks from randomization to relapse.
Abbreviation: COP, cyclophosphamide, Oncovin, prednisone.

promise does the future hold in the management of disseminated lymphoma? As Dr. Gamble (1970, see pages 285 to 294, this volume) has pointed out, the potential for increasing the rate and duration of remission may lie in combining chemotherapy and radiotherapy. The four-drug regimen used to produce remissions in patients with Hodgkin's disease has such a high rate of response that it seems unlikely that a better remission induction regimen for this disease will be devised in the near future. Since 50 per cent of the patients in the National Institutes of Health series relapsed, attention is being directed toward improving the quality of the complete remissions produced. We are currently trying two chemotherapeutic approaches. The first is to continue treating patients with the same drug regimen which produced the original remission. This approach is reasonable because it is obvious that the original regimen is effective and it may be possible that not enough courses of treatment have been given to completely eradicate the disease. However, it also may be possible that patients have developed resistance to the drugs in this regimen and that better remission consolidation can be achieved by utilizing different agents, ones to which the tumor, hopefully, is still sensitive. Both concepts are being investigated by us and by other members of the SWCCSG.

Attempts are being made to produce a higher rate of complete remission in patients with lymphosarcoma and reticulum cell sarcoma. Initially, the MOPP regimen was not used for these patients since the response rate of these diseases to nitrogen mustard and to procarbazine was not as good as to cyclophosphamide and to vincristine. There may, however, be something unique about the combination of drugs in the MOPP regimen, and it seems worthwhile to test the regimen in a group of patients with lymphosarcoma and reticulum cell sarcoma in the hope that a higher remission rate also can be produced in these patients.

As new drugs are developed and show promise in screening systems, they need to be applied to patients with lymphoma. Frequently, new drugs are tried in patients with a late stage of disease, and their true efficacy in patients who have previously received very little treatment is not noted. If they do show some promise, then they should be used in patients with earlier stages of disease. One such agent is bis-β-chloroethyl-nitrosourea (BCNU), which produces a 50 per cent total remission rate in patients with Hodgkin's disease who have relapsed on alkylating agents (Lessner, 1968). Although BCNU has been considered an alkylating agent, its effectiveness on alkylating agent-resistant lymphomas suggests that some other mechanism of action may also be operative. It is now being tried for remission maintenance and remission induction as well as for treatment of patients with far-advanced disease.

Clinical trials will continue along these lines. There is every reason to believe that total malignant cell elimination, *i.e.*, cure, will become routine and expected with chemotherapy alone or with chemotherapy plus radiotherapy in patients with disseminated malignant lymphomas.

REFERENCES

Burchenal, J. H.: Features suggesting curability in leukemia and lymphoma. In *Leukemia-Lymphoma.* A Collection of Papers Presented at the 14th Annual Clinical Conference on Cancer, 1969, at The University of Texas M. D. Anderson Hospital and Tumor Institute at Houston. Chicago, Illinois, Year Book Medical Publishers, Inc., 1970, pp. 93-104.

DeVita, V. T., Serpick, A., and Carbone, P. P.: Combination chemotherapy of advanced Hodgkin's disease: The NCI program, a progress report. (Abstract) *Proceedings of the American Association for Cancer Research,* 10:19, March 1969.

Freireich, E. J, Karon, M., and Frei, E., III: Quadruple combination therapy (VAMP) for acute lymphocytic leukemia of childhood. (Abstract) *Proceedings of the American Association for Cancer Research,* 5:20, March 1964.

Gamble, J. F., Fuller, L., and Shullenberger, C. C.: Combined use of chemotherapy and radiation therapy in the treatment of generalized Hodgkin's disease. In *Leukemia-Lymphoma,* A Collection of Papers Presented at the 14th Annual Clinical Conference on Cancer, 1969, at The University of Texas M. D. Anderson Hospital and Tumor Institute at Houston. Chicago, Illinois, Year Book Medical Publishers, Inc., 1970, pp. 285-294.

Lacher, M. J., and Durant, J. R.: Combined vinblastine and chlorambucil therapy of Hodgkin's disease. *Annals of Internal Medicine,* 62:468-476, March 1965.

Lessner, H. E.: BCNU (1,3,bis-β-chloroethyl)-1-nitrosourea: Effects on advanced Hodgkin's disease and other neoplasia. *Cancer,* 22:451-456, August 1968.

Skipper, H. E.: Leukocyte kinetics in leukemia and lymphoma. In *Leukemia-Lymphoma,* A Collection of Papers Presented at the 14th Annual Clinical Conference on Cancer, 1969, at The University of Texas M. D. Anderson Hospital and Tumor Institute at Houston. Chicago, Illinois, Year Book Medical Publishers, Inc., 1970, pp. 27-36.

Multiple Myeloma: A Nine-Year Experience with Melphalan Therapy at the M. D. Anderson Hospital*

RAYMOND ALEXANIAN, M.D.

Department of Medicine, The University of Texas M. D. Anderson Hospital and Tumor Institute at Houston, Houston, Texas

MULTIPLE MYELOMA is a disseminated malignant disease of plasma cells with major involvement of the bone marrow. In the past decade, this affliction has changed from one that caused severe disability for a short duration of life to a disease that is well tolerated for several years by increasing numbers of ambulatory patients. Earlier and more frequent diagnosis, superior management of life-threatening complications, and more effective chemotherapy for the malignant process have accounted for this improvement. This report reviews certain aspects of the natural history of this disease as influenced by melphalan chemotherapy at The University of Texas M. D. Anderson Hospital and Tumor Institute at Houston during the past nine years.

Methods of Study

From June 1960 to June 1969, 140 patients with multiple myeloma, previously untreated with an alkylating agent, were referred to this institution and treated with melphalan or a melphalan and prednisone combination under the auspices of the Southwest Cancer Chemotherapy Study Group (SWCCSG). All patients demonstrated symptoms of their disease and bone marrow plasmacytosis to more than 10 per cent of the cellularity. Electrophoresis demonstrated a monoclonal component in the serum and/ or urine of all but two of the 134 patients studied. Lytic bone lesions were

*This work was supported by United States Public Health Service Grants No. CA 06939 and No. CA 03195.

present in more than 70 per cent, and less than 10 per cent showed normal radiographic findings in the axial skeleton.

The age spectrum for all patients at the time of diagnosis ranged from the youngest, age 32 years, to the oldest, age 84. Four patients (3 per cent) were younger than 40. The median age was 61 years; patients between 60 and 70 years old formed the largest group (Fig. 1). This observation was similar to that of most reported series of myeloma patients, but contrasts with the Swedish experience (Waldenström, 1968), in which the patients between 70 and 80 years old formed the largest group. Whereas 42 per cent of the Swedish patients were older than 70, only 18 per cent of Anderson Hospital patients were this old. In view of the likelihood that the Swedish patients formed a more comprehensive sample, one might infer that myeloma patients over 70 years old were less likely than younger patients to be referred to Anderson Hospital. During the past year, 26 patients with multiple myeloma were referred from various parts of Texas to Anderson Hospital. If one assumes that the fraction of patients in each age decade has remained constant for the past nine years, one may calculate the number of patients of different ages referred by Texas physicians per 100,000 population. Figure 2 demonstrates the increasing incidence of such referrals for each age decade (an observation that closely parallels the Swedish

FIG. 1.—Age distribution of multiple myeloma patients referred to Anderson Hospital.

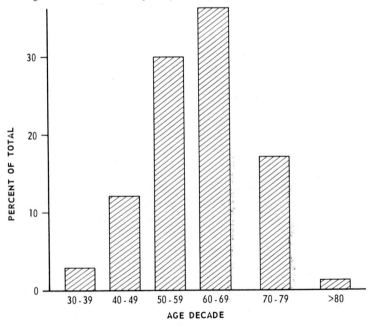

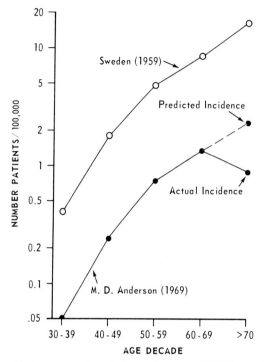

FIG. 2.—Age-specific incidence of multiple myeloma per 100,000 population in Sweden (-0-) in comparison with the frequency of Texans with myeloma referred to Anderson Hospital (-•-). The dotted line indicates the predicted incidence in Anderson Hospital patients, as extrapolated from the Swedish experience.

experience). However, the number of patients older than 70 referred to this institution was less than 50 per cent of that (14 per cent of 164/100,000) predicted by comparison with the lower age-decade groups and the Swedish experience. Presumably, this resulted from a combination of inadequate diagnosis and a decreased likelihood of the referral of elderly myeloma patients to this treatment center.

PROTEIN TYPE

The protein type of the monoclonal component was determined by immunoelectrophoresis in 134 of the 140 patients in this series. Table 1 outlines the breakdown of myeloma protein types in these patients as determined by Dr. Daniel Bergsagel (1967) and Dr. Philip Migliore, (1966) both formerly with Anderson Hospital. Except for the increased percentage of patients with only Bence Jones proteins, the distribution found was similar to that of other reported series. Only two patients (1 per cent) failed

TABLE 1.—Myeloma Protein Types in 134 Anderson Hospital Patients
(1960-1969)

Type	No. Patients	Anderson Hospital Series	% of Total Osserman and Takatsuki Series (1963)	Hobbs Series (1969)
γGK	47	35 ⎫		
		⎬ 51	53	53
γGL	21	16 ⎭		
γAK	9	7 ⎫		
		⎬ 21	22	25
γAL	18	14 ⎭		
K only	23	17 ⎫		
		⎬ 27	22	19
L only	14	10 ⎭		
No monoclonal peak	2	1	2	2
Miscellaneous (IgD, biclonal, etc.)	0	0	1	1

Abbreviations: K, kappa light chains; L, lambda light chains.

to show a peak in either serum or urine, and no patient with an IgD myeloma protein was found. In three of 35 patients showing no serum peak, electrophoresis of urine concentrated 100 times by dialysis was required to show a peak. In each of these three patients, the daily Bence Jones protein excretion was less than 500 mg. and kappa light chains were present. The median daily Bence Jones protein excretion was 6 g. (range, 0.2 to 27) in 23 patients with only kappa light chains, and 10 g. in 14 patients with only lambda light chains (range, 4 to 31). Only one of 14 patients with lambda light chains excreted less than 5 g. daily, in contrast to eight of 23 patients with kappa light chains. These observations emphasize the value of urine electrophoresis in confirming the diagnosis of myeloma in many patients and the importance of urine concentration in confirming the diagnosis in occasional patients. The larger quantities of light-chain proteins excreted by patients with only lambda light chains may have contributed to the higher frequency of renal failure, the resistance to melphalan chemotherapy, and the short survival of these individuals (Alexanian et al., 1969).

Criteria for Evaluation of Response to Chemotherapy

Serial evaluation of the patient and his laboratory abnormalities are required to document an objective response to chemotherapy. Nonevaluable patients included those who died within four months after treatment or those with inadequate documentation of essential laboratory parameters (*i.e.* no myeloma peak). Clinical response was confirmed when the level of serum myeloma protein fell by more than 50 per cent to less than 4 g./100 ml. and/or the daily excretion of Bence Jones protein fell by more than 90 per cent to less than 0.2 g. daily. In addition, responding patients must show control of certain disease complications caused by multiple myeloma and proved to be unrelated to other diseases. These included the maintenance of the hematocrit level above 30 volumes per cent without transfusions, of the serum albumin level above 3.0 g./100 ml., and of the serum calcium level below 12 mg./100 ml. There must be no progression in the size or number of lytic bone lesions and no decline of any normal immunoglobulins previously in the normal range; also, the product of the maximum diameters of all palpable plasmacytomas must have regressed by more than 50 per cent. With rare exceptions (*e.g.* paraplegia from cord compression), bone pain and impaired performance improved in all patients responding to treatment. Justification for these criteria for evaluating response to therapy has been presented elsewhere (Alexanian *et al.*, 1968).

MELPHALAN TREATMENT REGIMENS

From 1960 to the present, a variety of melphalan regimens have been used at this institution for the management of multiple myeloma. All were based on SWCCSG chemotherapy protocols and were coordinated either by Dr. D. Bergsagel (1960 through 1964) or by the author (1965 through 1969). An outline of these treatment regimens is presented in Tables 2 and 3. Table 2 demonstrates that the response rate to melphalan alone was similar (about 50 per cent) regardless of the dose regimen (schedules A,B,C, and D). Consequently, all of these patients were analyzed as a single group in Table 4.

From June 1965 to June 1969, an additional 49 patients were given melphalan in combination with prednisone. These patients were assigned at random to the treatment regimens (schedules E and F) outlined in Table 3 at the time when other patients were assigned to treatments C and D (Table 2) or to other combination regimens (to be reported elsewhere). In schedule E, melphalan was given in an intermittent schedule identical to that used for schedules B and D, but prednisone was given in a single morning dose of 1.0 mg./kg. on Monday, Wednesday, and Friday. In schedule F, prednisone was given concurrently with melphalan in large doses, but then tapered rapidly in dose, and stopped within four subsequent days. All intermittent courses of melphalan, with or without prednisone, were usualiy given at six-week intervals and continued indefinitely until death. In some patients, investigational drugs were tested when unresponsiveness to treat-

TABLE 2.—INCIDENCE OF RESPONSE TO TREATMENTS WITH MELPHALAN ALONE

TIME PERIOD	MELPHALAN REGIMEN	No. Patients		
		Treated	Evaluable	Responsive
A. June 1960 through April 1961	0.2 mg./kg./day for 14 days	11	7	3
B. May 1961 through May 1965	0.25 mg./kg./day for 4 days	49	41	22
C. June 1965 through November 1966	0.025 mg./kg./day	7	6	3
D. June 1965 through February 1968	0.25 mg./kg./day for 4 days	24	18	9
	Totals	91	72	37

TABLE 3.—INCIDENCE OF RESPONSE TO TREATMENTS WITH MELPHALAN PLUS PREDNISONE

TIME PERIOD	SCHEDULE	No. Patients		
		Treated	Evaluable	Responsive
E. June 1965 to November 1966	Melphalan 0.25 mg./kg./day for 4 days + prednisone 1.0 mg./kg. on M,W,F	6	6	4
F. December 1966 to June 1969	Melphalan 0.25 mg./kg./day for 4 days + prednisone 2.0 mg./kg./day for 4 days	43	38	29
	Totals	49	44	33

TABLE 4.—Response Rates from Melphalan Alone and Melphalan plus Prednisone

| | No. Treated | Not Evaluable | | No. Evaluable | No. Responding | Response Rate (%) | |
		Early Death	Incomplete Report			Evaluable	All
Melphalan alone	91	15	4	72	37	51	41
Melphalan and prednisone	49	5	0	44	33	75	67

ment was recognized. Because the response rates from both melphalan-prednisone combinations were similar, all of these patients were analyzed as a single group in Table 4.

RESPONSE RATE

The frequency of response was compared between all patients treated with melphalan alone and all patients treated with melphalan-prednisone combinations. The results are summarized in Table 4. Whereas 51 per cent of evaluable patients responded to melphalan alone, 75 per cent responded to combination chemotherapy with melphalan and prednisone. This difference was significant at the .05 level. These frequencies of response were about 15 per cent higher than those in patients given identical treatment regimens at neighboring SWCCSG institutions (Alexanian et al., 1969). Although an adequate explanation for this difference was not available, Anderson Hospital patients, who travel long distances, may present with less advanced disease. Also, these patients received more frequent courses of chemotherapy in larger doses. The frequency of early deaths during the initial treatment period declined slightly from 16 per cent between 1960 and 1965 to 10 per cent between 1965 and 1968. This improvement was attributed to the prevention and superior management of specific complications, particularly infection, hypercalcemia, and urate nephropathy, thus providing a better opportunity for some patients affected with severe complications to survive the early treatment period and respond to chemotherapy.

The response rates of Negroes and Caucasians to treatment with melphalan alone or with melphalan and prednisone were compared (Table 5). There was no significant difference between the races in their sensitivity to either treatment regimen. The lower response rate among Negroes to melphalan alone, reported in a previous evaluation of these patients by Bergsa-

TABLE 5.—EFFECT OF RACE ON RESPONSE RATE IN PATIENTS WITH MULTIPLE MYELOMA (RESULTS GIVEN IN PER CENT OF EVALUABLE PATIENTS)

| | RESPONSE RATE | |
	Negroes	Caucasians
Melphalan	33%	57%
Melphalan and prednisone	90%	71%
Total	56%	62%

TABLE 6.—EFFECT OF AGE ON RESPONSE IN PATIENTS WITH MULTIPLE MYELOMA (RESULTS GIVEN IN PER CENT OF EVALUABLE PATIENTS)

| | RESPONSE RATE | |
	65 and Older	Younger than 65
Melphalan	33%	53%
Melphalan and prednisone	83%	69%
Total	68%	58%

gel, Griffith, Haut, and Stuckey (1967), was confirmed. However, this difference disappeared when more patients treated with melphalan and prednisone were included in the analysis.

The response rate in patients 65 years and older (29 per cent of the total) was compared with the frequency of response in younger patients. As noted in Table 6, the incidence of objective remission was slightly higher in the older patients, although the difference was not significant. Thus, in contrast to recent experiences by Freireich, Bodey, Harris, and Hart (1967) suggesting a lower response rate to chemotherapy among older patients with acute leukemia, there was no apparent effect of age upon the frequency of response in patients with multiple myeloma. An adequate explanation for this difference was not available.

SURVIVAL

Survival was studied by the life-table method and was measured from the beginning of chemotherapy in all patients treated with melphalan or with a melphalan-prednisone combination. Dr. John Krall in the Department of Biomathematics completed this analysis. The median survival was about six months longer for patients receiving the combination regimen (27 months) than for patients treated with melphalan alone (21 months). This was attributed to a higher response rate and a superior degree of remission induced in patients responding to the melphalan-prednisone combinations (Alexanian et al., 1969). The median survival of responsive patients (38

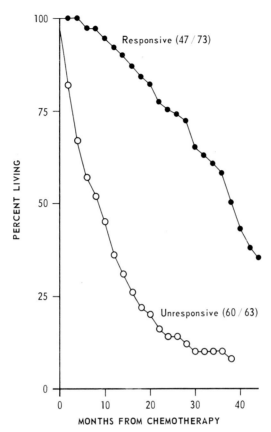

FIG. 3.—Survival of patients responsive to chemotherapy in comparison with unresponsive patients (including those dying early). Figures in parentheses indicate the number dead of total number of patients. Four patients whose responses were not evaluable because of inadequate data were excluded.

months) was more than two years longer than the survival of unresponsive patients, a group which included those dying early (Fig. 3). In previous studies, this prolongation of survival in responding patients had been accounted for by the duration of disease remission measured by the duration of suppression of the myeloma protein peak (Alexanian et al., 1968). About 20 per cent of responsive patients lived more than five years. These results indicate the superiority of combination chemotherapy with melphalan and prednisone in the treatment of patients with multiple myeloma and justify the search for new treatment regimens which will improve the degree and duration of remission. Similar combinations of drugs with independent toxicity also have been useful in patients with lymphoma, acute leukemia, and Hodgkin's disease.

CAUSE OF DEATH

An evaluation of the specific mechanism causing death was attempted for the 111 patients in this series who died. These data are summarized in Table 7. No specific cause of death was identified in 37 patients, mainly because detailed laboratory studies were not done shortly before death. In two thirds of the remaining 74 patients, bone marrow failure and immunoglobulin failure with infection were the major causes of death. Death was attributed to bone marrow failure when red blood cell transfusions were required for severe anemia, when the platelet count declined to less than 20,000, and when the granulocyte count decreased to less than 1,500. Immune failure was considered the major factor when the level of at least two normal (nonmyeloma) immunoglobulins fell to less than 20 per cent of normal (e.g. IgM <20 mg./100 ml. and IgA <40 mg./100 ml.) and the patient died of infection. Death caused primarily by renal failure was defined by progressive rise in the blood urea nitrogen (BUN) level to more than 100 mg./100 ml. in the terminal period. Table 8 indicates that all eight patients considered to have died from severe renal failure produced only Bence Jones proteins (2 kappa, 6 lambda), the median pretreatment excretion being 10 g./day (range, 5 to 31). No patient in this series with γG or γA myeloma proteins was considered to have died from renal failure. Hypercalcemia was confirmed when the calcium remained above 14 mg./100 ml. during the week before death. Death caused by cord compression was identified only when complete paraplegia and urinary retention requiring catheter drainage were present. When combinations of these complications were present, the more severe condition was chosen as the principal cause of death. Four patients died during remission from diseases unrelated to their myeloma. These conditions included acute tracheal obstruction, bronchogenic carcinoma, acute myelogenous leukemia, and carcinoma of the colon. From a careful postmortem study, Dr. Philip Migliore (unpublished

TABLE 7.—MAJOR CAUSES OF DEATH IN 74 PATIENTS WITH MULTIPLE MYELOMA

CAUSE OF DEATH	NO. PATIENTS	% OF TOTAL EVALUABLE
Bone marrow failure	26	35
Immunoglobulin failure	24	32
Renal failure	8	11
Hypercalcemia	7	10
Spinal cord compression	5	7
Unrelated diseases (during remission)	4	5
Total	74	100
Miscellaneous and unknown causes during relapse	37	

TABLE 8.–DEATH PRIMARILY FROM RENAL FAILURE
(BUN >100 MG./100 ML. BEFORE DEATH)

Kappa only	2/12 evaluable
Lambda only	6/9 evaluable
All other myeloma protein types	0/53 evaluable
BJP excretion (g./day) in patients	MEDIAN RANGE
dead from renal failure	10 5 to 31

Abbreviations: BJP, Bence Jones protein; BUN, blood urea nitrogen.

data) found that only two of 32 patients demonstrated histologic evidence of amyloidosis. In neither patient did the amyloidosis contribute to death.

Conclusions

A nine-year experience with melphalan therapy for 140 patients with multiple myeloma was reviewed. The likelihood of diagnosis and/or referral to this institution was less for multiple myeloma patients older than 70 years. Of the 140 patients, 99 per cent showed a monoclonal peak detected by electrophoresis of serum, urine, or urine concentrates. Criteria for the evaluation of clinical response to chemotherapy were based on significant changes in the myeloma protein level and control of major disease complications. Chemotherapy with intermittent courses of melphalan-prednisone combinations induced an objective response in 75 per cent of evaluable patients, in contrast to 51 per cent of those receiving melphalan alone. There was no relationship between response rate and either race or advanced age. Responsive patients lived more than two years longer than unresponsive patients, and patients treated with melphalan-prednisone combinations lived about six months longer than patients treated with melphalan alone. Bone marrow failure and immunoglobulin failure with severe infection were the most frequent causes of death. Death from renal failure occurred only in patients excreting large quantities of Bence Jones proteins.

REFERENCES

Alexanian, R., Bergsagel, D. E., Migliore, P. J., Vaughn, W. K., and Howe, C. D.: Melphalan therapy for plasma cell myeloma. *Blood, The Journal of Hematology,* 31:1-10, January 1968.

Alexanian, R., Haut, A., Khan, A. U., Lane, M., McKelvey, E. M., Migliore, P. J., Stuckey, W. J., Jr., and Wilson, H. E.: Treatment for multiple myeloma: Combination chemotherapy with different melphalan dose regimens. *Journal of the American Medical Association,* 208:1680-1685, June 2, 1969.

Bergsagel, D. E., Griffith, K. M., Haut, A., and Stuckey, W. J., Jr.: The treatment of plasma cell myeloma. *Advances in Cancer Research,* 10:311-359, 1967.

Freireich, E. J, Bodey, G. P., Harris, J. E., and Hart, J. S.: Therapy for acute granulocytic leukemia. *Cancer Research,* 27:2573-2577, December 1967.

Hobbs, J. R.: Immunochemical classes of myelomatosis: Including data from a therapeutic trial conducted by a Medical Research Council working party. *British Journal of Haematology,* 16:599-606, June 1969.

Migliore, P. J.: Immunoelectrophoresis and immunodiffusion techniques in diagnosis of neoplastic diseases. In *Recent Advances in the Diagnosis of Cancer,* A Collection of Papers Presented at the 9th Annual Clinical Conference on Cancer, 1964, at The University of Texas M. D. Anderson Hospital and Tumor Institute. Chicago, Illinois, Year Book Medical Publishers, Inc., 1966, pp. 158-169.

————: Unpublished data.

Osserman, E. F., and Takatsuki, K.: Plasma cell myeloma: Gamma globulin synthesis and structure. *Medicine,* 42:357-384, November 1963.

Waldenström, J. G.: *Monoclonal and Polyclonal Hypergammaglobulinemia.* Nashville, Tennessee, Vanderbilt University Press, and Cambridge, England, Cambridge University Press, 1968, 223 pp.

Survey of Current Therapy and of Problems in Chronic Leukemia*

CHARLES M. HUGULEY, JR., M.D.

Department of Medicine (Hematology),
Emory University School of Medicine, Atlanta, Georgia

Chronic Granulocytic Leukemia

THERE IS LITTLE NEW to be said about the current status of therapy for chronic granulocytic leukemia. For many years, we have had a variety of agents which will control the disease in its early stages rather easily and satisfactorily. Busulfan, introduced in 1953, has become the favorite drug. In about 25 per cent of cases, it has been possible to reduce the spleen and liver to normal size and restore the blood counts to normal values (Huguley *et al.*, 1963; Haut, Abbott, Wintrobe, and Cartwright, 1961). In another 65 per cent, somewhat less complete but nonetheless very good control of the disease has been achieved. Even unmaintained, these remissions sometimes last for many months. Many therapists prefer to give the drug intermittently, permitting a mild to moderate relapse between courses (Haut, Abbott, Wintrobe, and Cartwright, 1961). Others titrate the dose of busulfan to maintain approximately normal hematologic values with steady doses.

Newer agents, *e.g.*, dibromomannitol, have not been shown to be superior to busulfan (Silver, 1968).

With hematologic control, most manifestations of the disease return to normal and the patient is able to pursue his usual activities. The alkaline phosphatase activity of the granulocytes tends to become normal. Nevertheless, even with rather drastic treatment, the Philadelphia (Ph[1]) marker chromosome remains present in approximately all of the mitoses in the

---

*This investigation was supported by U. S. Public Health Service Research Grant No. CA-03227 from the National Cancer Institute, National Institutes of Health.

bone marrow (Carbone, Whang, Frei, and Tjio, 1964). The evidence is almost conclusive that all of the granulocytic, erythrocytic, and megakaryocytic precursor cells contain the Ph^1 chromosome; it has not been found in other cells. If this is a marker chromosome for a malignant cell, then it appears impossible to eliminate the malignant clone without complete ablation of the bone marrow (Trujillo, 1970, see pages 105 to 122, this volume). Theoretically, of course, it is possible to ablate the bone marrow, and techniques may eventually be available whereby normal bone marrow activity can subsequently be restored by transplantation. In the meantime, the outlook for cure of the disease is very pessimistic.

Despite very good control of the manifestations of disease usually obtained with busulfan, it has not been possible to demonstrate a significant increase in survival of patients with chronic granulocytic leukemia over that observed by Minot in the 1920's in a series of untreated patients (Haut, Abbott, Wintrobe, and Cartwright, 1961). Figure 1 illustrates the data collected by the End Results Evaluation Program of the National Cancer Institute for successive time periods over the past 25 years and represents all hospitals in Connecticut, half of those in California, and eight university hospitals scattered in other parts of the country (Cutler, Axtell, and Heise, 1967).

Why are there such poor survival rates in a disease which appears to be so easy to control?

There are little data as to what actually happens to patients with chronic granulocytic leukemia other than that their median survival is around three and a half years (Shullenberger, 1970, see pages 143 to 148, this volume). A small percentage of patients does not respond to treatment with busulfan initially and pursues a moderately rapid downhill course. Others become resistant. Occasionally, such patients may respond to 6-mercaptopurine (Huguley et al., 1963) or to hydroxyurea (Kennedy and Yarbro, 1966). More commonly, a change takes place in the disease after successful control for a period of several years. It can be demonstrated that some patients develop a steadily increasing degree of marrow failure and some eventually develop myelofibrosis with the resulting cytopenias. Prospective studies of this process are not advanced enough to say how often this happens.

The most common outcome is the development in 60 to 70 per cent of patients of the so-called blastic crisis of chronic granulocytic leukemia, a process indistinguishable from acute myeloblastic leukemia (Haut, Abbott, Wintrobe, and Cartwright, 1961; Shullenberger, 1970, see pages 143 to 148, this volume). Treatment of this acute process is even more disappointing than that for acute myeloblastic leukemia and very few reports cite a complete remission rate of more than 10 per cent.

Thus we see that the disease initially behaves almost as a benign prolifer-

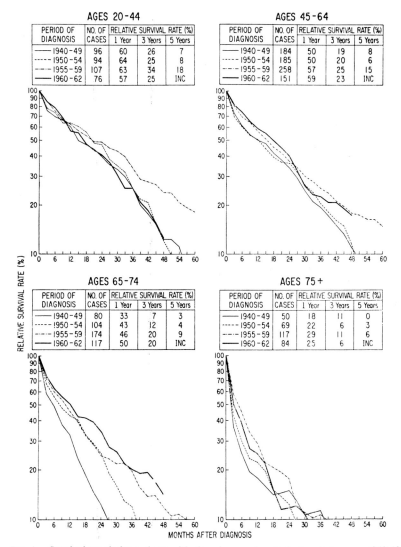

FIG. 1. —Survival trends for patients with chronic granulocytic leukemia by age—1940-1962. (Courtesy of Cutler, Axtell, and Heise, 1967.)

ative disease, the manifestations of which are well controlled in most patients for several years. The therapeutic problem is how to prevent the development of blastic crisis or of marrow failure with or without myelofibrosis or how to manage them if they develop. The deep pessimism of most investigators is reflected by the current scarcity of studies aimed at control of this disease.

Chronic Lymphocytic Leukemia

An aura of pessimism also pervades investigation of chronic lymphocytic leukemia. Because the average survival rate is a number of years and many patients do very well with minimal treatment and because previous attempts at vigorous therapy have not been notably successful, most clinicians use as little treatment as possible and direct their efforts primarily at symptomatic care (Boggs, Sofferman, Wintrobe, and Cartwright, 1966).

However, I believe this pessimism is unjustified. There is considerable new information about chronic lymphocytic leukemia which suggests that we should reorient our thinking about treatment of this disease and address ourselves more vigorously toward attempts at its control.

First, let us discuss the results of current therapy. Data collected in the End Results Evaluation Program show a very definite improvement in survival rates for patients with chronic lymphocytic leukemia ranging from age 20 to 44 and 45 to 64 during the periods 1955 to 1959 and 1960 to 1962 as compared with the preceding periods of 1940 to 1949 and 1950 to 1954 (Cutler, Axtell, and Heise, 1967) (Fig. 2). While this improvement has not been demonstrated in patients first diagnosed past the age of 65, of which there are an appreciable number, it does indicate that modern treatment improves survival rates. A valid point is that this improvement may be the result of better general medical care, the greater availability of blood products, and the advent of antibiotics effective against resistant staphylococci and gram-negative organisms (Boggs, Sofferman, Wintrobe, and Cartwright, 1966). Nevertheless, the improvement also coincides with the introduction of chlorambucil and subsequent chemotherapeutic agents effective in the control of this disease.

There are two attitudes toward treatment of chronic lymphocytic leukemia. Osgood has advocated initiating treatment as soon as the diagnosis is established and continuing it during the patient's lifetime on a regularly spaced, titrated basis (Osgood, Seaman, and Koler, 1956). Others prefer to defer treatment until evidence of active, progressive disease develops and then to treat intermittently (Boggs, Sofferman, Wintrobe, and Cartwright, 1966). There are, unquestionably, many patients with indolent, slowly progressing disease who do well for some years without treatment.

In recent years, the most popular agents have been chlorambucil and radiophosphorus. Prednisone has been used in patients with hemolytic anemia or thrombocytopenia and in those resistant to other therapy.

Figure 3 shows survival curves derived from the data of three reports (Osgood, Seaman, and Koler, 1956; Boggs, Sofferman, Wintrobe, and Cartwright, 1966; Cutler, personal communication). This last curve probably reflects well the survival of the average patient with this disease (Cutler, personal communication). The patients on the End Results Evaluation Pro-

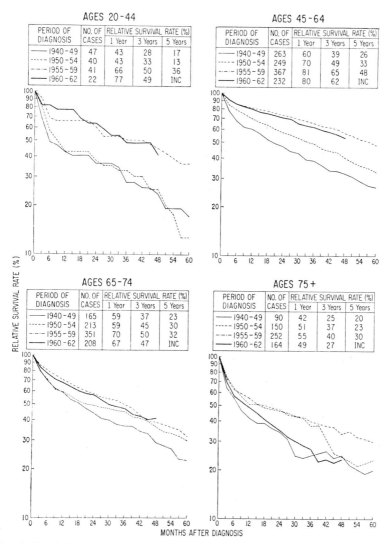

AGES 20-44

PERIOD OF DIAGNOSIS	NO. OF CASES	RELATIVE SURVIVAL RATE (%)		
		1 Year	3 Years	5 Years
——— 1940-49	47	43	28	17
----- 1950-54	40	43	33	13
---·- 1955-59	41	66	50	36
——— 1960-62	22	77	49	INC

AGES 45-64

PERIOD OF DIAGNOSIS	NO. OF CASES	RELATIVE SURVIVAL RATE (%)		
		1 Year	3 Years	5 Years
——— 1940-49	263	60	39	26
----- 1950-54	249	70	49	33
---·- 1955-59	367	81	65	48
——— 1960-62	232	80	62	INC

AGES 65-74

PERIOD OF DIAGNOSIS	NO. OF CASES	RELATIVE SURVIVAL RATE (%)		
		1 Year	3 Years	5 Years
——— 1940-49	165	59	37	23
----- 1950-54	213	59	45	30
---·- 1955-59	351	70	50	32
——— 1960-62	208	67	47	INC

AGES 75+

PERIOD OF DIAGNOSIS	NO. OF CASES	RELATIVE SURVIVAL RATE (%)		
		1 Year	3 Years	5 Years
——— 1940-49	90	42	25	20
----- 1950-54	150	51	37	23
---·- 1955-59	252	55	40	30
——— 1960-62	164	49	27	INC

RELATIVE SURVIVAL RATE (%)

MONTHS AFTER DIAGNOSIS

FIG. 2.—Survival trends for patients with chronic lymphocytic leukemia by age—1940-1962. (Courtesy of Cutler, Axtell, and Heise, 1967.)

gram represent all patients seen in a variety of general hospitals and treated in a variety of ways; all patients were previously untreated. Patients studied at a medical center specifically interested in leukemia might be expected to enjoy the benefits of closer follow-up and greater skill. In the Osgood series, all patients were treated from the time of diagnosis at one institution with regularly spaced, titrated radiophosphorus (Osgood, Seaman, and Koler,

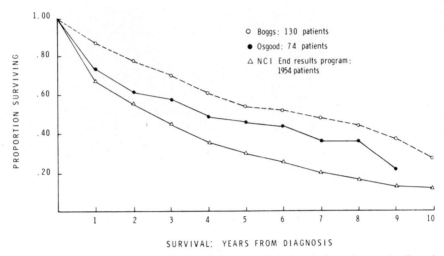

FIG. 3.—Survival of patients with chronic lymphocytic leukemia from three series. Boggs' patients were treated intermittently, usually with alkylating agents (Boggs, Sofferman, Wintrobe, and Cartwright, 1966). Osgood's series has been replotted to include only data on previously untreated patients (Osgood, Seaman, and Koler, 1957). These patients were treated with radiophosphorus in a regularly spaced, titrated dosage. The National Cancer Institute End Results Evaluation Program includes patients diagnosed from 1955 to 1964 and followed to 1968 (Cutler, personal communication). They were given varied treatment.

1956). This analysis is based only on the previously untreated patients from the Osgood series. The total group of patients had a better survival than that shown in Figure 3. The Boggs series also represents patients treated at one institution, but includes patients who previously had been treated elsewhere (Boggs, Sofferman, Wintrobe, and Cartwright, 1966). These patients were nearly all treated with chlorambucil or triethylenemelamine (TEM) administered intermittently. These authors did not believe there was a significant difference between their results and those reported by Osgood. However, the inference is that regularly spaced treatment with radiophosphorus is not necessarily the best form of treatment. The differences in these three survival curves probably reflect more the selection of patients and varying standards of medical care than the specific method of treatment.

In 1957, the Southeastern Cancer Chemotherapy Study Group (SECCSG) (unpublished data) initiated a long-term study of previously untreated patients with chronic lymphocytic leukemia. These patients were randomly assigned to one of three drugs (radiophosphorus, chlorambucil, or TEM) and to one of two regimens (regularly spaced, titrated therapy from the initiation of the study, or an intermittent therapy given only for specific manifestations of disease and continued only so long as necessary to produce a maximum response). Patients were defined as "symptomatic" if

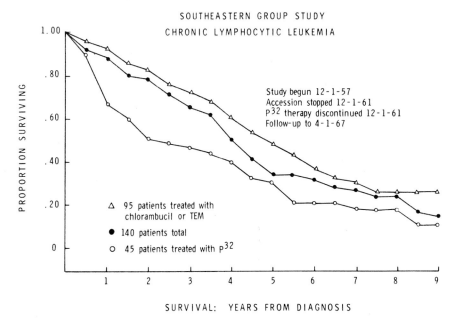

FIG. 4.—Survival of patients with chronic lymphocytic leukemia.

FIG. 5.—Survival of chronic lymphocytic leukemia patients treated on a regularly spaced, titrated dosage continuously from diagnosis.

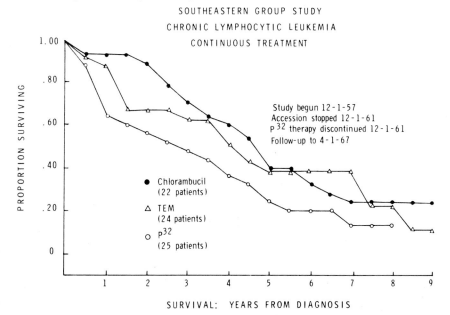

there was anemia, thrombocytopenia, progressive enlargement of nodes, spleen or leukemic infiltrates, painful leukemic infiltrates, otherwise un-explained fever persisting more than 10 days, otherwise unexplained weight loss of more than 10 per cent body weight over six months, or a fall in per-formance status (Karnofsky, 1961) of 20 per cent.

With one exception, the 140 patients entered in this study were followed to death or to early 1967. Patient accession was stopped after four years, at which time radiophosphorus therapy also was stopped because of poor results (Huguley, 1962).

Figure 4 illustrates the survival curve for the entire group and also the better survival of patients receiving an alkylating agent than of those re-ceiving radiophosphorus. These patients were followed in 10 different insti-tutions. The average age at diagnosis was 62 years, four years older than Osgood's (Osgood, Seaman, and Koler, 1956) and three years older than Boggs' (Boggs, Sofferman, Wintrobe, and Cartwright, 1966).

Figure 5 illustrates the survival of those patients treated on a continuous program with chlorambucil, TEM, and radiophosphorus. Figure 6 illus-trates results for those treated with the three drugs on an intermittent program. The difference between the alkylating agent and radiophosphorus groups is significant at three years for both regimens. No patient was con-

FIG. 6.—Survival of chronic lymphocytic leukemia patients treated only intermittently for specific complications of the disease.

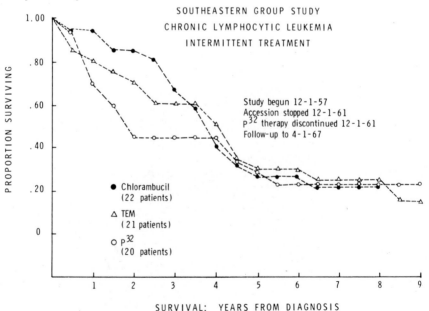

SURVIVAL: YEARS FROM DIAGNOSIS

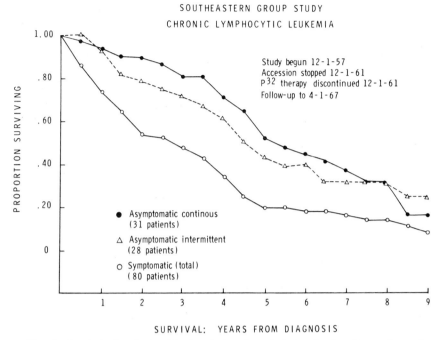

FIG. 7.—Survival of patients with chronic lymphocytic leukemia. Results are shown for continuous and intermittent regimens in asymptomatic patients and for all symptomatic patients.

tinued on radiophosphorus longer than four years since use of that agent was discontinued four years after the initiation of the study.

Figure 7 illustrates that there was a better survival curve for asymptomatic patients who were treated continuously than for asymptomatic patients whose treatment was deferred until morbidity. Upon analysis, the difference is not significant, but it does demonstrate that treatment is not bad for patients with slowly progressing disease. Symptomatic patients usually required almost continuous treatment even on the intermittent schedule and are illustrated separately.

It must be emphasized that although the patients with indolent disease at diagnosis enjoyed a better survival (median 52 months) than did those with active, progressive disease (median 27 months), their survival rate is not good enough to justify complacency. We must find ways to control the disease and treat the patients.

We are interested not only in survival with various treatments, but also in the ability to control the manifestations of the illness. Boggs, Sofferman, Wintrobe, and Cartwright (1966) indicated very poor success in controlling various manifestations of the disease other than leukocytosis by the use of chemotherapeutic agents. They encountered more success with prednisone, albeit short-lived. Similarly, the Southwest Cancer Chemotherapy Study Group (SWCCSG) in a preliminary report of their studies indicated a failure to effect much improvement in the over-all status of the patient by treatment (Sprague, 1962). The experience of the SECCSG has been different. We have defined improvement as being improvement from all manifestations of the disease. We have called the improvement "fair" if there was at least 25 per cent improvement from all manifestations and "good" if there was at least 50 per cent improvement. An "excellent" response indicated a "complete remission" or no evidence of the disease and bone marrow lymphocytosis of less than 30 per cent. By these criteria, we achieved 67 per cent responses of "fair" or better with chlorambucil and most of these responses were achieved within 12 weeks. Responses with TEM were not as good at 12 weeks but did improve to 57 per cent at six months. Responses to radiophosphorus were poorer and even at six months were only 31 per cent.

Patients who failed to achieve a response or who later developed severe thrombocytopenia or hemolytic anemia received prednisone. Following the use of prednisone, an additional 5 per cent of the chlorambucil-treated patients achieved a "fair" or better response, making a total response rate with chloambucil, with or without prednisone, of 72 per cent.

The entire experience of the SECCSG in utilizing chlorambucil therapy alone, which is detailed in Table 1, indicates a response rate of 69 per cent.

We do not know why we have achieved a better short-term response rate than have others. We believe it may be the result of a persistence in the administration of the drug to the point of minimal toxicity for long periods of time.

If we are to make progress in studying this disease, we must devise some way of predicting the long-term response of the patient from the response

TABLE 1.—EFFECTIVENESS OF CHLORAMBUCIL IN
CHRONIC LYMPHOCYTIC LEUKEMIA: SHORT-
TERM STUDIES OF SOUTHEASTERN CANCER
CHEMOTHERAPY STUDY GROUP
FROM 1957 TO 1964

| | PROJECT | | | | |
	I	II	VIII	301	TOTAL*
Response	17	28	6	20	71(69%)
No response	6	14	3	10	33
Total	23	42	9	30	104

*Twelve of these patients have achieved "complete remission."

observed over a short-term (three to six months) period of study. The SECCSG currently is analyzing the data in their series in the hope of finding a correlation between the status of various parameters of the disease at the time of diagnosis and the duration of survival. If this attempt is successful, we shall then attempt to determine whether improvement in any of these parameters during the initial period of therapy can be correlated with improvement in a survival rate over that predicted at diagnosis.

Experience with acute lymphocytic leukemia has indicated that the duration of survival is closely correlated to the attainment of a "complete remission." The question then arises as to whether it is possible to obtain such a remission in patients with chronic lymphocytic leukemia. This question must then be followed by a second question: Do "complete remissions," if obtained, result in prolongation of survival?

If the answers to both of these questions are affirmative, we obviously should consider an intensification of our efforts to achieve more complete control of the manifestations of chronic lymphocytic leukemia.

The literature contains reports of 25 patients who have obtained "complete remissions" (Schott, 1955, 1967; Walter, Szur, and Lewis, 1958; Reich, 1959, personal communication; Hickling, 1960, 1964, personal communication; Durant and Finkbeiner, 1964; Geller, 1964, personal communication; Bousser and Zittoun, 1965; Han, Ezdinli, and Sokal, 1967; Chervenick, Boggs, and Wintrobe, 1967; Johnson, Kagan, Gralnick, and Fass, 1967). To this the writer can add one patient of his own (Huguley, unpublished data). The results of this literature review are tabulated in Figure 8. Of these 26 remissions, the duration was recorded in 22 patients. The shortest duration was five months, the longest 217 months, and the median was 69 months. Ten patients are still in remission. The survival rates for the 22 patients ranged from more than 12 months to more than 300 months with a median of 117 months; 14 patients are still alive. Of the 26 patients having complete remissions, seven had severe disease, 16 had milder, active disease, and only three had indolent disease. Some of these remissions appeared to be spontaneous and often there was no clear relation to therapy. These data mean that "complete remissions" can be obtained and also indicate that when such remissions are obtained, even in severely ill patients, the prognosis is considerably better than is that for the average patient with the illness.

To these published data we can add several more from the studies of the SECCSG (Rundles et al., 1959, 1962; SECCSG, unpublished data). During the past 12 years, a total of 111 patients of the SECCSG have been treated with daily chlorambucil therapy in four successive protocols. Of these patients, 12 (10 per cent) obtained complete remission. The median remission for these patients was 21 months and varied from 12 to 96 months with one patient still in remission. The median survival was 84 months, varying from 39 to more than 132 months, with six patients still surviving.

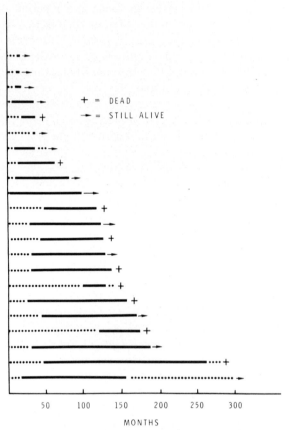

FIG. 8.—Survival of chronic lymphocytic leukemia patients reported to have achieved a "complete remission" (Schott, 1955, 1967; Walter, Szur, and Lewis, 1958; Reich, 1959, personal communication; Hickling, 1960, 1964, personal communication; Durant and Finkbeiner, 1964; Geller, 1964, personal communication; Bousser and Zittoun, 1965; Han, Ezdinli, and Sokal, 1967; Chervenick, Boggs, and Wintrobe, 1967; Johnson, Kagan, Gralnick, and Fass, 1967; Huguley, unpublished data).

For these two groups of patients totaling 38 patients, the median survivals are considerably better than those reported in the literature for all patients. Thus, there seems little question that complete remissions can be obtained and that, if obtained, the remissions usually last many months and result in increased survival. Certainly this evidence should spur us to a more vigorous treatment for chronic lymphocytic leukemia in the hope of increasing the percentage of complete remissions.

Are there other approaches which are possibly more effective?

Johnson has extended his previously reported observations on the value of whole-body irradiation given over a period of a few weeks (Johnson,

Kagan, Gralnick, and Fass, 1967; Johnson, personal communication). Of 17 patients so treated, none of whom had been previously treated and all of whom had active disease, eight obtained a complete remission.

In all of the four patients who were tested, the percentage of lymphocytes transformed by stimulation with phytohemagglutinin returned to normal. This finding suggests the possibility of two populations of cells, an abnormal population which had been drastically reduced by therapy and a normal population which remained. Hersh's data support a similar conclusion (Hersh, 1970, see pages 149 to 167, this volume).

Obviously, whole-body irradiation is a hopeful avenue for continued exploration.

To my knowledge, there has not been a study of intensive combination chemotherapy administered over many months. Presumably such a combination would include chlorambucil and prednisone, which appear to be the most effective chemotherapeutic agents currently available for chronic lymphocytic leukemia. This approach, too, demands study.

One of our current problems is that we do not know exactly what is the best schedule by which effective agents should be used. Knowledge of the cellular kinetics of the disease should influence our plans. Perry and his co-workers have studied the kinetics of lymphocytes in chronic lymphocytic leukemia and believe that their studies are consistent with the hypothesis that the disease reflects an accumulation of long-lived, nondividing lymphocytes (Zimmerman, Godwin, and Perry, 1968). This concept also has been discussed at length by Dameshek (1967).

The treatments known to be most effective for chronic lymphocytic leukemia are those which attack mature lymphocytes and which do not have a greater effect on proliferating cells than on nonproliferating cells. These agents destroy mature lymphocytes without having a greater effect on proliferating granulocytes, red cells, and platelets in the marrow. It is possible that the use of daily treatment may be more toxic to the normal bone marrow cells than some other treatment. It might be better to use intermittent treatment to gradually reduce the burden of slowly proliferating abnormal lymphocytes, permitting the normal cells to recuperate between doses. As Alexanian has pointed out, there is evidence that the intermittent use of phenylalanine mustard in plasma cell myeloma, a disease rather similar to chronic lymphocytic leukemia, may be more effective than the daily administration (Alexanian et al., 1969). The SECCSG has just begun a preliminary dose-seeking study of intermittent treatment with chlorambucil. Responses have been obtained, and the total dosage of the drug is much less when chlorambucil is given in relatively large doses every two weeks than when given daily. We have already observed hematologic recovery from the "packed marrow" syndrome after failure of prolonged daily chlorambucil.

There are other difficult therapeutic problems posed by the patient with chronic lymphocytic leukemia, notably, the poor immune response and the autoimmune phenomena which often develop. Our primary problem is better control of the body burden of abnormal cells. Unless we can solve this problem, there is little hope for much more than a symptomatic approach to the complications. If we can control the tumor cells, there is hope for a return to normal hemopoiesis and immunocompetence.

REFERENCES

Alexanian, R., Haut, A., Khan, A. U., Lane, M., McKelvey, E. M., Migliore, P. J., Stuckey, W. J., Jr., and Wilson, H. E.: Treatment for multiple myeloma. Combination chemotherapy with different melphalan dose regimens. *Journal of the American Medical Association,* 208:1680-1685, June 2, 1969.

Boggs, D. R., Sofferman, S. A., Wintrobe, M. M., and Cartwright, G. E.: Factors influencing the duration of survival of patients with chronic lymphocytic leukemia. *American Journal of Medicine,* 40:243-254, February 1966.

Bousser, J., and Zittoun, R.: Rémission spontanée prolongée d'une leucémie lymphoïde chronique. *Nouvelle Revue Française d'Hematologie,* 5:498-501, March 1965.

Carbone, P. P., Whang, J., Frei, E., III, and Tjio, J. H.: Cytogenetic studies in patients with chronic myelogenous leukemia (CML) undergoing intensive treatment. (Abstract) *Blood, The Journal of Hematology,* 24:833, 1964.

Chervenick, P. A., Boggs, D. R., and Wintrobe, M. M. : Spontaneous remission in chronic lymphocytic leukemia. *Annals of Internal Medicine,* 67:1239-1242, December 1967.

Cutler, S. J.: Personal communication.

Cutler, S. J., Axtell, L., and Heise, H.: Ten thousand cases of leukemia: 1940-62. *Journal of the National Cancer Institute,* 39:993-1026, November 1967.

Dameshek, W.: Chronic lymphocytic leukemia—an accumulative disease of immunologically incompetent lymphocytes. *Blood, The Journal of Hematology,* 29:566-584, April 1967.

Durant, J. R., and Finkbeiner, J. A.: "Spontaneous" remission in chronic lymphatic leukemia? *Cancer,* 17:105-113, January 1964.

Geller, W.: Chronic lymphocytic leukemia with hemolytic anemia. *Archives of Internal Medicine,* 114:444-448, September 1964.

————: Personal communication.

Han, T., Ezdinli, E. Z., and Sokal, J. E.: Complete remission in chronic lymphocytic leukemia and leukolymphosarcoma. *Cancer,* 20-243-253, February 1967.

Haut, A., Abbott, W. S., Wintrobe, M. M., and Cartwright, G. E.: Busulfan in the treatment of chronic myelocytic leukemia. The effect of long term intermittent therapy. *Blood, The Journal of Hematology,* 17:1-19, January 1961.

Hersh, E. M., Curtis, J. C., Harris, J. E., McBride, C., Alexanian, R., and Rossen, R.: Host defense mechanisms in lymphomas and leukemia. In *Leukemia-Lymphoma,* A Collection of Papers Presented at the 14th Annual Clinical Conference on Cancer, 1969, at The University of Texas M. D. Anderson Hospital and Tumor Institute at Houston. Chicago, Illinois, Year Book Medical Publishers, Inc., 1970, pp. 149-167.

Hickling, R. A.: Giant follicle lymphoma of the spleen: Recovery after splenectomy. *British Medical Journal,* 1:1464-1467, May 14, 1960.

————: "Giant follicle lymphoma of the spleen." A condition closely related to lymphatic leukaemia but apparently curable by splenectomy. *British Medical Journal,* 2:787-790, September 26, 1964.

————: Personal communication.

Huguley, C. M.: Long-term study of chronic lymphocytic leukemia: Interim report after 45 months. *Cancer Chemotherapy Reports,* 16:241-244, February 1962.

————: Unpublished data.

Huguley, C. M., Grizzle, J., Rundles, R. W., Bell, W. N., Corley, C. C., Jr., Frommeyer, W. B., Jr., Greenberg, B. G., Hammack, W., Herion, J. C., James, G. W., III, Larsen, W. E., Loeb, V., Leone, L. A., Palmer, J. G., and Wilson, S. J.: Comparison of 6-mercaptopurine and busulfan in chronic granulocytic leukemia. *Blood, The Journal of Hematology,* 21:89-101, January 1963.

Johnson, R.: Personal communication.

Johnson, R. E., Kagan, A. R., Gralnick, H. R., and Fass, L.: Radiation-induced remissions in chronic lymphocytic leukemia. *Cancer,* 20:1382-1387, September 1967.

Karnofsky, D. A.: Meaningful clinical classification of therapeutic responses to anticancer drugs. (Editorial) *Clinical Pharmacology and Therapeutics,* 2:709-712, November-December 1961.

Kennedy, B. J., and Yarbro, J. W.: Metabolic and therapeutic effects of hydroxyurea in chronic myeloid leukemia. *Journal of the American Medical Association,* 195:1038-1043, March 21, 1966.

Osgood, E. E., Seaman, A. J., and Koler, R. D.: Natural history and course of the leukemias. In *Proceedings of the Third National Cancer Conference,* Detroit, Michigan, 1956. Philadelphia, Pennsylvania, and Montreal, Canada, J. B. Lippincott Co., 1957, pp. 366-382.

Reich, C.: Apparent recovery in chronic lymphocytic leukemia. Report of a case with five-year remission and no clinical or hematological evidence of the disease. *Journal of the American Medical Association,* 170:169-171, May 2, 1959.

_____: Personal communication.

Rundles, R. W., Grizzle, J., Bell, W. N., Corley, C. C., Frommeyer, W. B., Jr., Greenberg, B. G., Huguley, C. M., Jr., James, G. W., III, Jones, R., Jr., Larsen, W. E., Loeb, V., Leone, L. A., Palmer, J. G., Riser, W. H., Jr., and Wilson, S. J.: Comparison of chlorambucil and Myleran in chronic lymphocytic and granulocytic leukemia. *American Journal of Medicine,* 27:424-432, September 1959.

Rundles, W., Grizzle, J., Bono, V. H., Jonsson, U., Huguley, C. M., Jr., and Corley, C. C., Jr.: Comparison of CB-1348 (chlorambucil, Leukeran) and CB-1364. *Cancer Chemotherapy Reports,* 16:223-230, February 1962.

Schott, M.: Ten-year recovery from chronic lymphocytic leukaemia. *British Medical Journal,* 1:877-879, April 9, 1955.

_____: Ten-year recovery from chronic lymphocytic leukaemia—twelve years later. (Letter to the editor) *British Medical Journal,* 3:433-434, August 12, 1967.

Shullenberger, C. C.: Natural history patterns in leukemia and lymphoma as related to clinico-pathologic classification. In *Leukemia-Lymphoma,* A Collection of Papers Presented at the 14th Annual Clinical Conference on Cancer, 1969, at The University of Texas M. D. Anderson Hospital and Tumor Institute at Houston. Chicago, Illinois, Year Book Medical Publishers, Inc., 1970, pp. 143-148.

Silver, R. T.: Dibromomannitol, a new agent for treating chronic granulocytic leukemia: Its effect compared with busulfan. (Abstract) *Abstracts of the Simultaneous Sessions. XII Congress International Society of Hematology,* 1968, p.13.

Southeastern Cancer Chemotherapy Study Group: Unpublished data.

Sprague, C. C.: Evaluation of the effectiveness of radioactive phosphorus and chlorambucil in patients with chronic lymphocytic leukemia. *Cancer Chemotherapy Reports,* 16:235-240, February 1962.

Trujillo, J. M., Fernandez, M. N., Shullenberger, C. C., Rodriguez, L. H., and Cork, A.: Cytogenetic contribution to the study of human leukemias. In *Leukemia-Lymphoma,* A Collection of Papers Presented at the 14th Annual Clinical Conference on Cancer, 1969, at The University of Texas M. D. Anderson Hospital and Tumor Institute at Houston. Chicago, Illinois, Year Book Medical Publishers, Inc., 1970, pp. 105-122.

Walter, L. H., Szur, L., and Lewis, S. M.: Prolonged remission in chronic lymphatic leukaemia. *British Medical Journal,* 1:859-862, April 12, 1958.

Zimmerman, T. S., Godwin, H. A., and Perry, S.: Studies of leukocyte kinetics in chronic lymphocytic leukemia. *Blood, The Journal of Hematology,* 31:277-291, March 1968.

The Treatment for Acute Leukemia in Adults*

GERALD P. BODEY, M.D.,†
VICTORIO RODRIGUEZ, M.D.,
JOHN P. WHITECAR, JR., M.D.,
JACQUELINE HART, M.D., AND
EMIL J FREIREICH, M.D.

*Department of Developmental Therapeutics, The University of Texas M. D. Anderson
Hospital and Tumor Institute at Houston, Houston, Texas*

THE TREATMENT OF CHILDREN with acute lymphocytic leukemia (ALL) has improved substantially in recent years. Similar progress has not been made in the treatment of adults with acute leukemia until recently. The majority of adults with this disease have acute myelogenous leukemia (AML), which has been much less responsive to therapy. Vincristine and prednisone, which are the most active agents against ALL, are only minimally effective in adults with AML. Single-agent therapy with methotrexate or 6-mercaptopurine seldom has induced remission in more than 20 per cent of adults (Acute Leukemia Group B, 1961; Vogler, Huguley, and Rundles, 1967).

A major advance in the treatment of children with acute leukemia was the introduction of combination chemotherapy with vincristine, prednisone, 6-mercaptopurine, and methotrexate (Karon, Freireich, and Carbone, 1965). This combination has been very effective in adults with AML who are under 35 years of age, but it has not been very useful in older patients.

Methylglyoxal bis(guanylhydrazone) was the first antileukemic agent which had greater activity in patients with AML than in patients with ALL.

*Supported in part by Grants No. CA 05831 and No. CA 10376 from the National Cancer Institute, National Institutes of Health, United States Public Health Service, Bethesda, Maryland.

†Dr. Bodey is a Scholar of The Leukemia Society of America, Inc.

This drug was capable of inducing remission in about 30 per cent of adults with AML (Freireich, Frei, and Karon, 1962). However, its extensive toxicity eliminated it as a useful agent for the management of this disease.

A major advance in the therapy of adults with acute leukemia occurred with the introduction of arabinosyl cytosine (Ara-C). This drug is a synthetic pyrimidine nucleoside which inhibits deoxyribonucleic acid (DNA) synthesis. It is active in several animal tumor systems, including murine leukemia L1210 (Evans, Musser, Bostwick, and Mengel, 1964; Wodinsky and Kensler, 1968).

At The University of Texas M. D. Anderson Hospital and Tumor Institute at Houston, studies of this agent in adults with acute leukemia were initiated in 1966. Eight patients with AML received single rapid intravenous injections of Ara-C daily in courses administered at two-week intervals. The duration of each course of therapy was gradually increased from three to five days, and the dosage was increased from 150 mg./m²/day to 450 mg./m²/day. Five of the eight patients received an adequate trial of Ara-C therapy. Only one patient achieved a complete remission, which lasted eight and one-half months.

Shortly thereafter, studies became available which indicated that the schedule of administration of Ara-C had a major influence on its therapeutic efficacy. In a tissue-culture system, the number of tumor cells destroyed was more dependent upon the duration of exposure to Ara-C than upon the dosage (Skipper, Schabel, and Wilcox, 1967). The dose of Ara-C required to destroy leukemic cells, as measured by spleen colony-forming units, was over 30-fold greater when the drug was administered by a single daily dose compared to multiple doses (Wodinsky, Swiniarski, and Kensler, 1967). Mice with leukemia L1210 could not be cured with single-dose therapy regardless of the amount of Ara-C administered. A majority of animals with early disease were cured when the drug was administered every three hours for 24 hours twice weekly (Skipper, Schabel, and Wilcox, 1967).

Subsequent studies in patients with metastatic cancer have demonstrated that the myelosuppressive effect of Ara-C is schedule dependent (Fig. 1) (Frei *et al.*, 1969). No myelosuppression was observed when a single intravenous injection of drug was administered, regardless of the dose. When the drug was administered as a 24-hour infusion, myelosuppression appeared at a dose of 600 mg./m². There was increasing myelosuppression with increasing doses up to 1,500 mg./m². There was no further increase in myelosuppression above this dosage. By using continuous intravenous infusions of 48- and 96-hour duration, myelosuppression began to be observed at a total dose of 450 mg./m² and increased progressively with increasing dosage.

After the unimpressive initial results with Ara-C in adults with leukemia, the schedule was changed to five-day continuous intravenous infusion ad-

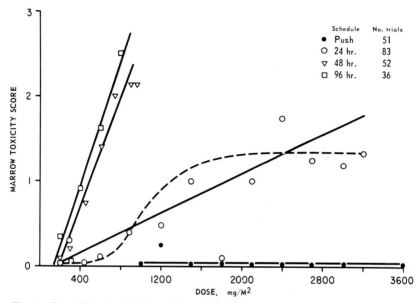

FIG. 1.—The effect of schedule and dose of Ara-C on marrow toxicity. Details regarding evaluation of marrow toxicity are reported elsewhere (Frei *et al.*, 1969).

FIG. 2.—Effect of Ara-C given by rapid intravenous injection and continuous infusion in a patient with AML. The patient failed to respond to rapid injection therapy, but achieved a partial remission after continuous infusion therapy.

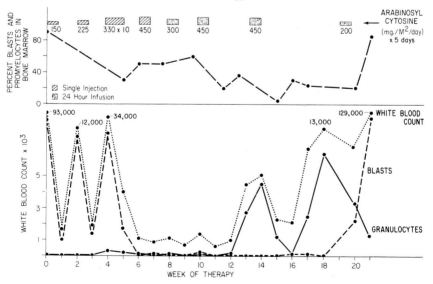

ministered at two-week intervals. The usual initial dose of Ara-C was 200 mg./m^2/day. A median of three courses of therapy was required to achieve remission. The dosage of subsequent courses was altered for some patients, based on their responses to the first course. The dosage was reduced by 25 to 35 per cent for patients whose marrow became very hypocellular with a major reduction in abnormal cells. The dosage remained the same for patients who demonstrated substantial improvement in the bone marrow without severe myelosuppression. The dosage was increased for those patients whose marrow showed no improvement. Patients who achieved remission received the same regimen, at the same or a lower dose, as maintenance therapy.

Patients were considered to be evaluable if they survived for at least two weeks after initiation of therapy. Most patients who died this early died of complications which were present before chemotherapy was initiated; none of these patients survived long enough to receive significant benefit from therapy. Patients were considered to have had an adequate trial if they received two courses of chemotherapy and survived at least four weeks. Complete remission was defined as less than 5 per cent blasts in the bone marrow with normal peripheral blood. Improvement was defined as return of the peripheral blood to normal without marrow improvement or with marrow improvement short of a complete remission.

The response of the first patient to receive Ara-C by continuous infusion is shown in Figure 2. This 18-year-old male with AML was treated while in a Life Island unit. His leukocyte count fell abruptly after the first two courses of Ara-C which were administered by rapid intravenous injection, but large numbers of abnormal cells reappeared promptly in the peripheral blood. He then received a 10-day course of Ara-C at a daily dose of 330 mg./m^2 and, subsequently, a five-day course at a daily dose of 450 mg./m^2, both administered by rapid intravenous injection. Abnormal cells disappeared from his peripheral blood, but his bone marrow failed to improve. After receiving three courses of Ara-C by continuous intravenous infusion, he achieved a partial remission which lasted one and one-fourth months.

Of the total of 16 patients entered in the Ara-C study, 13 received adequate trials (Table 1). Five patients achieved complete remission and four showed improvement.

Further studies of the effects of Ara-C on murine leukemia indicated that this drug prolonged life but did not cure animals with far-advanced disease (Schabel, 1968). However, the combination of Ara-C with nitrosourea or cyclophosphamide was synergistic and produced a high cure rate, even in animals with advanced disease. Biochemical evidence also supported this approach to therapy. Alkylating agents are active against preformed DNA, and Ara-C inhibits DNA synthesis, constituting a form of "complementary inhibition" (Sartorelli, 1965). Furthermore, the combination of a cycle-

TABLE 1.—RESULTS OF CHEMOTHERAPY IN ADULTS WITH
ACUTE LEUKEMIA

STATUS	No. PATIENTS RECEIVING		
	Ara-C	Ara-C + Ctx	COAP
Entered	16	40	33
Adequate trial	13	34	25
Complete remission	5	16	14
Improvement	4	5	6
Failure	4	13	5

sensitive agent (Ara-C) and a cycle-insensitive agent (alkylating agent) might be expected to have additive or synergistic effects (Bruce, Meeker, and Valeriote, 1966).

Studies on Ara-C in combination with cyclophophamide (Cytoxan [Ctx]) were undertaken (Bodey, Rodriguez, Hart, and Freireich, in preparation). Ctx was chosen because it is capable of inducing remissions in patients with acute leukemia when used alone (Fernbach, Sutow, Thurman, and Vietti, 1962). Both drugs were administered separately by rapid intravenous injection in four-day courses at two-week intervals. The usual initial daily dose of each drug was 150 mg./m^2 given in divided doses every eight hours. Dosage modifications were made as for Ara-C alone, but the same ratio of Ara-C to Ctx was maintained.

Of 40 patients entered in the study of Ara-C plus Ctx, 34 received adequate trials (Table 1). Sixteen patients achieved complete remission and five showed improvement.

After experience was gained with the combination of Ara-C and Ctx, vincristine (Oncovin) and prednisone were added to the regimen (this four-drug combination program is known as the COAP regimen). The latter two drugs are minimally effective as single agents in adults with AML. However, the experience with prednisone, Oncovin, methotrexate, and 6-mercaptopurine (Purinethol) (the POMP therapeutic regimen) indicated that these agents were synergistic with methotrexate and 6-mercaptopurine. Since Ara-C and Ctx were effective in the treatment of patients with AML, they were substituted for methotrexate and 6-mercaptopurine.

In the COAP regimen, the initial dose of Ara-C and Ctx was 120

TABLE 2.—RESPONSE OF ADULTS TO ANTILEUKEMIC THERAPY

STATUS	% OF PATIENTS RECEIVING		
	Ara-C	Ara-C + Ctx	COAP
Adequate trial/evaluable	87	94	86
Response/entered	56	53	61
Response/adequate trial	69	62	80
Complete remission/entered	31	40	42
Complete remission/adequate trial	38	47	56

TABLE 3.—SURVIVAL OF ADULTS RECEIVING ANTILEUKEMIC THERAPY

STATUS		ARA-C	ARA-C + CTX	COAP
Survival (months)	Median	3	7	5+
	Range	½-24	¼-22	¼-12½+
Duration of complete remission (months)	Median	10	5½	5+
	Range	2-21	1-16	1½-11+
Patients currently in complete remission		0	2	11
Patients currently living		0	2	14

mg./m²/day and was administered as in the Ara-C plus Ctx study. Vincristine was administered intravenously at a dose of 2 mg. on day 1 of each course. Prednisone was administered orally at a dose of 50 mg. four times daily for the four days of each course.

To date, 33 patients have been entered in the COAP study, and 25 have received adequate trials (Table 1). Fourteen patients achieved complete remission and six showed improvement.

Table 2 compares the results of the three therapeutic regimens. Over 85 per cent of the evaluable patients in each study received an adequate trial of chemotherapy; this indicates the minimal toxicity of the drugs and the benefits of improved supportive care. The response rate for all patients entered in study was highest for the COAP regimen. The addition of Ctx to Ara-C did not substantially improve the therapeutic results. However, these two studies are not strictly comparable since the schedule of administration of Ara-C was different. The superior results with COAP over the other two regimens are best exemplified by comparing the complete remission rates of patients receiving an adequate trial of chemotherapy. With each succeeding regimen, the complete remission rate improved by 9 per cent.

Survival data for the three regimens are shown in Table 3. The median survival for all patients entered in the study was least for Ara-C alone. The majority of patients who received COAP are still alive with their disease in remission; hence these data are not complete. The duration of complete remission was considerably longer for patients who received Ara-C alone than for patients who received Ara-C plus Ctx.

The major toxic effect caused by all three therapeutic regimens was myelosuppression. Table 4 indicates the amount of leukopenia observed in patients given Ara-C plus Ctx. The median lowest leukocyte count was usually below 1,500/mm³. Subsequent courses at the same drug dosage usually produced increased leukopenia. Substantial thrombocytopenia also was observed when this combination was used (Table 5). The median low-

TABLE 4.—LEUKOPENIA ASSOCIATED WITH
THE ADMINISTRATION OF ARA-C AND CTX

DOSAGE OF EACH DRUG (MG./M^2)	COURSE	NO. OF COURSES	NO FALL	LOWEST WBC COUNT × 10^3
50-75	Initial	10	0	2.0 (1.3-3.6)
	Subsequent	20	5	1.4 (0.2-3.7)
100-125	Initial	14	0	1.4 (0.5-3.9)
	Subsequent	16	1	1.3 (0.2-2.2)
150-175	Initial	11	0	2.0 (0.4-19.1)
	Subsequent	31	2	0.5 (0.1-3.3)
200-225	Subsequent	17	1	0.6 (0.1-2.6)

est platelet count was usually less than 30,000/mm^3. Similar myelosuppression was observed in patients given Ara-C alone and COAP. Substantial myelosuppression was necessary to achieve satisfactory therapeutic results.

An interesting phenomenon was observed in one patient given Ara-C therapy (Fig. 3). After she achieved complete remission, platelet rebound occurred following each course of remission maintenance therapy. Her platelet count fell after Ara-C infusions and then rose to over 1 million/mm^3. This phenomenon has been observed in other patients and has

TABLE 5.—THROMBOCYTOPENIA ASSOCIATED WITH
THE ADMINISTRATION OF ARA-C AND CTX

DOSAGE OF EACH DRUG (MG./M^2)	COURSE	NO. OF COURSES	NO FALL	LOWEST PLATELET COUNT × 10^3
50-75	Initial	7	1	21 (10-96)
	Subsequent	17	5	40 (9-138)
100-125	Initial	12	0	22 (5-94)
	Subsequent	12	1	24 (4-91)
150-175	Initial	8	1	14 (7-165)
	Subsequent	20	2	14 (2-102)
200-225	Subsequent	12	2	29 (10-42)

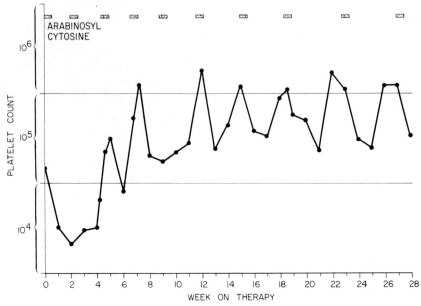

FIG. 3.—Platelet rebound following remission maintenance therapy with continuous infusions of Ara-C in a patient with AML.

resulted in thromboembolic complications (Frei *et al.*, 1969; Bodey, Freireich, Monto, and Hewlett, 1969).

Nausea and vomiting occurred in most patients during the infusion of Ara-C alone. Recovery was rapid upon cessation of therapy. The incidence of this toxic effect was greatly reduced in patients receiving combination chemotherapy.

Hepatotoxicity was observed following therapy with Ara-C plus Ctx (Table 6). The serum transaminase levels rose following 22 per cent of the therapeutic courses in patients in whom these levels were normal initially. However, no patient developed progressive hepatotoxicity that was clearly caused by the antileukemic therapy. Hemorrhagic cystitis caused by Ctx developed in four patients. The only additional toxic effects from COAP therapy were the expected side effects from vincristine and prednisone.

As effective chemotherapy for adult acute leukemia has become available, it has become possible to define those factors which are of major prognostic significance. As might be expected, the duration of survival is related to the therapeutic response (Fig. 4). The median survival time after initiation of therapy for patients who failed to respond to an adequate trial of one of the three therapeutic regimens was less than two months. None of these patients survived more than seven months. The median survival time

TABLE 6.—HEPATOTOXICITY ASSOCIATED WITH
THE ADMINISTRATION OF ARA-C AND CTX

| DOSAGE OF EACH DRUG | | DURING THERAPY | | |
(MG/M²)	TOTAL	Unchanged	Increased	Median
50-75	22	14	8	SGOT 85 (62-202) SGPT 104 (52-292)
100-125	17	11	6	SGOT 60, 99 SGPT 82 (57-138)
150-175	27	25	2	SGOT 135, 87 SGPT 245, 63
200-225	12	11	1	SGPT 61
250-300	3	2	1	SGOT 67 SGPT 108
Total	81	63	18	SGOT 86 (60-202) SGPT 82 (52-292)

Abbreviations: SGOT, serum glutamic oxalopyruvic transaminase; SGPT, serum glutamic pyruvic transaminase.

for patients who achieved a complete remission was 12 months, and over 20 per cent survived 18 months. Patients who improved short of complete remission had an intermediate survival rate.

The age of patients at diagnosis had a major effect on their survival (Fig. 5). The median survival time of patients over 65 years of age was approxi-

FIG. 4.—Survival of adults with acute leukemia related to therapeutic response. Patients who received continuous infusion Ara-C therapy, Ara-C plus Ctx, and COAP are included. Survival is dated from beginning of therapy. Patients who had inadequate trials are excluded from this analysis. Numbers in parentheses refer to number of patients in each group.

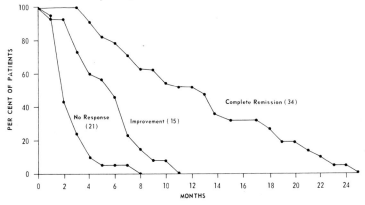

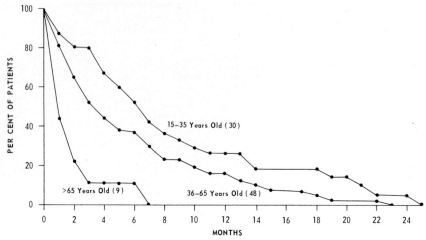

FIG. 5.—Survival of adults with acute leukemia related to age.

mately one month, compared to three months for patients 36 to 65 years old and over six months for patients 15 to 35 years old. The differences in survival time are the result of differences in therapeutic response. Only 22 per cent of the nine patients over 65 years old responded to therapy, compared to 51 per cent of the 49 patients 36 to 65 years old and 76 per cent of the 29 patients 15 to 35 years old.

The morphological type of acute leukemia also influenced the duration of survival (Fig. 6). The median survival time of patients with AML was three months, compared to five months for patients with ALL. More pa-

FIG. 6.—Survival of adults with acute leukemia related to morphological diagnosis.

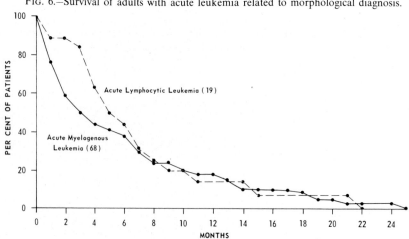

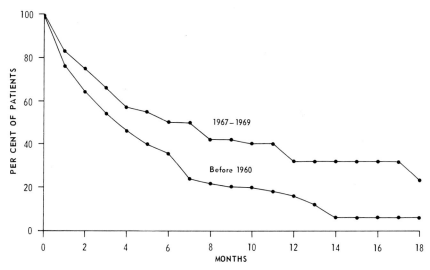

FIG. 7.–Improvement in survival of adults with AML in recent years. All adults with AML admitted to this institution from September 1967 to June 1969 are included. The data before 1960 were obtained from a previous report (Freireich, 1962).

tients with AML died during the first three months, but thereafter, the survival rate was nearly identical for the two groups.

The higher survival rate for patients with ALL was the result of the higher remission rate and younger age of these patients. The complete remission rate was 65 per cent for the 17 patients with ALL who received an adequate trial, compared to 43 per cent for the 53 patients with AML. However, 63 per cent of the patients with ALL were 15 to 35 years old, and none was over 65 years old. In comparing only patients 15 to 35 years old, the complete remission rate was 73 per cent for the 11 patients with ALL who received an adequate trial, compared to 77 per cent for the 13 patients with AML. This suggests that age is the most important factor in determining response to these three chemotherapeutic regimens.

Major progress has been made in the treatment of adults with acute leukemia in recent years (Fig. 7). The median survival time of patients with AML has increased from three and one-half months in the 1950's to seven months in the last two years (Freireich, 1962). Over 20 per cent of patients now survive more than 18 months, compared to less than 10 per cent 10 years ago. A major factor in this improved survival has been the introduction of Ara-C. Other factors include the availability of protected environment units, transfusion of blood products, and new, more effective antibiotics.

The present studies indicate that Ara-C, both alone and in combination with other agents, is an effective agent in the treatment of adults with acute leukemia. However, the optimum method of administering this agent has not been determined. Further studies are needed to demonstrate whether the addition of other agents will enhance the activity of Ara-C significantly. A random study of COAP versus Ara-C given by rapid intravenous injection every eight hours is currently in progress under the auspices of the Southwest Cancer Chemotherapy Study Group and should answer some of these questions.

REFERENCES

Acute Leukemia Group B (Frei, E., III, Freireich, E. J, Gehan, E., Pinkel, D., Holland, J. F., Selawry, O., Haurani, F., Spurr, C. L., Haynes, D. M., James, G. W., Rothburg, H., Sodee, D. B., Rundles, R. W., Schroeder, L. R., Hoogstraten, B., Wolman, I. J., Traggis, D. G., Cooper, T., Gendel, B. R., Ebaugh, F., and Taylor, R.): Studies of sequential and combination antimetabolite therapy in acute leukemia: 6-Mercaptopurine and methotrexate. *Blood, The Journal of Hematology,* 18:431-454, October 1961.

Bodey, G. P., Freireich, E. J, Monto, R. W., and Hewlett, J. T. (Writing Committee): Cytosine arabinoside (NSC-63878) therapy for acute leukemia in adults. *Cancer Chemotherapy Reports,* 53:59-66, February 1969.

Bodey, G. P., Rodriguez, V., Hart, J., and Freireich, E. J: Therapy of acute leukemia with the combination of arabinosyl cytosine and cyclophosphamide. (In preparation.)

Bruce, W. R., Meeker, B. E., and Valeriote, F. A.: Comparison of the sensitivity of normal hematopoietic and transplanted lymphoma colony-forming cells to chemotherapeutic agents administered in vivo. *Journal of the National Cancer Institute,* 37:233-245, August 1966.

Evans, J. S., Musser, E. A., Bostwick, L., and Mengel, G. D.: The effect of 1-β-D-arabino-furanosylcytosine hydrochloride on murine neoplasms. *Cancer Research,* 24:1285-1293, August 1964.

Fernbach, D. J., Sutow, W. W., Thurman, W. G., and Vietti, T. J.: Clinical evaluation of cyclophosphamide: A new agent for the treatment of children with acute leukemia. *Journal of the American Medical Association,* 182:30-37, October 6, 1962.

Frei, E., III, Bickers, J. N., Hewlett, J. S., Lane, M., Leary, W. V., and Talley, R. W. (Writing Committee): Dose schedule and antitumor studies of arabinosyl cytosine (NSC 63878). *Cancer Research,* 29:1325-1332, July 1969.

Freireich, E. J: Factors influencing patient selection for chemotherapy studies of acute leukemia. *Journal of Chronic Diseases,* 15:251-257, March 1962.

Freireich, E. J, Frei, E., III, and Karon, M.: Methylgyoxal bis (guanylhydrazone): A new agent active against acute myelocytic leukemia. *Cancer Chemotherapy Reports,* 16:183-186, February 1962.

Karon, M., Freireich, E. J, and Carbone, P. P.: Effective combination therapy of adult acute leukemia. (Abstract) *Proceedings of the American Association for Cancer Research,* 6:34, March 1965.

Sartorelli, A. C.: Approaches to the combination chemotherapy of transplantable neoplasms. *Progress in Experimental Tumor Research,* 6:228-288, 1965.

Schabel, F. M., Jr.: In vivo leukemic cell kill kinetics and "curability" in experimental systems. In *The Proliferation and Spread of Neoplastic Cells,* A Collection of Papers Presented at the 21st Annual Symposium on Fundamental Cancer Research, 1967, at The University of Texas M. D. Anderson Hospital and Tumor Institute at Houston. Baltimore, Maryland, The Williams and Wilkins Company, 1968, pp. 379-408.

Skipper, H. E., Schabel, F. M., Jr., and Wilcox, W. S.: Experimental evaluation of potential anticancer agents. XXI. Scheduling of arabinosylcytosine to take advantage of its S-phase specificity against leukemia cells. *Cancer Chemotherapy Reports,* 51:125-165, June 1967.

Vogler, W. R., Huguley, C. M., Jr., and Rundles, R. W.: Comparison of methotrexate with 6-mercaptopurine-prednisone in treatment of acute leukemia in adults. *Cancer,* 20:1221-1226, August 1967.

Wodinsky, I., and Kensler, C. J.: Activity of cytosine arabinoside (NSC-63878) in a spectrum of rodent tumors. *Cancer Chemotherapy Reports,* 47:65-68, August 1968.

Wodinsky, I., Swiniarski, J., and Kensler, C. J.: Spleen colony studies of leukemia L1210. II. Differential sensitivities of normal and leukemic bone marrow colony-forming cells to single and divided dose therapy with cytosine arabinoside (NSC-63878). *Cancer Chemotherapy Reports,* 51:423-429, December 1967.

Treatment for Acute Leukemia in Children*

J. R. WILBUR, M.D.,

W. W. SUTOW, M.D.,

M. P. SULLIVAN, M.D., AND

D. M. MUMFORD, M.D.,

Department of Pediatrics, The University of Texas M. D. Anderson Hospital and Tumor Institute at Houston, Houston, Texas

ELSEWHERE IN THIS MONOGRAPH, you have read about increasing success in the treatment of children with leukemia. This article reviews some of the new developments that contribute to an improving prognosis for children with acute leukemia. Advances in the progress of therapy for cancer include changes in drug therapy and immunotherapy, and improved techniques of supportive care.

Some of the most significant progress in the therapy for cancer has been made in the treatment of children with leukemia. Progress has not come from the discovery of a single "miracle drug," but rather from the tedious and careful study of many drugs by many investigators. The objectives of these studies have been to find agents that are effective against leukemic cells and that can be given with minimal toxicity. Pharmacologic sorting has been followed by the slow and gradual development of optimum techniques to utilize these drugs most effectively. An important adjunct to this progress has been the development of improvements in supportive care for the child with leukemia. The various clinical manifestations of the disease and the side effects of the new chemotherapy have required additional advances in supportive care.

*This investigation was supported in part by Public Health Service Grant No. CA-3713, Public Health Service Research Career Award Grant No. CA-2501 from the National Cancer Institute, and by the Clinical Center Grant No. CA-5831.

Evaluation of Therapy for Leukemia

Before discussing some of the new developments that contribute to an improving prognosis in acute leukemia, three aspects of their evaluation should be considered. First, the goals of therapy must be defined before evaluating therapeutic success. These goals may differ as each case progresses. Certainly, the primary objective should be to achieve prolonged disease-free survival and, hopefully, cure for the patient with leukemia. Secondary goals are utilized to evaluate the success of a single treatment program. These short-range steps are necessary to achieve our ultimate aim—eradication of all disease and prevention of recurrence. Remission of bone marrow disease is the first step, and is used as an initial evaluation of therapeutic success.

The next step is to achieve a full clinical remission that can be defined and measured. In this instance, the major problem is one of determining the extent to which the leukemic cell population has been reduced. At the present time, there are no methods available which are sensitive enough to measure this parameter or that can discriminate between long-term remission and "cure." Consequently a period of years is required before a definitive evaluation of a particular therapeutic program can be determined. As we achieve longer remissions, it takes a longer period of time to determine whether we have truly accomplished our ultimate goal of total eradication of neoplastic disease and prevention of recurrence.

VARIABLES IN THE EVALUATION OF THERAPEUTIC SUCCESS

A second and more complex aspect of the evaluation of therapeutic success involves the quantitative interpretation of the many variables inherent in any clinical trial during a particular course of treatment. One must consider numerous significant variables when evaluating even a single drug: the patient's age, histologic type of leukemia, stage of the disease at which the drug is being tested, previous therapy, length of time since the onset of disease, the extent of the disease, and the side effects that have been caused by the disease or previous therapy. One must also ascertain the most effective dose, schedule, and route of administration in the evaluation of a particular drug. Evaluation becomes even more complex when combinations of drugs are used.

A third important group of factors must be included when evaluating the relative success of a particular mode of therapy. This is an assessment of the side effects of that therapy. The price that the patient must pay in terms of painful procedures, length of hospitalization, and life-threatening side effects must be weighed against the long-term success achieved by that therapy.

Because of these inherent requirements, it has been possible to statistically screen only a limited number of combinations of drugs, doses, and schedules.

Current Chemotherapy for Childhood Leukemia

With these thoughts in mind, some aspects of current chemotherapy for acute lymphoblastic leukemia in children will be reviewed. Table 1 summarizes the drugs that are currently available and generally are considered useful, either singly or in combination. Some of these drugs, such as prednisone and vincristine, have been more effective in inducing remission. Once remission has been achieved, other drugs such as 6-mercaptopurine and methotrexate have been particularly effective in maintaining remission.

DRUG COMBINATIONS

Increased success in achieving remission has been accomplished with the use of combinations of drugs. Various investigators have reported bone marrow remission in approximately 90 per cent or more of patients receiving dual drug combinations such as prednisone and vincristine (George *et al.*, 1968), prednisone and 6-mercaptopurine (Saunders, Kauder, and Mauer, 1967), prednisone and methotrexate (Brubaker *et al.*, 1968), and multiple drug combinations such as prednisone, vincristine, and daunomycin (Mathé *et al.*, 1967; Bernard, Boiron, Jacquillat, and Weil, 1968), and the VAMP (vincristine, amethopterin, 6-mercaptopurine, and prednisone) (Freireich, Karon, and Frei, 1964) and POMP (prednisone, Oncovin, methotrexate, and Purinethol) (Henderson, 1967) schedules.

Another significant development has been the demonstration that the combined use of prednisone and vincristine can successfully reinduce remission for two, three, and even four or more times in some patients (Lane *et al.*, in press).

DEVELOPMENT OF NEW DRUGS

Other drugs which are currently being investigated are not included in Table 1. Two of the most recent additions, cytosine arabinoside and L-asparaginase, will be discussed. Each can be used to illustrate a problem in initially evaluating the effectiveness of a drug, its optimum dose and schedule, and toxicity.

CYTOSINE ARABINOSIDE.—Cytosine arabinoside, which has been discussed elsewhere in this book (Bodey *et al.*, 1970, see pages 333 to 345, this volume), has been particularly effective in the treatment of adults with acute granulocytic leukemia. Its value in the treatment of children with acute lymphocytic leukemia has not been completely evaluated. In one study (Howard,

TABLE 1.—DRUGS EFFECTIVE IN ACUTE
LYMPHOCYTIC LEUKEMIA IN CHILDREN

Prednisone
Methotrexate
6-Mercaptopurine (Purinethol)
Cyclophosphamide (Cytoxan)
Vincristine (Oncovin)
Cytosine arabinoside (Cytosar)
Daunomycin (rubidomycin)
Asparaginase

Albo, and Newton, 1968), it was reported that only two of 43 children who received the drug obtained a complete remission. Thirteen improved to a good partial remission. As previously mentioned, one must consider all of the variables involved. In using cytosine arabinoside, the dose and schedule of administration are especially critical. As discussed in his presentation, Skipper (1970, see pages 27 to 36, this volume), in a review of cell kinetics, showed that the effectiveness of this drug in mouse leukemia was very closely related to the schedule of administration. Thus, one would expect that the response to this drug in clinical trials might be both dose- and schedule-dependent.

Further preliminary studies utilizing various dosages and schedules, as well as the use of cytosine arabinoside in various combination chemotherapy studies, have been completed or are in progress. There is no question that this medication is one that can be valuable in the treatment of some children with acute leukemia. Current investigations of cytosine arabinoside are designed to determine its optimum use. Combination studies of this drug with cyclophosphamide indicate that the dose, which is primarily limited by bone marrow toxicity, and the frequency of therapy necessary to effectively control disease seem to differ in almost every patient. Close monitoring of the status of the bone marrow is a prime requirement in determining the ideal dose and schedule of the medication for each patient. At this time, more specific results of our studies are not available.

Other significant characteristics of cytosine arabinoside are its ability to cross the blood-brain barrier and its lack of toxicity when given intrathecally. Studies to evaluate its usefulness in the treatment of central nervous system leukemia are currently in progress.

L-ASPARAGINASE.—One of the most exciting new types of therapy developed in the last few years for patients with acute leukemia is a drug which causes degradation of an amino acid essential to the growth of the tumor cell. This mode of antitumor action has been utilized clinically with L-asparaginase. Initial patient studies (Hill *et al.*, 1967) indicated that asparaginase prepared from *E. coli* was capable of producing remission in patients with acute leukemia. Not only did L-asparaginase have a definite effect on leukemic cells, but it also represented an entirely different mechanism of action from that of other chemotherapeutic agents. Exogenous L-asparagine is apparently necessary for the optimal growth of leukemic cells. Thus, the antitumor effect of asparaginase appears to be related to the enzymatic degradation of circulating L-asparagine. The death of leukemic cells follows the absence of this amino acid essential for their growth. Since asparagine is a nonessential amino acid for a normal cell, asparaginase was initially thought to represent an example of ideal antileukemic therapy.

Studies by other investigators (Oettgen *et al.*, 1967) have established that asparaginase when used alone is an effective inducer of remission in approximately 50 to 60 per cent of the cases of acute lymphocytic leukemia in children. In our own experience at Anderson Hospital, 18 children with acute leukemia have received this medication in various dose and treatment schedules. Some have received asparaginase in combination with prednisone and vincristine. The therapeutic results of these studies, which have been similar to those reported by others (Tallal *et al.*, 1969) will not be summarized in detail here. Rather, a number of significant side effects that have been noted with the use of asparaginase will be reviewed.

Asparaginase toxicity.—Although asparaginase was initially thought to be a relatively nontoxic medication, a number of investigators have now reported many side effects (Table 2). The variability in the incidence of some of these effects may be the result of differences in the source and the lot of asparaginase used. The side effects are listed in the general order of the frequency in which they have occurred in our patients. However, this listing does not indicate the degree of severity of the side effects.

Although nausea and vomiting and weight loss were noted frequently, they were not incapacitating. Significant fever occurred in several patients;

TABLE 2.—ASPARAGINASE TOXICITY

Nausea and vomiting
Weight loss
Fever
Anemia
Liver dysfunction (hyperbilirubinemia, hypoalbuminemia)
Central nervous system toxicity (abnormal electroencephalograms, somnolence, tremor)
Clotting defect (hypofibrinogenemia)
Decreased kidney function (elevated blood urea nitrogen)
Hypersensitivity reactions
Pancreatitis (elevated amylase)

K.A. 72512

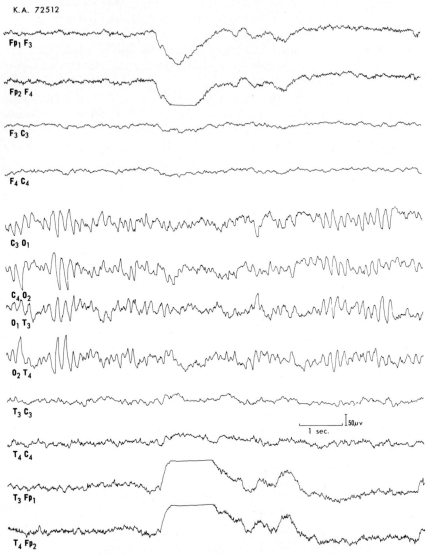

FIG. 1.—Electroencephalogram during asparaginase therapy. Diffusely slow in all regions.

this created a problem of distinguishing drug-induced fever from the fever of infection. Evidence of abnormal liver function, including hypoalbuminemia, was noted in most patients. Bilirubin elevations to a level greater than 5 mg./100 ml. occurred in five patients, but a direct cause-and-effect relationship with the asparaginase could not be established because of the

K.A. 72512

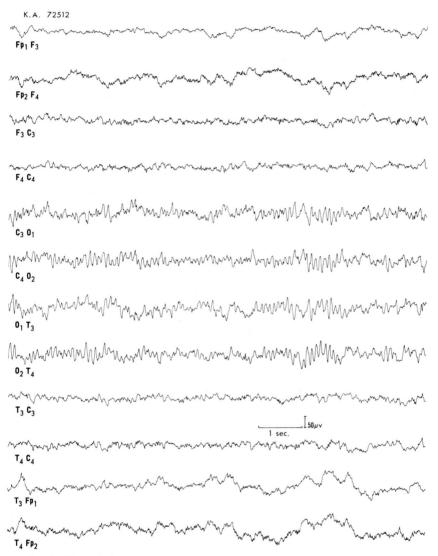

Fp₁ F₃

Fp₂ F₄

F₃ C₃

F₄ C₄

C₃ O₁

C₄ O₂

O₁ T₃

O₂ T₄

T₃ C₃

T₄ C₄

T₃ Fp₁

T₄ Fp₂

FIG. 2.—Normal electroencephalogram after completion of asparaginase therapy.

presence of other possible etiological factors, including sepsis and previous administration of blood products. An interesting observation in some of these patients was the presence of remarkably elevated serum ammonia levels, greater than 900 mcg./100 ml. in one case, and over 400 mcg./100 ml. in several cases. Clinical symptomatology usually associated with hyperammonemia was not present. Disorders in blood clotting, particularly a marked decrease in serum fibrinogen to levels of less than 10 mg./100 ml., were noted in several patients. These patients received fibrinogen prophylactically to help avoid hemorrhage.

The most disturbing side effects were associated with the central nervous system. Although some evidence of central nervous system toxicity had previously been reported in adults (Haskell *et al.*, 1969), we were surprised to find somnolence in many of our patients treated with asparaginase. This was associated with the development of confusion, lethargy, tremor, and marked changes in the electroencephalogram in six of our patients. These changes (Fig. 1) included diffuse slowing in all regions with loss of alpha activity; in some cases, there was complete disappearance of the normal pattern. The changes usually were reversible after cessation of therapy (Fig. 2). These effects may be partly the result of the particular lot of asparaginase used; however, side effects were noted to some degree with asparaginase produced by three different manufacturers. Another side effect that occurred twice was severe allergic response as manifested by an anaphylactoid reaction. One patient developed severe nonketotic hyperglycemia with a blood glucose of over 1,000 mg./100 ml. This gradually responded to insulin therapy.

In some patients, these toxic effects do not preclude the use of this drug. However, these examples illustrate that this new form of therapy has its limitations and dangers. Further studies are in progress utilizing various dosages and schedules of L-asparaginase and attempting to minimize side effects while achieving maximal antitumor effect. These studies also will determine if asparaginase can be more effectively used in combination with other drugs.

MULTIPLE DRUG THERAPY

Multiple drug combinations have been effective in achieving and prolonging an increased percentage of remissions. Hopefully, the use of intensive combination drug therapy will produce more long-term survivals. Thus far, it has not been determined which drug combination may prove to be most effective in achieving the largest number of long-term survivors as well as in prolonging the median survival time. At cancer centers throughout the world, investigative trials utilizing multiple drugs are in progress. The selection and scheduling of these drug combinations is based on the following principles: (1) to take maximum advantage of the antileukemic capability of each drug, (2) to utilize drugs with different mechanisms of action, and (3) to combine drugs which have different types of major toxicity.

Among the most encouraging results reported to date is the prolongation of median survival time to 33 months, achieved by the patients treated with the POMP program (Henderson, 1967). These data suggest the possibility of an increased number of prolonged disease-free survivals and possible cure of the disease. However, this can be confirmed only by continued observation of these patients.

Cancer Immunology

IMMUNOSUPPRESSION

The problems with suppression of the normal immune mechanism induced by prolonged and intensive chemotherapy have increased with the use of drug combinations. Therapy utilizing pulse techniques may be effective in preserving some of the patient's normal immunity. However, the problem of immunosuppression remains a serious one relative to the patient's defenses against infections and the relationship between the patient's immune system and his leukemic cells. More information about the effects of various therapeutic combinations and courses must be determined in order to minimize drug-induced immunosuppression. Immune profiles in children with malignant diseases are being studied before, during, and after chemotherapy (Mumford et al., in preparation).

IMMUNOTHERAPY

Immunotherapy of cancer is just beginning to develop as a possibly significant form of therapy. Although it has been known from animal models that tumors often contain tumor-specific antigens, the presence of similar tumor-associated antigens now has been demonstrated from some human malignant diseases (Dmochowski, 1970, see pages 37 to 52, this volume).

Current active immunotherapy clinical trials include those using some type of adjuvant therapy such as repeated BCG vaccination (Mathé et al., 1969). Other patients have been vaccinated from a pool of allogeneic leukemic lymphoblasts pretreated with formalin or irradiated in vitro. These two forms of therapy also have been combined. Recent immunotherapy trials include the transfer of leukemic cells from one patient with leukemia to immunize another leukemic patient. Subsequently, the donor passively receives the "immune" plasma and lymphocytes from the immunized patient. Using this scheme, initial success with some patients has been reported (Skurkovich, 1969), and further studies are in progress.

With certain neoplasms, common tumor-associated antigens can be demonstrated between the patient's own tumor and tissue cultures derived from his own or another patient's tumor. When this occurs, tissue culture material from either source can be reinjected in an *active* immunizing process.

This may prove particularly feasible when available tumor is limited in amount.

Current experimental results suggest that immunotherapy will be most effective when the number of tumor cells present is small (Southam, 1961, 1967). Therefore, immunotherapy should be utilized clinically in conjunction with other treatment modalities that reduce the number of viable tumor cells. In the use of such a combined approach, the timing of the immunotherapy in relation to the effect of chemotherapy on the patient's own immune system will be crucial.

It should be remembered that any attempt at the immunotherapy of cancer has both theoretical and real drawbacks. Three possible dangers deserve mention: (1) Instead of inducing immunity to the host tumor, the opposite phenomenon may occur; immunologic enhancement of tumor growth has been shown experimentally. (2) There is a real risk of inducing some form of autoimmune reaction with most of the procedures. (3) In many approaches, there is the possibility that undetected carcinogenic viruses may be transmitted. Despite these risks, we can expect to see the cautious continued development of immunotherapeutic studies in conjunction with different chemotherapeutic approaches. These combined treatment programs may increase the number of long-term survivors of both leukemia and other malignant diseases.

Supportive Care

The last area for consideration is a review of the improvements in the supportive therapy of children with leukemia. These improvements have played a major role in increasing the median survival time of patients, as well as in achieving a greater number of prolonged disease-free survivals. The success of intensive combination chemotherapy can, in large part, be credited to the improved supportive therapy that is available. During the period of intensive chemotherapy when severe side effects may be anticipated, the patient can best be cared for in a medical center by physicians experienced in the use of chemotherapeutic agents and in their side effects (Holland, 1969). The clinical oncologists in such a center will have available the latest techniques that have been developed to help manage these complications.

The two major causes of death in children with leukemia continue to be infection and hemorrhage. New developments in the prevention and management of both hemorrhage and infection have had a major role in the improved results reported with the use of intensive combination chemotherapy. The important role of platelet transfusion in the management of thrombocytopenia, whether secondary to disease or therapy, has been discussed (Freireich *et al.*, 1970, see pages 275 to 284, this volume). This therapy has greatly reduced the incidence of severe hemorrhage. However, infection continues to be a major complication. Several techniques are being studied to either prevent or control this complication of both the disease and the intensive chemotherapy.

ANTIBIOTIC THERAPY

Newer antibiotics, such as carbenicillin for *Pseudomonas* infections, are producing improved results in granulocytopenic patients (Bodey, Rodriguez, and Luce, 1969). Studies are underway to evaluate the role of prophylactic oral antibiotics, such as polymyxin-B, in preventing systemic infection (Sullivan, unpublished data). The use of protected environments, including both Life Island units and laminar air flow rooms (Bodey, Hart, Freireich, and Frei, 1968), has proved helpful in both adults and teenagers, but the feasibility of these techniques has not been tested adequately for younger children.

Other new developments in the area of supportive care, including therapy for infections occurring secondary to immunosuppression, can best be illustrated by the following case.

CENTRAL NERVOUS SYSTEM LEUKEMIA

In January of 1967, a six and one-half year-old girl was noted to have acute unclassified leukemia. She was started on therapy with prednisone and 6-mercaptopurine and went into a complete remission shortly after the initiation of therapy. With maintenance purinethol therapy, she did quite well for one and one-half years. In June of 1968, she developed central nervous system leukemia while still in bone marrow remission.

With the increasing numbers of long-term survivors with leukemia, an increasing number of patients develop central nervous system leukemia. In our experience, this is now approaching 50 per cent of the cases. The patient cited, following induction of remission of disease in the central nervous system with intrathecal methotrexate, was then started on a program of intrathecal methotrexate at a dose of 0.5 mg./kg. every six weeks. This schedule of therapy is being studied by the Southwest Cancer Chemotherapy Study Group to evaluate its effectiveness in preventing recurrence of central nervous system leukemia. At the present time, the patient is continuing on this program without evidence of recurrence of central nervous system leukemia or evidence of methotrexate toxicity. All six of the children entered on this schedule at Anderson Hospital have remained free of meningeal recurrence for periods of one year or longer. Three of the six patients are still alive and continue to show no evidence of their central nervous system leukemia from 14 to 18 months after initiation of this therapy.

Although this study is incomplete, thus far the results indicate that a scheduled treatment with intrathecal methotrexate may play an important role in the prevention of early recurrence of central nervous system disease.

INFECTIONS SECONDARY TO IMMUNOSUPPRESSION

This patient's history also illustrates other complications. She remained well until September 1, 1969, when she developed jaundice and intermittent high fever with associated respiratory distress. A fine granular infiltrate was apparent on her chest x-ray film (Fig. 3). Our clinical impression was cytomegalovirus pneumonia. Further evidence suggesting the diagnosis of

FIG. 3.—Diffuse inflammatory changes throughout both lung fields consistent with cytomegalovirus pneumonia (September 3, 1969).

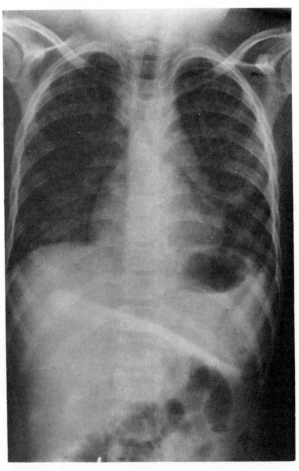

cytomegalovirus infection was the finding of a characteristic inclusion body in the urinary sediment. This patient was started on therapy with 5-FUdR in a dose of 10 mg./kg. daily, intravenously, for five days and concomitant therapy with prednisone, 2.2 mg./kg./day. Within 12 hours, her high swinging fever returned to normal and remained normal. In addition, she felt better within the first 24 hours. Her rapid respiration decreased and chest findings on auscultation, which previously had been minimal, now revealed widespread rales.

CYTOMEGALOVIRUS PNEUMONIA.—We now have had 23 patients who have shown clinical symptoms compatible with cytomegalovirus pneumonia. With the 12 most recent patients, we have given therapy with 5-FUdR. Remarkable clinical improvement has been associated with the administration of 5-FUdR in cytomegalovirus pneumonia (Cangir, Sullivan, Sutow, and Taylor, 1967). Laboratory confirmation of the diagnosis of cytomegalovirus infection was not always obtainable by culture of the virus, comple-

FIG. 4.—Patchy pneumonic infiltrates noted prior to needle biopsy of the lung (September 15, 1969).

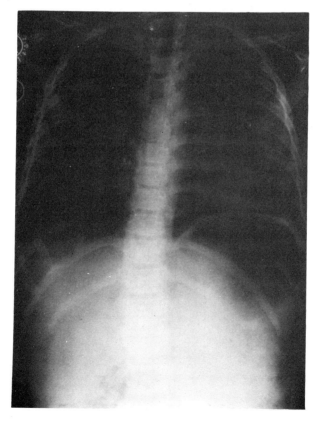

ment-fixation antibody titer changes, or observation of the inclusion bodies in the urine. However, the x-ray findings and clinical course were similar to that described in this patient. Eleven of 12 patients survived the acute episode. Improvement resulting from 5-FUdR therapy followed a characteristic pattern. This consisted of rapid dissolution of the fever, usually within 12 hours, decrease in respiratory rate, and improved lung aeration within the first 24 to 48 hours. Included in this group of patients are one child who had strong evidence of a second episode of cytomegalovirus infection and two children who had suggestive evidence of a second episode of the disease some months after their initial infection.

PNEUMOCYSTIS CARINII.—Within one week after initial, marked improvement of the cytomegalovirus pneumonia, this particular patient again appeared ill. Fever and increasing respiratory distress developed, and

FIG. 5.—Almost complete clearing of the lungs noted two days following completion of pentamidine isothionate therapy for pneumonia caused by *Pneumocystis carinii* (October 1, 1969).

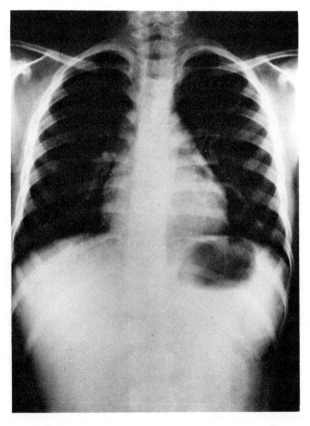

pulmonary infiltrates were seen on her chest x-ray film (Fig. 4). The pattern of this infiltrate was quite different from that seen with her cytomegalovirus pneumonia. She underwent a needle biopsy of the lung. Examination of the specimen revealed the presence of *Pneumocystis carinii*, the cause of her new pneumonia. She was started on therapy with pentamidine isothionate using a dose of 4 mg./kg./day intramuscularly for 14 days. Though critically ill, she gradually improved, and a chest x-ray film taken two days after completion of therapy (Fig. 5) shows marked clearing of the pulmonary infiltrate. Subsequently, the patient was discharged from the hospital, and she is continuing to do well. She remains in her initial bone marrow remission, with no evidence of activity of her central nervous system disease.

Summary

Recent advances in the therapy of acute leukemia in children include the following:

1. The use of combination drug regimens to achieve a higher "kill" of leukemic cells; in association with this, more long-term survivors without evidence of disease are being reported.

2. The use of prednisone and vincristine to induce multiple remissions when necessary.

3. The utilization of new drugs such as cytosine arabinoside and L-asparaginase as specific chemotherapeutic agents.

4. The study and application of immunotherapeutic techniques to neoplasms of man, both to manage existing disease and to prevent recurrence.

5. The refinement of the use of platelet transfusions to support patients during episodes of thrombocytopenia.

6. Improved capacity to deal with bacterial infections in granulocytic patients, particularly since the development of new antibiotics; the use of prophylactic oral antibiotics; and the utilization of protected environments, including Life Island and laminar air flow systems.

7. Progressive improvement in the treatment of central nervous system leukemia, including evaluation of the possible role of regularly scheduled intrathecal methotrexate injections to prevent recurrence of central nervous system disease activity.

8. The effective utilization of new drugs for the management of infections occurring secondary to immunosuppression, exemplified by 5-FUdR for cytomegalovirus infection and pentamidine isothionate for *Pneumocystis carinii* pneumonia.

These advances in therapy have been achieved by the combined efforts of many investigators throughout the world and have brought about a continually improving opportunity for long-term survival in children with acute leukemia.

Acknowledgments

The Parasitic Disease Drug Service, through the National Communicable Disease Center, Atlanta, Georgia, provided the pentamidine isothionate, and Hoffmann-LaRoche, Inc., Nutley, New Jersey, through the National Cancer Institute, provided the 5-FUdR.

REFERENCES

Bernard, J., Boiron, M., Jacquillat, C., and Weil, M.: Rubidomycin in 400 patients with leukemias and other malignancies. (Abstract) *Abstracts of the Simultaneous Sessions XII Congress International Society of Hematology,* 1968, p. 5.

Bodey, G. P., Hart, J., Freireich, E. J, and Frei, E., III: Studies of a patient isolator unit and prophylactic antibiotics in cancer chemotherapy. General techniques and preliminary results. *Cancer,* 22:1018-1026, November 1968.

Bodey, G. P., Rodriguez, V., and Luce, J. K.: Carbenicillin therapy of gram-negative bacilli infections. *American Journal of the Medical Sciences,* 257:408-414, June 1969.

Bodey, G. P., Rodriguez, V., Whitecar, J. P., Jr., Hart, J., and Freireich, E. J: The treatment for acute leukemia in adults. In *Leukemia-Lymphoma,* A Collection of Papers Presented at the 14th Annual Clinical Conference on Cancer, 1969, at The University of Texas M. D. Anderson Hospital and Tumor Institute at Houston. Chicago, Illinois, Year Book Medical Publishers, Inc., 1970, pp. 333-345.

Brubaker, C. A., Gilchrist, G. S., Hammond, D., Hyman, C. B., Shore, N. A., and Williams, K. O.: Induction of remission in acute leukemia with prednisone and intravenous methotrexate. *The Journal of Pediatrics,* 73:623-625, October 1968.

Cangir, A., Sullivan, M. P., Sutow, W. W., and Taylor, G.: Cytomegalovirus syndrome in children with acute leukemia. Treatment with floxuridine. *Journal of the American Medical Association,* 201:612-615, August 21, 1967.

Dmochowski, L.: Current status of the relationship of viruses to leukemia, lymphoma, and solid tumors. In *Leukemia-Lymphoma,* A Collection of Papers Presented at the 14th Annual Clinical Conference on Cancer, 1969, at The University of Texas M. D. Anderson Hospital and Tumor Institute at Houston. Chicago, Illinois, Year Book Medical Publishers, Inc., 1970, pp. 37-52.

Freireich, E. J, Bodey, G. P., de Jongh, D. S., Curtis, J. E., and Hersh, E. M.: Supportive therapeutic measures for patients under treatment for leukemia-lymphoma. In *Leukemia-Lymphoma,* A Collection of Papers Presented at the 14th Annual Clinical Conference on Cancer, 1969, at The University of Texas M. D. Anderson Hospital and Tumor Institute at Houston. Chicago, Illinois, Year Book Medical Publishers, Inc., 1970, pp. 275-284.

Freireich, E. J, Karon, M., and Frei, E., III: Quadruple combination therapy (VAMP) for acute lymphocytic leukemia of childhood. (Abstract) *Proceedings of the American Association for Cancer Research,* 5:20, March 1964.

George, P., Hernandez, K., Hustu, O., Borella, L., Holton, C., and Pinkel, D.: A study of "total therapy" of acute lymphocytic leukemia in children. *The Journal of Pediatrics,* 72: 399-408, March 1968.

Haskell, C. M., Canellos, G. P., Leventhal, B. G., Carbone, P. P., Serpick, A. A., and Hansen, H. H.: L-Asparaginase toxicity. (Letter to the editor) *Cancer Research,* 29:974-975, April 1969.

Henderson, E. S.: Combination chemotherapy of acute lymphocytic leukemia of childhood. *Cancer Research,* 27:2570-2572, December 1967.

Hill, J. M., Roberts, J., Loeb, E., Khan, A., MacLellan, A., and Hill, R. W.: L-Asparaginase therapy for leukemia and other malignant neoplasms. Remission in human leukemia. *Journal of the American Medical Association,* 202:882-888, November 27, 1967.

Holland, J. F.: Who should treat acute leukemia? *Journal of the American Medical Association,* 209:1511-1513, September 8, 1969.

Howard, J. P., Albo, V., and Newton, W. A., Jr.: Cytosine arabinoside: Results of a cooperative study in acute childhood leukemia. *Cancer,* 21:341-345, March 1968.

Lane, D. M., Haggard, M.E., Lonsdale, D., Sullivan, M. P., and Starling, K.: Second course vincristine-prednisone combination for remission induction in acute leukemia. *Cancer Chemotherapy Reports.* (In press.)

Mathé, G., Amiel, J. L., Schwarzenberg, L., Schneider, M., Cattan, A., Schlumberger, J. R., Hayat, M., and de Vassal, F.: Active immunotherapy for acute lymphoblastic leukemia. *Lancet,* 1:697-699, April 5, 1969.

Mathé, G., Hayat, M., Schwarzenberg, L., Amiel, J. L., Schneider, M., Cattan, A., Schlumberger, J. R., and Jasmin, C.: Acute lymphoblastic leukaemia treated with a combination of prednisone, vincristine, and rubidomycin: Value of pathogen-free rooms. *Lancet,* 2:380-382, August 19, 1967.

Mumford, D. M., Wilbur, J. R., Sullivan, M. P., Sutow, W. W., and Taylor, H. G.: Selected immune profiles of children with solid tumors during treatment. (In preparation.)

Oettgen, H. F., Old, L. J., Boyse, E. A., Campbell, H. A., Philips, F. S., Clarkson, B. D.,Tallal, L., Leeper, R. D., Schwartz, M. K., and Kim, J. H.: Inhibition of leukemias in man by L-asparaginase. *Cancer Research,* 27:2619-2631, December 1967.

Saunders, E. F., Kauder, E., and Mauer, A. M.: Sequential therapy of acute leukemia in childhood. *The Journal of Pediatrics,* 70:632-635, April 1967.

Skipper, H. E.: Leukocyte kinetics in leukemia and lymphoma. In *Leukemia-Lymphoma,* A Collection of Papers Presented at the 14th Annual Clinical Conference on Cancer, 1969, at The University of Texas M. D. Anderson Hospital and Tumor Institute at Houston. Chicago, Illinois, Year Book Medical Publishers, Inc., 1970, pp. 27-36.

Skurkovich, S. V., Kisljak, N. S., Machonova, L. A., and Begunenko, S. A.: Active immunization of children suffering from acute leukemia in acute phase with "live" allogeneic leukaemic cells. *Nature,* 223:509-511, August 2, 1969.

Southam, C. M.: Applications of immunology to clinical cancer. Past attempts and future possibilities. *Cancer Research,* 21:1302-1316, October 1961.

————: Cancer immunology in man. In Busch, H., Ed.: *Methods in Cancer Research.* New York, New York, and London, England, Academic Press, 1967. Vol. II, pp. 1-43.

Sullivan, M. P.: Unpublished data.

Tallal, L., Tan, C., Oettgen, H., McCarthy, M., Helson, L., and Murphy, L.: L-Asparaginase in 111 children with leukemias and solid tumors. (Abstract) *Proceedings of the American Association for Cancer Research,* 10:92, March 1969.

Perspectives in
Leukemia-Lymphoma Research

EMIL FREI, III, M.D.

*Department of Developmental Therapeutics, The University of Texas M. D. Anderson
Hospital and Tumor Institute at Houston, Houston, Texas*

IT IS CLEAR from this conference that substantial progress has been made on a broad front in leukemia and lymphoma research. There is increasing knowledge at the experimental and, to a limited extent, at the clinical level concerning the causes of these diseases; cytokinetic, immunologic, clinical, and other studies have substantially increased knowledge concerning their pathogenesis and natural history; and major progress has been made in the radiotherapy, chemotherapy, and supportive care of patients with hematologic malignant diseases. It is essential that activity in these areas be sustained and increased, since effective control of localized lymphoma is possible and definitive treatment of patients with some forms of disseminated lymphoma and leukemia should be increasingly possible.

ETIOLOGY

There are several congenital diseases associated with immunologic abnormalities wherein an increased risk of lymphoid neoplasms occurs (Good et al., 1969). In addition, there is evidence that the sustained immunosuppression during and following organ transplantation may increase the risk of lymphoid neoplasias (Penn, Hammond, Brettschneider, and Starzl, 1969). These observations are consistent with the immunologic surveillance hypothesis. Another explanation for the increased incidence of lymphoid neoplasias in patients receiving organ transplants is the possible carcinogenic effects of antitumor agents and/or antilymphocytic serum. In addition, it is possible that the chronic host-*vs.*-graft reaction that follows many organ transplantations may ultimately "escalate" the immunologic reaction to a neoplasia as may occur in experimental systems (Schwartz,

André-Schwartz, Armstrong, and Beldotti, 1966). These observations have a number of theoretical and basic implications and some clinical implications. There is a need to look at other, perhaps more subtle, abnormalities of immune response that may allow lymphocytic neoplasia to occur. The increasing use of antitumor agents, many of which are immunosuppressive, in diseases other than neoplastic diseases (e.g. collagen diseases, advanced psoriasis, etc.) must be pursued cautiously with continuing evaluation with respect to carcinogenicity.

It has been observed that congenital and induced cytogenetic abnormalities commonly increase the risk of lymphoid neoplastic transformation. This is true for trisomy 21 (mongolism) and for the Bloom and Fanconi syndromes, which are associated with an increased number of nonspecific lymphoid cytogenetic abnormalities (Swift and Hirschhorn, 1966). Skin fibroblasts of such patients have an increased susceptibility in vitro to neoplastic transformation with SV40 viruses (Todaro, Green, and Swift, 1966). Preliminary studies suggest that relatives of such patients are intermediate in terms of this in vitro test and thus are heterozygous. These cytogenetic and immunologic observations indicate that small populations with an increased risk of cancer can be identified and that, with further research, this may become increasingly possible.

The conclusive evidence that viruses are a causal agent for leukemia and lymphoma in a variety of subhuman mammalian species indicates that it probably plays a causal role in some forms of human neoplasia. Electron microscopic studies have provided suggestive but not conclusive evidence in this regard (Dmochowski and Grey, 1957). The extraordinary progress in immunological, tissue culture, and molecular biological techniques will certainly increase our understanding of the relationship of viruses and human neoplasia. Of particular current interest are the relationships of the Epstein-Barr (EB) virus to Burkitt's lymphoma, related tumors, and infectious mononucleosis and of the Moloney sarcoma virus to osteogenic sarcoma (Rauscher, 1968; Soehner and Dmochowski, 1969).

TREATMENT

Progress in the therapy for leukemia and lymphoma has been substantial and accelerating. In view of this, it seems likely that future progress will involve both new therapeutic modalities as well as progress along the lines which have proved successful in the recent past. Some of the factors responsible for progress in the treatment of patients with leukemia and lymphoma are listed in Table 1.

NEW AGENTS.—An increasing number of new agents are introduced into the clinic each year, and an increasing number of such agents are found to be effective. Thus, more clinically useful chemotherapeutic agents have

TABLE 1.—Selected Factors Contributing to Progress
in the Treatment of Hematologic Neoplasias

1. New agents
2. Improved dose schedules and combination therapy
3. Treatment during remission
4. Immunotherapy
5. Supportive care
6. Interaction of clinical investigators with those from the bridging and basic sciences, pharmacology, cytokinetics, molecular biology, *etc.*

been introduced in the last 10 years than in all prior time. For lymphoma, the introduction of vincristine, vinblastine, procarbazine, arabinosylcytosine, and the identification of the antilymphoma activity of prednisone has occurred during the past 10 years. For the acute leukemias, vincristine, arabinosylcytosine, asparaginase, cyclophosphamide, and daunomycin have been introduced in recent years. Much of this has resulted from increased support for such activities in government, industry, and universities. Substantial progress has been made in the development and application of experimental systems which predict antitumor activity in man (Goldin, Serpick, and Mantel, 1966). Thus, while a relatively precise predictive system such as obtains for many of the infectious diseases remains to be developed, several transplanted rodent tumor systems such as the L1210 correlate reasonably well with some forms of neoplastic disease in man. Increasing knowledge of comparative pharmacology and cytokinetics has resulted in further development and interpretation of these predictive systems and correlations. The development of a spontaneous, virus-induced leukemia (AKR) for quantitative screening is particularly promising. This tumor is cytokinetically much more similar to clinical leukemia and lymphoma than the transplanted leukemias and in preliminary studies would appear to predict effectively for leukemia (Skipper, 1970, see pages 27-36, this volume).

Such predictive systems are improving our ability to select from the increasing number of agents developed from many sources (natural or synthetic) by techniques ranging from (and usually combining) the empiric method to those of basic molecular biology. It is reasonable, therefore, to anticipate an increasing number of active agents with greater tumor selectivity.

Dose schedules and combination chemotherapy.—The development of improved dose schedules and combination cancer chemotherapy has contributed in a major way to therapeutic progress. Much of the progress that has been made in the management of childhood acute leukemia, in terms of improved survival, has resulted from such studies (Holland, 1969).

The major increase in the complete remission rate in acute leukemia and lymphoma has resulted largely from combination chemotherapy (Frei and Freireich, 1965). Studies of the biomedical significance of the complete remission state and of the significance of unmaintained remissions have provided major leads. The major increase in remission duration has resulted from the use of optimal dose schedules, combination chemotherapy, sequential and cyclic chemotherapy, and "reinduction" chemotherapy during remission (Acute Leukemia Group B, 1961; Frei and Freireich, 1965; Acute Leukemia Group B, 1965; Chevalier and Glidewell, 1967; Zuelzer, 1964).

It is commonly believed that chemotherapy is effective only against "rapidly growing" tumors. The major objective and subjective improvement and survival prolongation in myeloma that results from treatment with L-phenylalanine mustard, alone or combined with prednisone belie this axiom (Alexanian *et al.,* 1969).

Lymphoma Staging and Radiotherapy

The clinical staging, histopathologic classification, and radiotherapeutic management of patients with lymphoma are evolving rapidly. Lymphangiograms have greatly improved such staging (Wallace, 1970, see pages 223-239, this volume). More recently, laparotomies performed in patients with clinically localized disease have provided new insight into the frequency and distribution of disease below the abdomen and into the mechanism of spread of Hodgkin's disease. The evidence that the histopathologic types of Hodgkin's disease are associated with different patterns of anatomic distribution and spread has major implications with respect to the diagnostic work-up and management. The evidence is unequivocal that radiotherapy, properly applied, will cure the majority of patients with localized lymphoma (stages I and II) (Fuller, Gamble, and Butler, 1970, see pages 241-259, this volume; Peters, 1970, see pages 261-274, this volume). There is also evidence that "total lymphoid" radiotherapy may improve the long-term survival and perhaps cure rate in patients with certain types of localized disease and that such radiotherapy applied to patients with stage IIIA disease will produce a significant proportion of long-term, relapse-free survivors (Kaplan, 1968; Johnson, 1969). Radiotherapy can provide more than palliative management in patients with some types of disseminated Hodgkin's disease, and there is evidence that chemotherapy may provide more than palliative treatment for some types of localized lymphoma. Thus, a substantial proportion of patients with stages I and II Burkitt's lymphoma in Africa and in the United States receiving intermittent cyclophosphamide therapy have long-term, tumor-free survival (up to 10 years) (Burchenal, 1970, see pages 93-104, this volume). Similarly, patients with localized Hodgkin's disease in Central Africa, where radiotherapeutic equipment is lacking, have had long-term, tumor-free response to chemotherapy. Combined chemotherapy of stage IV Hodgkin's disease has produced a high complete remission rate and prolonged remissions. Clearly, the staging of lymphoma will continue to change and improve. Similarly, a fixation on the principle that radiotherapy exclusively should be applied to localized disease with curative intent and that chemotherapy primarily should be applied to disseminated disease with palliative intent is no longer appropriate. Combined application of optimal chemotherapy and optimal radiotherapy to the intermediate stages (stage IIB to stage IIIB) is indicated and initial studies suggest that it can be done safely (Gamble, Fuller, and Shullenberger, 1970, see pages 285-294, this volume). Depending upon the results, application to other forms of lymphoma and perhaps to selected categories of more localized and stage IV Hodgkin's disease will be indicated. Thus, one predictable outcome is the increased and effective interaction of chemotherapists and radiotherapists in the treatment of patients with lymphoma.

Of great significance is the awareness in recent years that, for some forms of neoplastic disease, cure is a reasonable target of chemotherapy. Thus, chemotherapy is curative for a substantial proportion of patients with trophoblastic tumors and Wilms' tumor and also probably is curative for a small proportion of patients with Burkitt's lymphoma, acute lymphocytic leukemia, and Hodgkin's disease (Burchenal, 1970, see pages 93-104, this volume).

Tumor Immunity and Immunotherapy

The conclusive evidence that virus and chemical carcinogen-induced tumors regularly have tumor-specific transplantation antigens and that this is also true for at least some forms of spontaneous tumors in experimental systems has major implications concerning the diagnosis, pathogenesis, and management of neoplastic disease (Klein, 1968). The rapid improvement in techniques such as indirect membrane and cytoplasmic immunofluorescence, mixed hemagglutination, colony inhibition, etc., allows for the development of evidence for such tumor-specific transplantation antigens in noninbred mammalian systems including man (Hellström, Pierce, and Hellström, 1969; Morton, Malmgren, Holmes, and Ketcham, 1968). These studies have prompted a number of immunotherapeutic attempts in experimental systems, some of which have proved successful. Some have been extended to the clinic. After complete remission induction and consolidation with chemotherapy in children with acute leukemia, a significant prolongation of remission has been achieved with immunotherapy (Mathé et al., 1969). This immunotherapy consisted of nonspecific immune stimulation (with BCG) and active immunization with pooled human leukemic lymphoblasts. This active immunization assumes the existence of similar tumor-specific transplantation antigens for leukemias in man. Such antigens for leukemias induced by the common leukemogenic viruses are known to exist in rodents. Experimental techniques involving the adoptive transfer of immunologic information including tumor immunity with lymphocytes and lymphoblasts have proved successful. There is increasing knowledge concerning the efficiency with which immunologic information can be transferred in man by adoptive immunologic techniques. A major limitation of this approach relates to histocompatability and the risk of graft vs. host disease. The isolation of a clone of lymphocytes particularly targeted for the human tumor-specific transplantation antigen involved is possible. Increasing data concerning the mechanisms whereby lymphocytes impart information such as through migration inhibitory factor (MIF) and particularly transfer factor have major implications for future immunotherapy. Thus, it ultimately may be possible to transfer tumor immunity with noncellular low-molecular-weight substances such as transfer factor (Lawrence, 1969).

Most experimental studies indicate that immunotherapy has the potential for greater tumor tissue selectivity than chemotherapy, whereas chemotherapy has greater cytotoxic potency. There is evidence that chemotherapy is particularly likely to be curative when there is host immunity to the tumor, which occurs in patients with gestational choriocarcinoma and Burkitt's lymphoma. For these reasons, the setting in which immunotherapy is most likely to be effective (and perhaps curative) is when it is directed against "minimal residual neoplastic disease" that may follow surgical therapy, radiotherapy, and/or chemotherapy.

SUPPORTIVE CARE

The morbidity and mortality of patients with cancer and particularly of patients with the hematologic malignant diseases result from the complications rather than from the direct effect of the disease. This is often caused by bone marrow failure with resultant hemorrhage and infection. Widely practiced and definitive bone marrow element replacement therapy should be possible in the not-too-distant future. This is attributed in part to improved acquisition of peripheral blood elements (particularly white blood cells) by using the vein-to-vein, continuous centrifuge (IBM-NCI) (Freireich et al., 1970, see pages 275-284, this volume). This has proved to be an important clinical research and therapeutic tool. Improved techniques for the short- and long-term storage of platelets, white blood cells, and bone marrow and particularly tissue culture techniques for the growth of normal stem cells and possibly of the more differentiated progeny may be possible. Finally, a major contribution to current and particularly future progress in this area relates to histocompatibility typing. The selection of a proper donor already has led to immunologic reconstruction in patients with the DeGeorge syndrome (absence of cellular immunity). Preliminary studies indicate that bone marrow transplantation in patients with acute and/or chronic bone marrow failure employing appropriate immunosuppression and histocompatibility typed donor stem cells is possible. Finally, tissue matched platelet (and probably granulocyte) transfusions have a superior recovery and survival in the recipient (Grumet, Yankee, and Rogentine, 1969).

BRIDGING SCIENCES

Much of the above progress has resulted from interaction between clinical scientists, scientists in the "bridging" disciplines such as biochemical pharmacology and cytokinetics, and scientists in the basic scientific disciplines, most particularly those in molecular biology. This constitutes an important evolution that has occurred relatively recently. Fifteen to 20 years ago a clinician focusing on cancer tended to be isolated not only from biomedical scientists in the bridging and basic disciplines but also, to some extent, from other clinical disciplines. This reflected for the most part the hopelessness that existed at the time with respect to gaining knowledge concerning the basic nature of the neoplastic problem and particularly with respect to the systemic treatment of patients with disseminated neoplasia. Only one example of the interaction of bridging scientists with clinical scientists will be given.

The cell population kinetics of normal and neoplastic cells have been increasingly studied in experimental systems. This knowledge and the knowledge that chemotherapeutic agents affect cells during different stages of the mitotic cycle and that many agents affect only proliferating cells have provided a number of therapeutic hypotheses. Arabinosylcytosine (Ara-C) is a cell cycle-specific agent affecting cells only during the S (DNA synthesis) phase of the mitotic cycle. Employing this knowledge and cytokinetic and biological knowledge concerning the duration of the mitotic cycle and the rate of recovery from DNA synthesis inhibition of L1210 leukemia cells and normal stem cells (bone marrow and gastrointestinal tract), a dose schedule program for Ara-C was developed for L1210 mouse leukemia which had a greatly improved therapeutic index compared to conventional daily treatment (Skipper, Schabel, and Wilcox, 1967). With appropriate modification for leukemia and bone marrow stem cell cytokinetics in man, the schedule was applied and found to produce a complete remission rate of 30 per cent compared to 15 per cent for conventional daily treatment (Bodey, Freireich, Monto, and Hewlett, 1969; Bickers and Freireich, un-

372 / FREI

published data). This is only one of many examples of how clinical scientists, using information from the basic and bridging sciences can improve treatment of patients with cancer.

REFERENCES

Acute Leukemia Group B (Frei, E., III, Freireich, E. J, Gehan, E., Pinkel, D., Holland, J. F., Selawry, O., Haurani, F., Spurr, C. L., Hayes, D. M., James, G. W., Rothberg, H., Sodee, D. B., Rundles, R. W., Schroeder, L. R., Hoogstraten. B., Wolman, I. J., Traggis, D. G., Cooper, T., Gendel, B. R., Ebaugh, F., and Taylor, R.: Studies of sequential and combination antimetabolite therapy in acute leukemia: 6-Mercaptopurine and methotrexate. *Blood, The Journal of Hematology,* 18:431-454, October 1961.
Acute Leukemia Group B (Selawry, O. S., Hananian, J., Wolman, I. J., Abir, E., Chevalier, L., Gourdeau, R., Denton, R., Gussoff, B. D., Levy, R., Burgert, O., Jr., Mills, S. D., Blom, J., Jones, B., Patterson, R. B., McIntyre, O. R., Haurani, F. I., Moon, J. H., Hoogstraten, B., Kung, F. H., Sheehe, P. R., Frei, E., III, and Holland, J. F.): New treatment schedule with improved survival in childhood leukemia: Intermittent parenteral vs daily oral administration of methotrexate for maintenance of induced remission. *Journal of the American Medical Association,* 194:75-81, October 4, 1965.
Alexanian, R., Haut, A., Khan, A. U., Lane, M., McKelvey, E. M., Migliore, P. J., Stuckey, W. J., Jr., and Wilson, H. E.: Treatment for multiple myeloma: Combination chemotherapy with different melphalan dose regimens. *Journal of the American Medical Association,* 208:1680-1685, June 2, 1969.
Bickers, J., and Freireich, E. J: Unpublished data.
Bodey, G. P., Freireich, E. J, Monto, R. W., and Hewlett, J. S. (Writing Committee): Cytosine arabinoside (NSC-63878) therapy for acute leukemia in adults. *Cancer Chemotherapy Reports,* 53:59-66, February 1969.
Burchenal, J. H.: Features suggesting curability in leukemia and lymphoma. In *Leukemia-Lymphoma,* A Collection of Papers Presented at the 14th Annual Clinical Conference on Cancer, 1969, at The University of Texas M. D. Anderson Hospital and Tumor Institute at Houston. Chicago, Illinois, Year Book Medical Publishers, Inc., 1970, pp. 93-104.
Chevalier, L., and Glidewell, O.: Schedule of 6-mercaptopurine and effect of inducer drugs in prolongation of remission maintenance in acute leukemia. (Abstract) *Proceedings of the American Association for Cancer Research,* 8:10, March 1967.
Dmochowski, L., and Grey, C. E.: Electron microscopy of tumors of known and suspected viral etiology. *Texas Reports on Biology and Medicine,* 15:704-753, Fall 1957.
Frei, E., III , and Freireich, E. J: Progress and perspectives in the chemotherapy of acute leukemia. *Advances in Chemotherapy,* 2:269-298, 1965.
Freireich, E. J, Bodey, G. P., de Jongh, D. S., Curtis, J. E., and Hersh, E. M.: Supportive therapeutic measures for patients under treatment for leukemia or lymphoma. In *Leukemia-Lymphoma,* A Collection of Papers Presented at the 14th Annual Clinical Conference on Cancer, 1969, at The University of Texas M. D. Anderson Hospital and Tumor Institute at Houston. Chicago, Illinois, Year Book Medical Publishers, Inc., 1970, pp. 275-284.
Fuller, L. M., Gamble, J. F., and Butler, J. J.: Results of definitive radiotherapy in localized Hodgkin's disease, as related to both clinical presentation and pathological classification. In *Leukemia-Lymphoma,* A Collection of Papers Presented at the 14th Annual Clinical Conference on Cancer, 1969, at The University of Texas M. D. Anderson Hospital and Tumor Institute at Houston. Chicago, Year Book Medical Publishers, Inc., 1970, pp. 241-295.
Gamble, J. F., Fuller, L., and Shullenberger, C. C.: Combined use of chemotherapy and radiation therapy in the treatment for generalized Hodgkin's disease. In *Leukemia-Lymphoma,* A Collection of Papers Presented at the 14th Annual Clinical Conference on Cancer, 1969, at The University of Texas M. D. Anderson Hospital and Tumor Institute at Houston. Chicago, Illinois, Year Book Medical Publishers, Inc., 1970, pp. 285-294.
Goldin, A., Serpick, A. A., and Mantel, N.: A commentary: Experimental screening procedures and clinical predictability value. *Cancer Chemotherapy Reports,* 50:173-218, May 1966.

Good, R. A., Finstad, J., Cain, W. A., Fish, A., Perey, D. Y., and Gatti, R. A.: Models of immunologic diseases and disorders. *Federation Proceedings*, 28:191-205, January-February 1969.

Grumet, F. C., Yankee, R. A., and Rogentine, G. N.: Compatible platelet donor selection and histocompatibility. (Abstract) *Proceedings of the American Association for Cancer Research*, 10:33, March 1969.

Hellström, I., Pierce, G. E., and Hellström, K. E.: Human tumor specific-antigens. *Surgery*, 65:984-989, June 1969.

Holland, J. F.: Who should treat acute leukemia? *Journal of the American Medical Association*, 209:1511-1513, September 8, 1969.

Johnson, R. E.: Modern approaches to the radiotherapy of lymphoma. *Seminars in Hematology*, 6:357-375, October 1969.

Kaplan, H. S.: Clinical evaluation of radiotherapeutic management of Hodgkin's disease and the malignant lymphomas. *New England Journal of Medicine*, 278:892-899, April 18, 1968.

Klein, G.: Tumor-specific transplantation antigens: G. H. A. Clowes Memorial Lecture. *Cancer Research*, 28:625-635, April 1968.

Lawrence, S.: Transfer factor and cellular immunity. *Hospital Practice*, 4:40-43, 49-50, 55-58, December 1969.

Mathé, G., Amiel, J. L., Schwarzenberg, L., Schneider, M., Cattan, A., Schlumberger, J. R., Hayat, M., and de Vassal, F.: Active immunotherapy for acute lymphoblastic leukemia. *Lancet*, 1:697-699, April 5, 1969.

Morton, D. L., Malmgren, R. A., Holmes, E. C., and Ketcham, A. S.: Demonstration of antibodies against human malignant melanoma by immunofluorescence. *Surgery*, 64:233-240, July 1968.

Penn, I., Hammond, W., Brettschneider, L., and Starzl, T. E.: Malignant lymphomas in transplantation patients. *Transplantation Proceedings*, 1:106-112, March (Part 1) 1969.

Peters, M. V.: Changing concepts in radiotherapy for the lymphomas. In *Leukemia-Lymphoma*, A Collection of Papers Presented at the 14th Annual Clinical Conference on Cancer, 1969, at The University of Texas M. D. Anderson Hospital and Tumor Institute at Houston. Chicago, Illinois, Year Book Medical Publishers, Inc., 1970, pp. 261-274.

Rauscher, F. J., Jr.: Virologic studies in human leukemia and lymphoma: The herpes-type virus. *Cancer Research*, 28:1311-1318, July 1968.

Schwartz, M., André-Schwartz, J., Armstrong, M. Y. K., and Beldotti, L.: Neoplastic sequelae of allogenic disease. I. Theoretical considerations and experimental design. *Annals of the New York Academy of Sciences*, 129:804-821, December 30, 1966.

Skipper, H. E.: Leukocyte kinetics in leukemia and lymphoma. In *Leukemia-Lymphoma*, A Collection of Papers Presented at the 14th Annual Clinical Conference on Cancer, 1969, at The University of Texas M. D. Anderson Hospital and Tumor Institute at Houston. Chicago, Illinois, Year Book Medical Publishers, Inc., 1970, pp. 27-36.

Skipper, H. E., Schabel, F. M., Jr., and Wilcox, W. S.: Experimental evaluation of potential anticancer agents. XXI. Scheduling of arabinosylcytosine to take advantage of its S-phase specificity against leukemia cells. *Cancer Chemotherapy Reports*, 51:125-141, June 1967.

Soehner, R. L., and Dmochowski, L.: Induction of bone tumours in rats and hamsters with murine sarcoma virus and their cell-free transmission. *Nature*, 224:191-192, October 11, 1969.

Swift, M. R., and Hirschhorn, K.: Fanconi's anemia: Inherited susceptibility to chromosomal breakage in various tissues. *Annals of Internal Medicine*, 65:496-503, September 1966.

Todaro, G. J., Green, H., and Swift, M. R.: Susceptibility of human diploid fibroblast strains to transformation by SV40 virus. *Science*, 153:1252-1254, September 9, 1966.

Wallace, S.: Newer radiodiagnostic contributions to the study of the lymphoma patient. In *Leukemia-Lymphoma*, A Collection of Papers Presented at the 14th Annual Clinical Conference on Cancer, 1969, at The University of Texas M. D. Anderson Hospital and Tumor Institute at Houston. Chicago, Year Book Medical Publishers, Inc., 1970, pp. 223-239.

Zuelzer, W. W.: Implications of long-term survival in acute stem cell leukemia of childhood treated with composite cyclic therapy. *Blood, The Journal of Hematology*, 24:477-494, November 1964.

Management of Patients with Lymphoma

CLINICOPATHOLOGICAL PANEL DISCUSSION*

Arranged by the Department of Pathology of The University of Texas M. D. Anderson Hospital and Tumor Institute at Houston and Co-sponsored by Texas Society of Pathologists

THE FINAL SESSION of The University of Texas M. D. Anderson Hospital and Tumor Institute at Houston Fourteenth Annual Clinical Conference on Cancer was a half-day panel discussion on Management of Patients with Lymphoma. Case histories of patients treated at this institution were presented, featuring clinical and pathologic correlation, relating the type of lymphoma to the therapy selected, the results of treatment, and general prognosis. Choice of therapy relative to type of disease was featured because selection of appropriate therapy is assuming increasing importance with the advances in the various modalities used individually, or in combination, particularly cytotoxic drugs.

The program of the Annual Clinical Conference provides a wide range of information on lymphoma and leukemia, related to pathologic diagnosis and therapy, as well as pathogenetic and immunologic aspects. The panel discussion by physicians responsible for patient care provides a viewing of

*Panel moderators (from whom reprints may be obtained) and members are as follows:

Moderators
WILLIAM O. RUSSELL, M. D., Head, Department of Pathology, The University of Texas M. D. Anderson Hospital and Tumor Institute at Houston
GEORGE J. RACE, M.D., President, Texas Society of Pathologists, Director of Laboratories and Chief of Pathology, Baylor University Medical Center, Dallas, Texas

Staff Members of The University of Texas M. D. Anderson Hospital and Tumor Institute at Houston

JAMES J. BUTLER, M.D.	JAMES K. LUCE, M.D.
LILLIAN M. FULLER, M.D.	C. C. SHULLENBERGER, M.D.
JESS F. GAMBLE, M.D.	SIDNEY WALLACE, M.D.

the clinical applications of the information presented in the preceding sessions of the Conference. Those attending the Clinical Conference thus have opportunity for sharing their own personal experiences in discussions related to patient treatment.

Because the pathologist is the physician who initially establishes the diagnosis of cancer, communicating this to the patient's physician, he occupies a key position in patient care. Therefore, the panel discussions relating the various applications of therapy to the type of disease are of particular significance to the pathologist. In consultation with the attending physician, the pathologist's opinion of the tumor will aid in achieving the best possible decisions regarding selection of therapy. Awareness of this responsibility for cancer patient care prompted the Texas Society of Pathologists to join with the Anderson Hospital staff in co-sponsorship of this panel discussion. This activity symbolizes the educational and scientific interests of the Texas Society of Pathologists in enhancing the role of pathologists in cancer patient treatment. The panel members represent the clinical specialties involved in the problems of diagnosis, individual selection of therapy, and management of lymphomatous diseases. By providing this spectrum of clinical expertise, the variables and problems involved in all aspects of patient treatment are clearly demonstrated. The benefits of a team approach to cancer patient care are further emphasized and provide additional stimulus to physicians at the community level to solve their problems of patient treatment in a similar manner.

The following pages contain a summary of each case presented with brief excerpts of the major points discussed.

CASE 1.—*Nodular lymphoma, mixed type,* was diagnosed by biopsy in a 27-year-old male in 1957 and again in 1964. He initially presented with generalized lymphadenopathy which regressed with chemotherapy; local recurrences in 1964 and 1968 responded promptly to local irradiation. He was asymptomatic when last seen in September 1969, 12 years after the initial onset of disease.

Clinical resume.—This patient noticed painless enlargement of his left inguinal lymph nodes in May 1957. In August, similar nodes appeared in the left side of the neck and both axillae. A right axillary lymph node biopsy in February 1958 revealed mixed type nodular lymphoma.

On the initial evaluation, the posterior-anterior and lateral radiographs of the chest were negative and the routine hematological survey was normal. He received a course of Leukeran with regression of all lymph nodes by mid-April.

The patient remained free of disease until December 1963, when he noticed a tender, fluctuating swelling behind the right mandible. When seen for follow-up examinations in April 1964, a 3-cm. lymph node was present in the tail of the right parotid gland. Examination of the nasopharynx revealed excessive lymphoid tissue. Biopsy of the lymph node and the nasopharynx showed mixed type nodular lymphoma. The patient was treated with ^{60}Co irradiation to the nasopharynx, both sides of the neck, and the supraclavicular fossae, at the rate of 1,000 rads tumor dose per week to a total of approximately 3,000 rads.

The patient was well until December 1967, when he developed an infection in the left popliteal area. At the time, he noted enlarged, tender left femoral lymph nodes. When seen in April 1968, the left femoral node was enlarged, and a mass was questioned in the left inguinal region. In June, an ill-defined mass was palpable in the left iliac fossa. A lymphangiogram in August revealed extensive involvement of the left inguinal, iliac and para-aortic nodes. ^{60}Co irradiation was administered to the pelvis and upper abdomen in sequence, the tumor dose being approximately 3,000 rads delivered in four weeks. The patient was asymptomatic when last seen in September 1969.

This case illustrates the course, prognosis, and response to therapy in most patients with nodular lymphoma. Although nodular lymphoma is generally considered a systemic disease which involves the entire reticuloendothelial system, it may manifest itself as a localized process initially. Whatever the manner of presentation, the disease usually responds well to chemotherapy or radiotherapy. For localized disease, radiotherapy is the treatment of choice. In this case, chemotherapy was administered initially because the disease was extremely generalized. Radiotherapy was reserved for localized exacerbations.

Nodular lymphomas of all cell types may maintain the same histological pattern throughout the course of the disease, in which event survival is usually prolonged as in this patient. In other patients, there is a transition from the nodular pattern to a diffuse lymphoma of the same cell type. Although survival is somewhat dependent upon the cell type, *i.e.*, whether poorly differentiated lymphocytic or histiocytic reticulum cell sarcoma, the persistence of, or failure to maintain, the nodular pattern is more important and thus prognostically significant. Repeat lymph node biopsies with exacerbations are recommended when practical.

CASE 2.—*Hodgkin's disease with nodular sclerosis* in a 15-year-old girl was manifested by enlarged supraclavicular lymph nodes and a mediastinal mass which regressed with irradiation therapy; subsequently, local recurrence in the cervical lymph nodes and extension to the left lung were managed successfully with local irradiation therapy; subsequently, local recurrence in the cervical lymph nodes and extension to the left lung were managed successfully with local irradiation. Nine years after onset, the patient has no evidence of disease.

Clinical resume.—This patient first noted a small, tender lump in the left lower neck in July 1958. When antibiotic therapy failed to produce any change, a lymph node biopsy was performed on July 25. The diagnosis was Hodgkin's disease with nodular sclerosis. She was referred to Anderson Hospital for treatment. Physical examination revealed enlarged bilateral supraclavicular lymph nodes. The chest x-ray film showed a small anterior-superior mediastinal mass. The mediastinum, neck, and both axillae were treated intensively with ^{60}Co irradiation.

The patient was well until September 1959, when she noted recurrence of a small node in the right supraclavicular area, and a small right axillary node. When these nodes increased in size over a two-month period, she was retreated to both sides of the neck and to the right axilla.

A chest x-ray film taken in December 1959, while she was receiving her second course of irradiation, showed an ill-defined density in the lingula of the left lung. Histoplasmin and tuberculin tests were negative. Over the next four years, the lesion gradually increased in size, but the patient continued to feel well. A chest x-ray film taken in June 1964 showed massive involvement of the upper two thirds of the left lung. Tomograms of the mediastinum failed to show recurrent adenopathy. She received 4,000 rads to the upper two thirds of the lung over a period of four weeks and has been asymptomatic since that time.

This case illustrates several clinically important points. Nodular sclerosing Hodgkin's disease is a disease of young persons, particularly young females. Involvement of the mediastinum is more frequent in this type of Hodgkin's disease than in all other types combined. For this reason, prophylactic irradiation therapy usually is given to the mediastinum in patients presenting with this type of disease in the lower cervical lymph nodes even without demonstrable mediastinal disease. The mediastinum is not treated prophylactically when Hodgkin's disease is restricted to the upper neck. Axillary involvement often develops in patients with mediastinal disease within two years. Patients who present with axillary involvement, whatever the histologic type, usually do not develop mediastinal involvement; when they develop additional disease, the abdomen usually is the next site of involvement.

Nodular sclerosing Hodgkin's disease may be associated with stable, or with progressive, disease. No histological parameters exist which would predict the course. The clinical stage is the most reliable indicator. Patients presenting with either clinical stage I or stage II disease of this type usually have long survival. Direct extension to the lung, secondary to nodular sclerosing Hodgkin's disease, should be considered as a localized process. Depending upon the location, removal may be the treatment of choice. If surgical resection is not possible because of proximity to the previously irradiated hilum, irradiation therapy is employed.

CASE 3.—*Well-differentiated lymphocytic lymphoma* was diagnosed in a 53-year-old male who presented with cervical lymph node enlargement, which disappeared with irradiation therapy administered before referral. He subsequently had local recurrences, treated with irradiation and chemotherapy. Eventually, the patient developed chronic lymphocytic leukemia. In September 1969, he had no clinical symptoms referrable to his disease.

Clinical resume.—This patient noted enlarged cervical lymph nodes in January 1962. In August 1962, a left cervical lymph node was removed; the diagnosis was well-differentiated lymphocytic lymphoma. He received irradiation therapy to both sides of the neck and then was referred to this hospital.

When seen three weeks after completion of irradiation therapy, he had barely palpable lymph nodes in the left jugular area of the neck. Enlarged nodes were present in both axillae. Both tonsils were enlarged. The spleen and liver were not palpable. The blood counts were normal. The chest x-ray films showed only cardiomegaly; an intravenous pyelogram was normal. When seen one week later, the previously palpable lymph nodes had regressed. The patient was followed at regular intervals with no change until December 1963, when a 2-cm. right submental node appeared. At this time, the white blood cell count was 8,300 with 54 per cent lymphocytes. By July 1964, the submental node measured 3 cm. in diameter and the tonsils appeared larger. On July 21, 1964, a left tonsillectomy was performed. The diagnosis was well-differentiated lymphocytic lymphoma. The white blood cell count at this time was 14,630 with 60 per cent lymphocytes. The patient was treated with irradiation therapy to the tonsillar areas and both sides of the neck for relief of local symptomatology. Lymphangiography showed enlarged pelvic and para-aortic nodes. In January 1965, bilaterally enlarged inguinal and femoral nodes were present. By March 1965, a 4-cm. node had appeared in the left axilla. The white blood cell count was 6,400 with 37 per cent lymphocytes. A course of Leukeran was initiated which resulted in partial regression of the adenopathy. However, repeated courses of Leukeran were necessary for continued control of recurring adenopathy. After the last course of chemotherapy in March 1969, the white blood cell count was 9,000 with 67 per cent lymphocytes. When seen in September 1969, the patient was asymptomatic. However, he gave a history of having had a recent episode of herpes zoster involving the right thigh. His white blood cell count at this time was 19,200 with 87 per cent lymphocytes. His hemoglobin was 13.5 g.; his platelet count was 189,000.

Patients with well-differentiated lymphocytic lymphoma respond to either irradiation therapy or chemotherapy. The type of therapy depends on the extent of involvement and on whether lymphocytic leukemia has developed. With clinically localized disease in a nonleukemic patient, irradiation therapy would be the treatment of choice. If leukemia developed during the course of treatment, radiotherapy would usually be completed unless the patient's general condition deteriorated or the white blood cell and platelet counts fell to unsatisfactory levels. Irradiation therapy would be attempted in a leukemic patient if threatened with advancing localized disease in an anatomically critical area such as Waldeyer's ring or the retroperitoneum. Chemotherapy usually would be employed for generalized disease or in leukemic patients except as noted. Chemotherapy is given intermittently to minimize the appearance of resistant cell strains.

Lymphocytic leukemia is another manifestation of lymphocytic lymphoma and is not evidence of a different disease.

CASE 4.—*Hodgkin's disease with nodular sclerosis* was diagnosed in this 16-year-old boy who presented with an axillary mass which was removed surgically. The area was irradiated; shortly afterwards, systemic symptoms appeared and involvement of the bone marrow and spleen was proved. With subsequent chemotherapy, his condition improved.

Clinical resume.—This patient was examined one year after the gradual onset of a mass in the right axilla accompanied by a 5-lb. weight loss, but no other symptoms. The examination was normal except for a 10-cm. movable firm mass in the right axilla. Laboratory examination showed: hemoglobin 11.8, white blood cell count 6,700, polymorphonuclear granulocytes 84, lymphocytes 10, monocytes 5, and eosinophiles 1; Bromsulphalein (BSP) 3 per cent retention; protein electrophoresis showed an albumin of 3.6 g. with a slightly elevated alpha$_2$ peak. Serum copper was 205 mcg./ml. (normal 69 to 133 mcg./ml.). The chest x-ray film, lymphangiogram, and intravenous pyelogram were normal. Bone marrow biopsy was normal. The mass was excised and revealed Hodgkin's disease with nodular sclerosis. He received intensive ^{60}Co irradiation via a mantle technique to the neck, supraclavicular areas, mediastinum, and both axillae.

One month after completion of radiotherapy, the boy developed fever to 103°C daily. Physical examination was otherwise normal. The laboratory examination showed: hemoglobin 11.0, *white blood cell count 2,200,* platelets 130,000 polymorphonuclear granulocytes 55, lymphocytes 40, and monocytes 5. *The BSP was 17 per cent.* The sequential multiple analyzer (SMA) 12/60 showed an alkaline phosphatase of 115 (normal 30 to 80), lactic dehydrogenase (LDH) 230 (normal 80 to 200), and serum glutamic oxalopyruvic transaminase (SGOT) 70 (normal 40 to 50). The protein electrophoresis showed an albumin of 2.4 g. and a total protein of 5.8 g. The alpha$_2$ peak was not elevated. Liver biopsy and bone marrow examination showed infiltration by Hodgkin's disease. The patient was treated with antibiotics including ampicillin, carbenicillin, and kanamycin but the fever persisted. He was then started on chemotherapy with a combination of nitrogen mustard, vincristine, procarbazine, and prednisone, after which he became afebrile.

The notable decrease in the white blood cell count with irradiation therapy to the lymph node-bearing area of the upper torso should have suggested undiscovered bone marrow involvement. This change in the blood count would not have been surprising if the patient had received abdominal irradiation. Since Hodgkin's disease involves the bone marrow, liver, and spleen in a nodular pattern, it is common for a needle biopsy, such as the initial bone marrow biopsy in this case, to fail to demonstrate evidence of disease.

Serum copper levels are used to follow the clinical course of patients rather than as a diagnostic test. Untreated and relapsing patients with lymphoma or Hodgkin's disease have high levels of serum copper. Satisfactory clinical response to treatment has been equated with a decrease to normal in serum copper levels. Serum copper levels have been observed to rise well above normal values before symptoms or the laboratory findings indicate relapse. In this patient, the serum copper levels correlated quite well with disease activity.

BSP retention and alkaline phosphatase levels are the most sensitive tests to indicate liver involvement by Hodgkin's disease and lymphoma as well as other focal processes such as granulomas.

CASE 5.—*Histiocytic reticulum cell sarcoma* was diagnosed in this 69-year-old woman who presented with tumors of the scalp and enlarged cervical lymph nodes which responded initially to irradiation therapy. Chemotherapy was eventually required for progression of disease. The patient has been followed seven years.

Clinical resume.—This patient noted the gradual appearance of three scalp masses. Ten months later, these lesions were excised. Tumor was found to penetrate the outer table of the skull. Pathologically, however, the material showed only atypical cells in fibrous tissue.

Six months later, a subdigastric node was enlarged. Biopsy revealed malignant lymphoma of the histiocytic reticulum cell sarcoma type. The patient was treated with ^{60}Co irradiation to the head and neck with a tumor dose of 3,000 rads in four weeks. To avoid exceeding the tolerance of the underlying brain tissue, additional treatment was administered to residual scalp masses with a superficial x-ray unit. Four years after the initial onset of her disease, a small left supraorbital mass appeared and this mass was irradiated.

Five and one-half years after the onset of the disease, a right submaxillary mass was retreated with irradiation. Shortly thereafter, scalp masses began to reappear and a repeat biopsy again revealed malignant lymphoma of the histiocytic reticulum cell type. Laboratory examination at this time showed a slightly hypocellular bone marrow. The hemoglobin was 13.5 g., white blood cell count 5,200, and platelets 412,000. The BSP showed 14 per cent retention. The alkaline phosphatase was 2.5 Bessey-Lowry units. She was started on a combined chemotherapy program of cyclophosphamide, vincristine, and prednisone, administered intermittently. The scalp masses and cervical nodes regressed completely within two weeks and have not reappeared. Treatment was continued for four months, at which time she fractured her hip. Two years later, exacerbations of disease were heralded by right pleural effusion and enlargement of a right submaxillary node. Needle biopsy of the node showed connective tissue with fibrosis, chronic inflammation, and degenerating glands. The pleural fluid was negative for tumor cells on two occasions. However, the third aspiration showed an exudate containing a few cells that were suspect for lymphoma. The fluid was negative for acid-fast bacilli and fungi.

Over a period of seven years, the patient has gradually developed signs of cerebellar degeneration, which are considered to be secondary to either old age or reticulum cell sarcoma, rather than to treatment with irradiation or chemotherapy.

Although histiocytic reticulum cell sarcoma usually is rapidly progressive, treatment of these patients should be aggressive since a few, such as this patient, will show a good response. Irradiation therapy was used initially for very extensive but clinically localized disease. Chemotherapy was instituted when she developed several recurrences in a previously irradiated area.

A lymphangiogram was not performed on this patient because of her age, and the absence of dorsalis pedis pulses. Had retroperitoneal lymph node involvement been demonstrated by lymphangiography, irradiation therapy would not have been the treatment of choice for two reasons: very few older patients can tolerate intensive abdominal irradiation, and reticulum cell sarcoma is a relatively radioresistant tumor. Abdominal involvement can seldom be eradicated with irradiation therapy because of limited tolerance of the surrounding structures. In younger persons, a preliminary trial of a combination of chemotherapy and irradiation therapy for abdominal involvement seems to be more effective.

CASE 6.—*Poorly differentiated lymphocytic lymphoma* was diagnosed in this 42-year-old woman who presented with stage IV disease manifested by generalized adenopathy, massive abdominal involvement, and infiltration of the bone marrow. Initially, irradiation therapy was administered sequentially to all peripheral lymph node-bearing areas and the abdomen. Subsequent exacerbations responded to chemotherapy. However, because of inadequate bone marrow reserve, the total dosage of chemotherapy that could be achieved with any given agent was limited. The patient died within two years of onset of her disease.

Clinical resume.—This 42-year-old white woman noted the onset of easy fatigability and generalized maculopapullar rash associated with pruritus in May 1966. She saw her physician who found enlarged lymph nodes in the neck, one of which was biopsied. The diagnosis was poorly differentiated lymphocytic lymphoma.

When the patient was seen at Anderson Hospital in June 1966, only a 1-cm. posterior occipital lymph node was palpable. The spleen extended 3 cm.

below the left costal margin. A separate epigastric mass extending 8 cm. below the left costal margin was palpated to the right of the spleen. The chest x-ray film revealed prominent hilar adenopathy. An upper gastrointestinal series demonstrated that the larger abdominal mass was secondary to lymphomatous involvement of the stomach and small intestine. Barium enema revealed involvement of the colon. A nasopharyngeal tumor survey confirmed the presence of a large soft tissue mass arising from the superior posterior aspect of the nasopharynx. The white blood cell count was 3,570 with 57 polymorphonuclear granulocytes, 31 lymphocytes, 7 monocytes, and 5 eosinophiles. The hemoglobin was 9 g. and the platelet count was 348,000. A bone marrow examination revealed involvement by lymphoma.

In July and August, she received sequential intensive irradiation to the upper abdomen, pelvis, both sides of the neck, and the nasopharynx. Although the major abdominal mass regressed after irradiation therapy, the spleen remained palpable 3 to 4 cm. below the left costal margin. An upper gastrointestinal series in January 1967 revealed a persistent, but less extensive involvement of the stomach. The blood count had changed very little. Tests for hemolytic anemia were negative. Because serum iron levels were low, she received intramuscular iron with some improvement in the hemoglobin.

By August 1967, the patient had evidence of progression of disease with further enlargement of the spleen and the popliteal nodes. The latter were successfully treated with irradiation. In October, pruritus became a problem. In addition, the left eye was slightly protruberant. Femoral and iliac nodes were palpable. A decision was made to treat the patient with a combination of prednisone and cyclophosphamide, but this treatment was unsuccessful, and by December a mass filled the left lacrimal fossa. Irradiation was given for palliation. In February, severe edema, which was thought to be secondary to blockage of the lymph drainage by enlarging lymphomatous masses, had developed in both legs. She received a combination of chlorambucil and prednisone, but treatment had to be discontinued because of leukopenia of 1,900 and thrombocytopenia. The differential count showed a leukemic pattern; 25 per cent of the cells were immature lymphocytes. From April until her death in August 1968, the disease continued to progress and was complicated by rectal bleeding. Supportive therapy was given. Further attempts at therapy included reduced doses of chlorambucil, vincristine, and Purinethol. Her condition continued to deteriorate and she died at home in August 1968.

Involvement of the stomach by lymphocytic lymphoma may present as diffuse enlargement of the gastric folds, as in this patient, or as localized nodular or ulcerated masses or linitis plastica. The abnormal cells in the bone marrow, which were characterized by nuclear indentations and a narrow rim of cytoplasm, were designated as lymphosarcoma or leukosarcoma cells, an older terminology for poorly differentiated lymphocytes. Although this patient initially was treated with radiotherapy, chemotherapy might have been better from the standpoint of conservation of treatment time and bone marrow reserve. However, massive abdominal disease often does not respond to the most aggressive chemotherapy.

Poorly differentiated lymphocytic lymphoma usually runs a rapid course. However, exceptions do occur. Since patients with well-differentiated lymphocytic lymphoma are occasionally mistakenly included in this group, clearer definitions of the subdivisions of lymphocytic lymphoma might change the prognostic index.

CASE 7.—*Histiocytic reticulum cell sarcoma* of the testis with associated para-aortic lymph node involvement in a 52-year-old male was managed with irradiation therapy. Subsequent spread to the neck responded to irradiation. However, recurrence in the abdomen was not influenced by chemotherapy. The patient died one year after onset.

Clinical resume.—This patient noted enlargement of the right testis associated with discomfort but no pain beginning in April 1965. Over the next three months, the testis grew to three times its normal size. In June, an orchiectomy was performed in another hospital. The patient subsequently was referred to Anderson Hospital. The histological diagnosis of seminoma was confirmed at this institution.

Physical examination was unremarkable except for the absence of the right testis. The intravenous pyelogram was normal, but the lower limb lymphangiogram showed disease in the right para-aortic region. He subsequently received irradiation therapy on the ^{60}Co unit to the deep iliac and para-aortic lymph node chains, followed by prophylactic irradiation to the mediastinum and the left supraclavicular region. Subsequently, the patient developed a painful mass in the posterior right cervical area. Biopsy revealed histiocytic reticulum cell sarcoma. On review of the testicular tumor, the diagnosis was revised to histiocytic reticulum cell sarcoma. The patient received irradiation to the mass in the right neck. The therapy was completed in December 1965.

In January 1966, physical examination revealed a large right axillary node and a small right suprapubic lymph node. One week later, he developed nausea and vomiting secondary to compression of the duodenum. On February 7, 1966, he underwent an exploratory laparotomy with a gastrojejunostomy, for massive retroperitoneal lymph node enlargement with obstruction and compression of the duodenum. Postoperatively, he received chemotherapy which was ineffective. Subsequently, he developed herpes zoster on the right leg and buttocks. He died at home on April 29, 1966.

This case emphasized the difficulty in the differential histologic diagnosis of seminoma and histiocytic reticulum cell sarcoma and the importance of the histologic diagnosis as related to selection of therapy. The tumor dose recommended for seminoma is not sufficient for histiocytic reticulum cell sarcoma involving the abdomen. Neither are the inverted "Y" shaped fields appropriate for this disease since it tends to be more diffuse. If this patient were seen today with known histiocytic reticulum cell sarcoma involving the abdomen, he would be treated with a preliminary course of chemotherapy followed by intensive irradiation to the whole abdomen. Once an aggresive neoplasm such as histiocytic reticulum cell sarcoma spreads beyond the abdomen to the neck, further dissemination generally is rapid.

Seminoma can be differentiated from histiocytic reticulum cell sarcoma by the glycogen contained in the seminoma cells. Glycogen is not present in the cells of histiocytic reticulum cell sarcoma. Glycogen is best demonstrated with the periodic acid-Schiff (PAS) stain with and without prior digestion of the unstained slide with diastase or saliva; glycogen is removed by the digestion, whereas other substances staining with the PAS stain are not removed.

In advanced malignant lymphoma and Hodgkin's disease, the incidence of herpes zoster is much higher than in nonlymphomatous patients. It can be a very serious disease in these patients and may even cause death.

Index